Seminars in Psychosexual Disorders

College Seminars Series

Series Editors

Professor Hugh Freeman, Honorary Professor, University of Salford, and Honorary Consultant Psychiatrist, Salford Health Authority

Dr Ian Pullen, Consultant Psychiatrist, Dingleton Hospital, Melrose, Roxburghshire

Dr George Stein, Consultant Psychiatrist, Farnborough Hospital, and King's College Hospital

Professor Greg Wilkinson, Editor, *British Journal of Psychiatry*, and Professor of Liaison Psychiatry, University of Liverpool

Other books in the series

Seminars in Alcohol and Drug Misuse. Edited by Jonathan Chick & Roch Cantwell

Seminars in Basic Neurosciences. Edited by Gethin Morgan & Stuart Butler

Seminars in Child and Adolescent Psychiatry. Edited by Dora Black & David Cottrell

Seminars in Clinical Psychopharmacology. Edited by David King

Seminars in General Adult Psychiatry. Edited by George Stein & Greg Wilkinson

Seminars in Practical Forensic Psychiatry. Edited by Derek Chiswick & Rosemarie Cope

Seminars in Psychiatric Genetics. By Peter McGuffin, Michael J. Owen, Michael C. O'Donovan, Anita Thapar & Irving Gottesman

Seminars in the Psychiatry of Learning Disabilities. Edited by Oliver Russell

Seminars in Psychology and the Social Sciences. Edited by Digby Tantam & Max Birchwood

Forthcoming titles
Seminars in Psychiatry for the Elderly. Edited by Brice Pitt & Mohsen Naguib

Seminars in Psychotherapy. Edited by Sandra Grant & Jane Naismith

Seminars in Psychosexual Disorders

Series editors

Hugh Freeman
Ian Pullen
George Stein
Greg Wilkinson

GASKELL

British Library Cataloguing-in-Publication Data
A catalogue record for this book is available from the British Library.

ISBN 1-901242-03X

Distributed in North America
by American Psychiatric Press, Inc.
ISBN 0-88048-581-7

Gaskell is an imprint of the Royal College of Psychiatrists,
17 Belgrave Square, London SW1X 8PG
The Royal College of Psychiatrists is a registered charity, number 228636

The views presented in this book do not necessarily reflect those of the Royal College of Psychiatrists, and the publishers are not responsible for any error of omission or fact. College Seminars are produced by the Publications Department of the College; they should in no way be construed as providing a syllabus or other material for any College examination.

Printed by Bell & Bain Ltd, Thornliebank, Glasgow

Contents

List of contributors   vi
Foreword   vii

Section I

1. The neuroendocrine basis of sexuality and organic dysfunction. *Michael Murphy* — 1
2. Gender development. *Susan Golombok and Robyn Fivush* — 30
3. Sexology and male sexuality: a history of socio-medical attitudes towards sexual behaviour. *Sue Collinson* — 44
4. Sexual therapy and the couple. *Michael Crowe* — 59
5. Physical treatments for sexual dysfunctions. *Kevan R. Wylie* — 84
6. Child abuse. *Gerry Doyle* — 101
7. Psychiatric aspects of HIV infection and disease. *Massimo Riccio* — 114
8. Problems of sexuality among people in mental health facilities. *Donald J. West* — 124

Section II

9. The paraphilias: an evolutionary and developmental perspective. *Raymond E. Goodman* — 142
10. Transgenderism and the psychiatrist. *Jed Bland* — 156

Section III

11. Counselling and sex therapy for couples with psychosexual problems. *Jane Roy* — 172
12. An investigation of partnership problems in sex therapy. *Patricia Gillan* — 184
13. A counsellor's work with clients presenting with paraphilias. *Christopher F. Headon* — 193

Bilbliography. *P. De Silva* — 206
Index — 209

Contributors

Dr Jed Bland, Counsellor and Trustee of the Beaumont Trust

Dr Sue Collinson, Lecturer, Department of Medical and Dental Education, St Bartholomew's and the Royal London School of Medicine and Dentistry, West Smithfield, London EC1A 7BE

Dr Michael Crowe, Consultant Psychiatrist, The Maudsley Hospital, Denmark Hill, London SE5 8AZ

Dr P. De Silva, Consultant Psychiatrist, Buckrose Ward, Bridlington and District Hospital, Bridlington YO16 4QP

Dr Gerry Doyle, Senior Registrar in Child Psychiatry, Child and Family Psychiatry Unit, Queen Elizabeth Hospital, Sheriff Hill, Gateshead, Tyne & Wear NE9 6SX

Dr Robyn Fivush, Department of Psychology, Emory University, Atlanta GA 30322, US

Dr Patricia Gillan, Consultant Psychologist/Psychotherapist, 10 Hanley Street, London W1N 1AA, and North Wales Medical Centre, Queen's Road, Llandudno, Gwynedd LL30 1UD

Professor Susan Golombok, Family and Child Psychology Research Centre, City University, Northampton Square, London EC1V 0HB

Dr Raymond E. Goodman, Consultant in Psychosexual Medicine, Department of Medicine, University of Manchester, BUPA Hospital Manchester, Russell Road, Whalley Range, Manchester M16 8AJ

Christopher F. Headon, Therapist, The Albany Trust, at Art of Health and Yoga, 280 Balham High Road, Tooting, London SW17 7AL

Dr Michael Murphy, Consultant, Queen Mary's University Hospital, Roehampton

Dr Massimo Riccio, Consultant, The Priory Group, Priory Lane, Roehampton, London SW15 5JJ

Dr Jane Roy, 10 Faraday Drive, Shenley Lodge, Milton Keynes MK5 7DA

Professor Donald J. West, Emeritus Professor of Clinical Criminology, Cambridge Institute of Criminology, 32 Fen Road, Milton, Cambridge CB4 6AD

Dr Kevan Wylie, Consultant, Community Mental Health Care Directorate, Whilteley Wood Clinic, Woofindin Road, Sheffield S10 3TL

Foreword

Series Editors

The publication of *College Seminars*, a series of textbooks covering the breadth of psychiatry, is very much in line with the Royal College of Psychiatrists' established role in education and in setting professional standards.

College Seminars are intended to help junior doctors during their training years. We hope that trainees will find these books useful, on the ward as well as in preparation for the MRCPsych examination. Separate volumes will cover clinical psychiatry, each of its subspecialities, and also the relevant non-clinical academic disciplines of psychology and sociology.

College Seminars will also make a contribution to the continuing professional development of established clinicians.

Psychiatry is concerned primarily with people, and to a lesser extent with disease processes and pathology. The core of the subject is rich in ideas and schools of thought, and no single approach or solution can embrace the variety of problems a psychiatrist meets. For this reason, we have endeavoured to adopt an eclectic approach to practical management throughout the series.

The College can draw on the collective wisdom of many individuals in clinical and academic psychiatry. More than a hundred people have contributed to this series; this reflects how diverse and complex psychiatry has become.

Frequent new editions of books appearing in the series are envisaged, which should allow *College Seminars* to be responsive to readers' suggestions and needs.

Hugh Freeman
Ian Pullen
George Stein
Greg Wilkinson

1. The neuroendocrine basis of sexuality and organic dysfunction

Michael Murphy

The sexual brain • Spinal mechanisms and pathways • Peripheral pathways • Sex steroids • Sex, drugs and neurotransmitters • Medical and surgical causes of sexual dysfunction • Conclusions

The neuroendocrine mechanisms subserving sexual appetite/motivation and copulation in male mammals have been extensively investigated in the last two decades; likewise the biological mechanisms of human penile erection. This research has increased our understanding of the pathophysiology of sexual dysfunction in men. But a dearth of research and the inadequacy of animal models for the human female leaves us questioning how far these findings can be generalised to women. Descriptions of the 'sexual response', like Kaplan's triphasic model of desire–arousal–orgasm, and classifications of sexual dysfunctions, e.g. DSM–IV (American Psychiatric Association, 1994), emphasise the similarities between the sexes. Thus, erectile dysfunction is the prototype of 'impaired sexual arousal', but there is little information on whether organic causes of erectile dysfunction also impair genital responses in women.

While the physiology of erection has been empirically investigated since the mid 19th century, the female genitals were subjected to the mythical physiology of psychoanalysis. The phallocentric physiologist kept his probes and electrodes a proprietous distance from the clitoris and vagina until Masters and Johnson (1966) described the "female sexual response'. Since then pathophysiological researchers have almost all reverted to studying penile erection.

In this chapter we review the biology of sex and examine how disease, drugs and other physical factors cause sexual dysfunction. Since most cases of sexual dysfunction seen in psychiatric practice are caused by psychotropic drugs, pharmacology will be emphasised.

The sexual brain

Sexual responses to non-tactile erotic stimuli and fantasy (initiated through central processes independently of somatic and visceral sensation) presumably begin with neocortical neural activity. But there is no identified

1

area of the neocortex subserving specifically sexual behaviour or experience. However, neural systems involved in the expression of desire (appetitive behaviour), arousal, copulation and orgasm have been identified in telencephalic limbic, diencephalic, mesencephalic and medullary regions of the mammalian brain.

Electrical stimulation of the genital sensory receiving area of the parietal cortex during neurosurgery with conscious subjects, for example induces genital sensations devoid of any erotic quality. In contrast, stimulation of the amygdala, the septal area and certain thalamic nuclei can elicit erotic thoughts, feelings, erection and orgasm.

Animal researchers distinguish between sexual appetitive and consummatory behaviour. Appetitive behaviour is anthropomorphically assumed to reflect motivation, desire or drive. Consummatory behaviour in this context means copulation. The validity of the distinction is supported by the demonstration of different neurobiological systems at work in each of the behaviours.

Sexual desire, motivation, drive and appetite

People develop problems with coitus (e.g. erectile failure or anorgasmia) without any loss of sexual appetite. Others experience diminished desire, but can have normal coitus. It may be clinically relevant in such cases that the neural basis and neuroendocrine mechanisms regulating sexual appetitive behaviour are distinct from those regulating copulation.

The terms desire, motivation, drive and appetite are often used interchangeably. They may also be used more precisely, for example in the context of incentive-motivational theory or drive-reduction theory. Regardless of the psychological model, two components of the biological substrate of desire are important: steroidal hormones and ventral striatal dopamine-dependent mechanisms. The latter affect appetitive sexual behaviour without direct influence on copulatory behaviour, while sex steroids are involved differentially in both.

Barry Everitt and his colleagues have demonstrated the role of the amygdala in the acquisition of sexual appetitive behaviour. Previously neutral environmental stimuli become sexually salient and elicit appetitive sexual responses through their predictive association with sexual reinforcement. Such conditioning requires the interaction of the basolateral amygdala with dopamine-dependent events in the ventral striatum. Activity at both these sites increases on exposure to cues that have acquired sexual motivational significance. Copulation, on the other hand, depends on the hypothalamus and the adjacent medial pre-optic area (MPOA). Everitt sees a major challenge to the neuroscience of sex in establishing the way in which elements of the telencephalic limbic system, the striatum and pre-optic area, and the actions of sex steroids, interact to produce an integrated pattern of sexual behaviour (for review see Everitt, 1990).

Consummatory sexual behaviour – arousal

The most important neural structures generating and integrating consummatory sexual behaviour are located in the medial pre-optic anterior hypothalamic continuum. The roles of specific groups of neurones within this region are different for males and females, and anatomical differences (sexual dimorphism) has been established in several mammalian species including humans.

The MPOA is critical in the expression of male copulatory behaviour. This has been demonstrated by numerous methods (hormone, peptide and pharmacological manipulations; surgical and selective neurotoxic lesions; electrical stimulation and single neurone recording studies) in rodents and primates. To give an example, electrical stimulation of the MPOA in primates elicits copulatory behaviour. This is not simply the generation of a pattern of motor responses, since it will only occur in the presence of a female in heat, and does not occur in the presence of a female not in heat. Simon LeVay (1993) at Harvard argues that the MPOA generates an inner state in which incentive cues from the female elicit mounting and pelvic thrusting. He does not suggest that sexual feelings are localised in the MPOA, but that activity in the area activates other brain areas and is a crucial node in the neural circuits for sexual behaviour.

Oomura and his colleagues (1988) in Japan have recorded single neurone discharges from MPOA and hypothalamic cells in male and female monkeys. The highest rates of activity in the male MPOA occurred as the female was brought into the male's range and coincided with penile erection and the initiation of consummatory behaviour. The discharge rate dropped during copulation and activity virtually ceased after ejaculation. Increased neuronal activity in the adjacent dorsomedial nucleus of the hypothalamus (DMH) persisted until ejaculation.

Similarly, changes in the female MPOA were related to the commencement of sexual consummatory behaviour, but after that there was a difference. Sustained activity occurred in the ventromedial hypothalamic nucleus (VMH), not the DMH.

To understand the role of the MPOA at the onset of sexual arousal we need to know its afferent and efferent connections (Fig. 1). In the 1960s Paul MacLean and his colleagues, who had pioneered the limbic system, turned their attention to the cerebral localisation of erection (for review see Murphy, 1993*a*). Points in the brain where electrical stimulation elicited erection in monkeys (positive loci) suggested a pathway for erection. Positive loci in the septal area tracked into the MPOA and anterior hypothalamus. The septal area and its outflow have also been electrically stimulated in conscious men and induced erection, sexual thoughts and feelings (Heath, 1964).

In the hypothalamus, positive loci run into the paraventricular nucleus (PVN), a centre integrating autonomic, neuroendocrine and behavioural

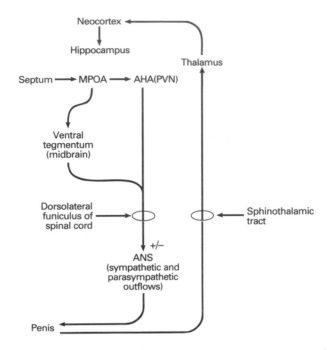

Fig. 1.1 Diagram showing central nervous system structures and pathways likely to be involved in erection. MPOA, anterior hypothalamic area; AHA, anterior hypothalamic area; PVN, paraventricular nucleus of the hypothalamus; MFB, medial forebrain bundle; ANS, autonomic nervous system. Adapted from Gregoire & Pryor (1993), with permission.

responses, in particular those involving eating, sexual activity, and breast-feeding – three consummatory behaviours whose overlapping neural substrate might have interested Freud. Some PVN neurones project to the neurohypophysis and secrete a pulse of oxytocin into the circulation at orgasm in man (Murphy *et al*, 1987). Other PVN oxytocin-containing neurones project to autonomic centres in the spinal cord regulating bloodflow to the genitals, and others to spinal motor neurones supplying pelvic striated muscles involved in genital arousal and orgasm. Thus the PVN and its projections appear to be involved in integrating genital reflexes with other aspects of copulation under hypothalamic control (Murphy, 1993*a*).

   Animal studies show that oxytocin release into the blood during coitus is associated with central release and there is a wealth of research on the importance of oxytocin in social bonding. But the ability of oxytocin to induce sexual arousal in a woman has just recently been reported. The woman was taking the peptide by intranasal spray to facilitate breast-feeding. The effects were dramatic. Two hours after ingestion, she noticed vaginal transudate trickling down her leg and intense subjective arousal (data suggest the intranasal route can bypass the blood–brain barrier).

She initiated intercourse and reported an intensification of vaginal and uterine contractions along with heightened pleasure at orgasm. She repeated the experience a second time, but on a third occasion the spray was without effect. The apparent reason: she had stopped the progestagenic pill which she was taking on the two previous occasions, and steroidal priming determines the activational effects of oxytocin. If this observation is replicated it will be additional evidence for the pivotal integrative role of oxytocin in the sexual response.

While the hypothalamus has the major role in organising the sexual response, integration of the visceral response with psychological and somatic aspects of sexual behaviour occurs on multiple levels above and below the hypothalamus. After leaving the hypothalamus, for example, the effector pathway for erection travels through the midbrain and pons where further influences from limbic, extrapyramidal and neocortical outflows may be integrated.

Spinal mechanisms and pathways

During normal sexual activity the brain mechanisms described above interact with the spinal reflexes controlling the vascular, secretory and neuromuscular events characteristic of genital responses seen during arousal in both sexes. The brain exerts both excitatory and inhibitory influences on the spinal mechanisms regulating erection. Vasocongestion as a result of increased parasympathetic outflow leads to erection in the male, and swelling of the external genitalia and increased vaginal transudate in the female. Most research concerns penile erection, but it appears that the spinal sexual circuitry involved is similar in both sexes and that coital reflex events are generated by a hormone-insensitive spinal pattern generator.

Entirely reflex erection can be observed in men with complete spinal cord lesions above the sacral segments. In such men there is obviously no sensation and erection depends on a sacral cord mechanism in isolation from the rest of the central nervous system. The receptors for the reflex are concentrated in the glans, frenulum and the corpora cavernosa. The afferent pathway is in the dorsal nerve of the penis and the pudendal nerve. Afferent impulses activate spinal interneurones, which in turn activate the parasympathetic preganglionic neurones at the S2 and S3 level.

The pathways transmitting information between the brain and spinal centres are not yet clearly identified. Bilateral anterolateral cordotomy at the upper thoracic level for pain relief is followed by variable effects on sexual function. Most men show loss of erectile ability, while others retain erections and ejaculation but lose erotic sensations and orgasm. As touch and two-point discrimination remain unaffected by this procedure, it seems likely that the erotic quality of genital stimulation depends on ascending fibres that run with the spinothalamic pathways for pain and temperature. This is supported by studies on monkeys in which the relevant fibres could be traced to the caudal thalamic intralaminar nuclei, which may be the receiving area for erotic genital sensation. Electrical stimulation of these nuclei in humans has been reported to cause erotic feelings and orgasm.

The brain-stem exerts a tonic descending inhibitory influence on spinal mechanisms activated during coitus, including reflexes for penile erection, vasocongestion of the female genitals (the cause of increased vaginal transudate) and the involuntary neuromuscular concomitants of orgasm. A group of neurones in the ventral medulla (the paragigantocellular reticular nucleus) projecting to pelvic efferent neurones and interneurones mediate this inhibition in rats.

Peripheral mechanisms

Genital arousal

Three peripheral neural mechanisms regulate erection:

(1) a parasympathetic vascular mechanism
(2) a sympathetic inhibitory mechanism
(3) a somatomotor muscular mechanism.

The two autonomic systems act in opposition to one another to regulate smooth muscle tone in the arterioles and trabeculae of the penis. The somatomotor mechanism involves activation of the bulbocavernosus and ischiocavernosus muscles via the pudendal nerve. This is usually activated reflexly, but can be influenced by voluntary action.

Since the same three types of neural input control the bloodflow and striated muscle activity of the female genitals, it is likely that similar mechanisms operate in genital arousal in women. However, there are few investigations of female genital arousal, which can be assessed by measuring vaginal bloodflow with photoplethysmography. This technique shows significant increases in vaginal bloodflow in response to erotic stories.

The parasympathetic vascular mechanism

Parasympathetic activity causes dilatation of the arterioles supplying erectile tissue and relaxation of the trabecular smooth muscle, thus expanding the corporal space. The effect is to increase bloodflow through both the corpora cavernosa and corpus spongiosum and glans. The vessels supplying the erectile tissue remain dilated for the duration of the erection.

In addition, occlusion of the veins draining the penis must occur for an erection to be maintained. These veins are compressed between the distended sinusoidal walls and the non-compliant tunica albuginea during full erection (Fig. 2). However, some researchers believe that venous occlusion is not entirely mechanical, and that outflow resistance is under neural control. Both inadequate arterial blood supply and veno-occlusive dysfunction cause erectile dysfunction, as do lesions and pathology of the nerves carrying the parasympathetic fibres.

Although acetylcholine is involved in mediating parasympathetic effects on penile tumescence, muscarinic blockade with atropine does not impair erection in normal volunteers. Acetylcholine may have effects on erection via nitric oxide release and prostaglandin synthesis (discussed below), but muscarinic transmission is not required for erection in the way that many psychiatrists currently believe (judging by the frequency with which antimuscarinic effects of psychotropic drugs are blamed for causing erectile dysfunction). Several lines of evidence suggest that vasoactive intestinal polypeptide (VIP) is the most important neurotransmitter in erection (Fig. 3). Ultrastructural examination of human penile tissue shows that VIP-containing vesicles are colocalised with acetylcholine vesicles and VIP has been identified in pelvic ganglion cell bodies that have cholinergic projections to the penis. Elevated concentrations of VIP have been found in penile venous blood during erection in men, and VIP relaxes adrenergically contracted cavernosal smooth muscle *in vitro*. A reduction in nerve fibres containing VIP has been demonstrated in men with erectile dysfunction regardless of cause, suggesting that fibre loss is secondary to other causes.

Neural stimulation
|
Neurotransmitters
|
Smooth muscle relaxation
(arterial and cavernosal)
|
Dilatation of vascular spaces
(decrease in peripheral resistance)
| |
Vasodilatation   Compression of venules
| |
Increase in arterial flow   Decrease in venous return
| |
Increase in intracorporeal pressure
|
Contraction of ischiocavernosus muscles
|
Rigidity

Fig. 1.2 Mechanisms of erection. From Gregoire & Pryor (1993), with permission.

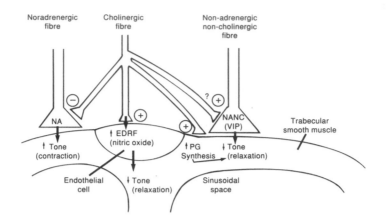

Fig. 1.3 Peripheral neurochemical control of trabecular muscle tone: relaxation is associated with erection, contraction with flaccidity and detumescence. NA, noradrenaline; EDRF, endothelium-derived relaxing factor; PG, prostaglandin; NANC, nonadrenergic, noncholinergic; VIP, vasoactive intestinal polypeptide; $\oplus$, excitatory effect; $\ominus$, inhibitory effect; $\uparrow$, increases; $\downarrow$, decreases. From Gregoire & Pryor (1993), with permission.

The sympathetic mechanism

Sympathetic output from the eleventh thoracic to the third lumbar (T11–L3) segments of the spinal cord tonically inhibits erection and causes detumescence (there is individual variation in segmental supply). The flaccid state is maintained through the activation of postsynaptic alpha$_1$-adrenoceptors which causes contraction of cavernosal and vascular smooth muscle, thus restricting bloodflow. Thus, alpha-antagonists such as phenoxybenzamine induce penile tumescence when injected intra-cavernosally.

Anxiety can impair a man's ability to achieve or maintain an erection (especially in specific situations). Increased sympathetic tone may contribute to such erectile dysfunction through this pathway.

The somatomotor mechanism

Penile sensory fibres belong to spinal segments S2, S3 and S4 and travel in the dorsal nerve of the penis, a branch of the pudendal nerve (Fig. 4). They form the afferent pathway for reflex erection. The motor neurones supplying the ischiocavernosus and bulbocavernosus (penile striated muscles) form a ventrolateral group in the anterior grey column of the cord known as "the nucleus of Onufrowicz" or Onuf's nucleus. The significance of the somatomotor system in erection is still unclear. Contractions of the penile muscles increase the rigidity of a full erection.

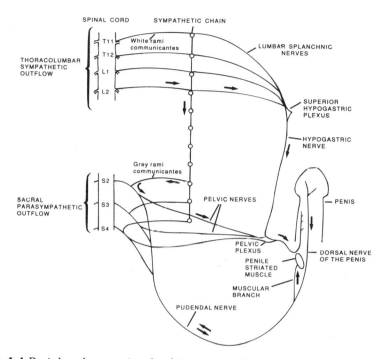

Fig. 1.4 Peripheral nerves involved in erection. Arrows denote direction of neural conduction. From Gregoire & Pryor (1993), with permission.

During full erection, intracavernous pressure is just below systolic blood pressure; with striated muscle contraction there is a further rise in intracavernous pressure above systolic blood pressure, resulting in a 'rigid erection'. The rise in intracavernosal pressure results from the ischiocaverosus muscles compressing the proximal ends of the corpora cavernosa. It has been suggested that rigid erection occurs during sexual activity when tactile stimulation of the penis triggers the bulbocavernosus reflex. While this reflex might facilitate penetration, it is not essential. On the other hand, its absence has been associated with primary anorgasmia in men and women. The reflex is sometimes used in the neurological assessment of patients with erectile dysfunction. It is elicited by pinching the glans and palpating the perineum or anus for contraction. However, it is clinically detectable in only 70% of men with normal sexual function.

Indirect chemical mechanisms – nitric oxide and prostaglandins

The vasodilatory effect of acetylcholine is not directly mediated by muscarinic neuromuscular junctions, but rather by an endothelium derived relaxing factor. In the penis, as elsewhere, this factor is nitric oxide. It causes relaxation of both vascular and cavernosal muscle by increasing intracellular cyclic guanosine monophosphate. A study of cavernosal tissue from diabetic men with erectile dysfunction suggests that impairment of this endothelium-mediated mechanism may partly account for their dysfunction (Saenz de Tejada *et al*, 1989). It might also explain the increased rate of erectile dysfunction in men with hypertension not receiving antihypertensive drugs.

Prostaglandins relax cavernosal muscle and induce erection after intracavernosal injection in men with erectile failure of non-vasculogenic origin. Human cavernosal tissue can synthesize various prostaglandins including large amounts of prostacyclin (PG12). Like PGE1, which is used in the diagnosis and treatment of erectile dysfunction, prostacyclin is a potent vasodilator. Furthermore, prostacyclin synthesis in penile tissue can be stimulated by muscarinic agents. Not surprisingly, these findings have led to speculation that prostacyclin is involved in erection.

Ejaculation and orgasm

Ejaculation occurs in three stages:

(1) emission of semen into the posterior urethra
(2) closure of the bladder neck and internal urethral sphincter
(3) anterograde ejaculation due to contraction of the urethra and striated muscles of the penis.

Urethral stimulation in male rats elicits ejaculation and rhythmic contractions of the striated perineal muscles. In females, striated muscle contraction is accompanied by vaginal and uterine contractions. These responses are similar to those occurring at orgasm in humans. This response, the urethrogenital reflex, is unaffected in either sex by gonadectomy. As in genital arousal (vasocongestion) the urethrogenital reflex is produced by a spinal pattern generator and under tonic descending inhibition from the brain-stem. It is thought that these recent findings may be a model for experimental study of the neural mechanisms of sexual function in both sexes.

Sex steroids

In animals, many elements of sexual behaviour depend on androgens. In humans, however, the relationship between sexual behaviour and plasma hormone levels rarely show straightforward correlations. In men with normal gonadal function, for example, there is no correlation between circulating testosterone levels and measures of sexual interest, activity or erectile function. In women, testosterone can increase sexual appetite, but not always.

In animals, some elements of sexual behaviour persist for weeks or months after castration, depending on the species. In man, erections may continue for years. In all mammals, sexual behaviour continues after testosterone and its metabolites have disappeared from the circulation. Likewise, there is a delay before testosterone replacement gradually restores male sexual behaviour after chronic androgen deficiency.

Studies of hypogonadal and castrated men suggest that lack of androgens leads to reduced sexual interest and activity. John Bancroft and his colleagues in Edinburgh have studied the complex relationship between androgens and erectile function (Bancroft, 1989). In one experiment, erectile responses of hypogonadal men to erotic films were unaffected by androgen withdrawal and replacement. However, androgens affected how well these men developed erections with sexual fantasy. These findings suggest that androgens have more effect on the brain systems involved in the cognitive and affective aspects of sex than they do on peripheral mechanisms. Sleep erections, on the other hand, are impaired by androgen withdrawal, and testosterone increases the rigidity of sleep erections in normal men.

The effects of sex steroids on women's sexual behaviour are more subtle, complex and difficult to unravel. Oophorectomy reduces oestrogen and androgen production by 50%, yet has little effect on either desire or arousal in most women. Other postsurgical results show that androgens are more important than oestrogens in determining a woman's sexual appetite; there is a striking loss of sexual appetite after the adrenalectomy in oophorectomised women. The endocrine effect of this combined procedure is total androgen depletion and sexual appetite is restored by androgen replacement. Testosterone has also produced increased sexual appetite in women receiving hormonal treatment for breast cancer and gynaecological disorders. Trials comparing oestrogen alone with oestrogen plus testosterone in oophorectomised and postmenopausal women show significantly greater enhancement of sexual desire and arousal in those given testosterone in addition to oestrogen (Sherwin & Gelfand, 1987). Moreover, these changes covaried with plasma testosterone but not with plasma oestradiol. Rates of coitus and orgasm were also higher in those treated with the combination. Thus, while oestrogens can enhance sexual function in postmenopausal women by reversing atrophic changes in the vaginal mucosa, these findings imply that androgens are more important for maintaining optimal sexual function in postmenopausal women.

Several studies of female sexual behaviour across the menstrual cycle show that both female-initiated and male-initiated sexual activities are more likely around the time of ovulation. Frequency of intercourse has been shown significantly to correlate with mid-cycle testosterone levels. Many women report increased sexual arousal and sexual pleasure as they progress from the menses to the late luteal phase. These data have been interpreted as the result of hormonal fluctuations, but cognitive factors associated with the menstrual cycle could also be important.

Steroid effects on sexual behaviour are mediated at many sites. These include the MPOA and anterior hypothalamus where high densities of androgen and oestrogen receptors have been visualised. Castration reduces the responsiveness of MPOA neurones and leads to cessation of copulatory behaviour in male rats. Copulatory behaviour can then be restored by minute testosterone implants in the MPOA.

Some of the neural effects of testosterone are not the result of testosterone *per se*, but rather of its metabolites, oestradiol and dihydrotestosterone (DHT). There is evidence that the nerve cells of the MPOA aromatise testosterone to oestradiol, which then stimulates the cellular processes leading to activation of male copulatory behaviour. Testosterone is therefore both a hormone and prohormone and its effects are determined by the enzyme activity of target tissue. Thus, testosterone, as well as activating androgen receptors, acts in tissues with a high aromatase level as an oestrogen via the oestrogen receptor. Furthermore, the other main metabolite of testosterone, DHT, also binds to the oestrogen receptor and thereby can act as an inhibitor of oestrogen action. In short, different metabolites of testosterone affect different components of sexual behaviour through actions at different sites.

Sex, drugs and neurotransmitters

Psychopharmacology

It is often stated that dopamine facilitates, while serotonin inhibits sexual behaviour. This has proved to be an overgeneralisation: drugs acting on both transmitter systems often have dose-dependent biphasic effects and some inhibit one component of sexual behaviour while enhancing another. Noradrenaline acting on central $alpha_2$-adrenoceptors increases sexual activity in rats, while several neuropeptides have been shown to induce erection. The interactions of neurotransmitter systems with other factors, including environmental context and gonadal steroids, has also been elucidated.

While psychotropic medication is by far the commonest cause of sexual dysfunction in psychiatric practice, there is little systematic research on this problem. It is likely that sexual side-effects significantly reduce compliance with treatment. Knowledge of the neurotransmitters involved in sexual physiology can help clinicians find alternative drug regimes when sexual dysfunction interferes with a patient's treatment. Drug-induced sexual problems can be due to either central or peripheral actions. The work reviewed below suggests that central effects are considerably more important than is generally accepted.

Dopamine

Apomorphine, a dopamine agonist, induces erection in man unaccompanied by any other sign of arousal or effect on desire. It shows little therapeutic promise because of its side-effects. The effect is mediated by central D2 receptors and is blocked by haloperidol.

Microinjection studies with dopamine D2 and D1 receptor agonists and antagonists suggest that interactions between D1 and D2 receptors on hypothalamic PVN neurones are involved in the integration of genital reflexes. Low doses of D2 agonist induce intense erections, while high doses facilitate seminal emission and inhibit erection. The effect on seminal emission is potentiated by the D1 antagonist.

Both appetitive and consummatory behaviours are disrupted by dopamine receptor antagonists in male rats, but appetitive sexual behaviours are the more sensitive. Infusions of haloperidol into specific brain areas demonstrate that inhibition of sexual appetite results from dopamine blockade in the nucleus accumbens (part of the ventral striatum, but an endfield of the mesolimbic dopamine system). Haloperidol's effects in the MPOA are on both appetitive and consummatory measures.

Antipsychotic drugs

Loss of sexual desire as a result of dopamine blockade is common in both sexes, and withdrawal of antipsychotic drugs is associated with the return of sexual interest and activity. *In vivo* animal studies indicate that dopaminergic transmission in the ventral striatum increases dramatically on exposure to sexual cues. This applies to primary unconditioned incentive stimuli (the odour of a on-heat female) and learned cues (a light that has been paired with an on-heat female to become a conditioned stimulus). When dopamine receptor antagonists are infused into the ventral striatum, sexual appetitive behaviour is dramatically diminished without impairing the ability to copulate.

Antipsychotic drugs may thus impair sexual appetite by disrupting the limbic-striatal interaction discussed above. These drugs also interfere with many other aspects of sexual function including erection and ejaculation through a variety of neurotransmitter mechanisms. However, when patients report they can still have coitus or masturbate to orgasm, it remains important to ask about effects on desire, frequency of intercourse and the hedonic quality of arousal and orgasm. Some patients will reveal that despite their ability to consummate sex, they are unhappy with the effect their medication has on their sex-drive and that they default from treatment because of this effect. It is sometimes possible through dose reduction to ameliorate this side-effect and avoid non-compliance without precipitating relapse into psychosis.

Diverse effects on ejaculation are common with antipsychotic drugs which are unlikely to be the result of dopamine blockade. Failure to ejaculate at orgasm (aspermia) has been reported in a third of patients on thioridazine. This may be related to its potent alpha-blocking effect as aspermia is occasionally seen with other alpha-adrenoceptor antagonists. There must, however, be additional mechanisms specific to thioridazine-induced aspermia to explain the frequency of this effect, which is not as common with other antipsychotic drugs despite their alpha-blocking effect. There are conflicting findings on the mechanism of aspermia; retrograde ejaculation into the bladder and failure of emission (release of semen into the posterior urethra prior to bladder neck closure and anterograde ejaculation) have both been implicated. Fluphenazine is reported to reduce the quantity of ejaculate and produce changes in the quality or ability to achieve orgasm.

Antipsychotic drug-induced sexual dysfunction can sometimes be alleviated by switching to agents with dissimilar pharmacological effects without jeopardizing adequate control of a patient's psychotic symptoms.

L-dopa enhances sexual desire and performance independently of its effect on mobility in Parkinson's disease. There is some evidence that it may have this effect in non-parkinsonian subjects, but this putative aphrodisiac effect of L-dopa has been widely disputed (see Segraves, 1989).

Serotonin (5-HT)

Inhibiting serotonin synthesis in male rats causes a dramatic increase in sexual activity. Conversely, drugs that increase central serotonergic neurotransmission reduce sexual activity. The extent to which these observations reflect effects on general behavioural arousal is unresolved.

Spinal serotonergic receptors are involved in modulating penile reflexes. In rats, stimulation of these receptors suppresses erection while facilitating seminal emmission. But some serotonin agonists induce erection in man after intravenous injection. Since there are at least seven subtypes of serotonin receptor these different effects are not hard to explain. Erectogenic effects are mediated by 5-HT1C and/or 5-HT2 receptors in the central nervous system (CNS).

Selective serotonin reuptake inhibitors (SSRIs)

Clinical reports suggest that SSRIs have adverse effects on sexual function in over a third of patients (Jacobsen, 1992; Balon *et al*, 1993). Anorgasmia and retarded ejaculation are most frequently reported, but diminished desire and erectile dysfunction also occur. Less commonly, improvements in erectile function and clitoral engorgement are described.

Clomipramine, a heterocyclic antidepressant that predominantly increases synaptic concentrations of serotonin, abolished orgasm in 96% of men and women, often within days of starting treatment (Monteiro *et al*, 1987). The mechanism for this is unclear, but since anorgasmia occurs with the other serotonin reuptake blockers and is reversed by treatment with cyproheptadine or amantadine (antiserotonergic drugs), it is probably mediated by effects on serotonin receptors. Fluoxetine does not cause anorgasmia as frequently as clomipramine, but sexual dysfunction (including erectile difficulties and decreased sexual desire) affects a third of patients after commencement of 20–40 mg of the drug. Monoamine reuptake inhibitors that act predominantly on noradrenergic systems can be substituted when anorgasmia is a problem with SSRIs. However, these may cause sexual side-effects of their own (e.g. lofepramine can cause painful ejaculation).

Ecstasy

3,4-methylenedioxymethamphetamine (MDMA; 'ecstasy') is a potent serotonin agonist with effects on sexual behaviour. Users report enhancement of the sensuous aspects of sex, but inhibition of ejaculation and orgasm. At high doses it has neurotoxic effects on serotonergic nerve terminals in the CNS in both rodents and primates. Repeated systemic administration of MDMA to sexually active male rats transiently disrupts copulatory behaviour. MDMA-treated males that continue to copulate show delayed ejaculation compared with controls. After one week, despite continued MDMA treatment and marked depletion of serotonin in the striatum and hippocampus, the copulatory behaviour of MDMA-treated rats returns to normal.

Noradrenaline

The role of peripheral alpha-adrenoreceptors in the penis is well established. The activation of these receptors on cavernosal and vascular smooth muscle maintains tonic muscular contraction. Most drugs that cause priapism do so by blocking peripheral alpha-adrenoceptors.

Heterocyclic antidepressants and MAOIs

There are numerous case reports of these drugs causing erectile dysfunction, but few systematically collected data. Sexual side-effects are frequently seen with amitriptyline, imipramine, amoxapine, protriptyline, phenelzine and tranylcypromine. In most reports, erectile difficulties have occurred within weeks of treatment and recovery is rapid on stopping the drug or reducing the dose.

A study comparing phenelzine and imipramine with placebo reported sexual impairment in 80% of males and 57% of females treated with phenelzine, and 50% of males and 27% of females treated with imipramine (Harrison *et al*, 1986). The placebo had adverse sexual effects in 8% of males and 16% of females. Since these drugs increase peripheral as well as central adrenergic neurotransmission, they may impair genital responses by enhancing the adrenergically mediated contraction of vascular and erectile smooth muscle. Most antidepressants are also anticholinergic, and although muscarinic blockade alone does not clinically impair erection in normal men, it may aggravate difficulties due to increased adrenergic tone in depressed, anxious or psychologically stressed men (see Fig. 3).

Antidepressants may lead to an improvement in erectile function in some men. This can be the result of improvement in the patient's mental state, but in the case of trazodone it appears to be a direct action. Trazodone has led to recovery of erectile function, the development of prolonged erections and priapism.

Opioid peptides and opiates

Opiate drugs and beta-endorphin inhibit copulatory behaviour in male rats. This occurs acutely and is reversed by naloxone, and is specific, i.e. stimulation of opioid receptors disrupts copulatory behaviour at doses which do not affect other motor or social behaviours. The opiate antagonist naloxone has more variable effects on copulation. Some have found no effect and others have described facilitatory effects in sexually active rats. Naloxone has also induced copulation in rats normally sexually inactive (Murphy, 1993*b*).

Experimental tests on animals show that morphine acutely inhibits reflex erections in a dose-related fashion. Seminal emission is even more sensitive and is suppressed by the smallest doses of morphine. Thus, in addition to the inhibitory effects of opiates on sexual drive, their acute effects on genital reflexes may play a role in the sexual dysfunction seen with opiate use. Studies of penile reflexes in rats treated chronically with morphine found that erectile ability was relatively well preserved. This suggests that the decline in sexual behaviour seen with long-term regular opiate use is primarily due to a failure of sexual arousal, and not of erectile ability.

In healthy men, the acute effects of opiate antagonists have varied, but include a report of spontaneous penile erections with naltrexone. This effect is likely to result from reduction of tonic opioid-mediated inhibition of spinal reflexes. Studies of naloxone-induced erections in anaesthetised animals suggest considerable interindividual variation in the degree of this inhibitory control.

In a randomised, double-blind, cross-over laboratory study of naloxone's effect on the sexual responses of normal male volunteers to visually erotic stimuli, naloxone attenuated the pleasure experienced with arousal and at orgasm (Murphy *et al*, 1990). Naloxone also inhibited the surge in plasma oxytocin normally seen at orgasm, a possible epiphenomenon of impaired processing of sensory information in the amygdala, rather than a direct effect on the hypothalamo-neurohypohyseal system on which opioids have an inhibitory effect.

The combination of naloxone with yohimbine has been reported to cause sustained and full erection in healthy volunteers. A high dose of naloxone (1mg/kg) alone induced partial erection in half the subjects, while yohimbine alone had no effect. The combination produced a full erection, lasting for at least 60 minutes in all subjects. There was no effect on sexual appetite, but the combination caused marked anxiety, the extent of which limits clinical application. This synergistic effect raises the possibility of a physiological relationship between central opioid and noradrenergic systems in the neural control of erection, as is seen in other neural systems.

The chronic use of opiates is associated with a generalised decline in sexual function with loss of desire, erectile ability and anorgasmia. These features are part of a broad picture of psychophysiological disturbance and tell us little about the direct role of endogenous opioid peptides in sexual function.

Benzodiazepines and GABA

Benzodiazepines are agonistic at the benzodiazepine-GABA receptor complex. Stimulation of GABA receptors in the lumbosacral spinal cord inhibits erectile reflexes in rats. There are, however, several subtypes of GABA receptor, and effects depend on which subtype is being stimulated. Chlordiazepoxide, for example, has been shown experimentally to enhance penile spinal reflexes. To add to the complexity of data, chlordiazepoxide has an opposing effect on erection via its action in the hypothalamus where it inhibits apomorphine-induced erections in rats. Clinically, benzodiazepines are associated with impaired appetite and arousal, which usually presents as erectile dysfunction in men.

Antihypertensives

Antihypertensive drugs are frequently blamed for causing impotence. However, many patients with hypertension have arterial disease which can cause erectile dysfunction *per se*. There is evidence that untreated hypertensive men without erectile difficulties have subclinically reduced penile bloodflow which may precede vasculogenic erectile dysfunction. Bulpitt *et al* (1976) found that erectile failure was reported by 17% of untreated hypertensives compared with 7% of normotensive controls. The difference did not reach statistical significance. In hypertensives on treatment the difference became significant (25% v. 7%).

The two most frequently used first-line drugs in hypertension are thiazide diuretics and beta-blockers. Thiazides have been found to cause erectile dysfunction more frequently than beta-blockers in an MRC study of 9000 men, which was single-blind and based in general practice (Medical Research Council, 1981). Erectile dysfunction was the commonest reason for withdrawal from active treatment and was significantly more common with bendrofluazide than with propranolol. Compared with placebo, the difference was significant at the $P<0.001$ level for both drugs. It is difficult to ascribe much meaning to this last figure in a single-blind design, since doctors are unlikely to attribute dysfunction to a placebo. However, the difference between the two drugs is unlikely to be the consequence of the study's design. The mechanism of bendrofluazide's effect is unknown. In most of those affected, erectile function recovered within a few weeks of stopping bendrofluazide.

Ganglion blocking drugs interfere with neurotransmission through both sympathetic and parasympathetic autonomic ganglia. It is not surprising that they often prevent erection; however, they are seldom used today. Methyldopa interferes with noradrenaline synthesis and adrenergic transmission in peripheral and central neurones. It is still used, particularly in the elderly. Its main effect is loss of sexual appetite.

Most of the newer antihypertensive drugs are also thought to cause or aggravate erectile dysfunction. ACE inhibitors, such as captopril, are possible exceptions. Many antihypertensives also interfere with ejaculation. It is not clear how or what predisposes some men more than others to this effect.

Erectile dysfunction is unlikely to be the result of simply lowering blood pressure, since some drugs are more likely to cause it than others, suggesting other pharmacological mechanisms are involved. This is clinically important, because drug-induced dysfunction may be alleviated by switching to a drug from another class.

Propranolol seems more likely than other beta-blockers to cause erectile dysfunction. Although beta-adrenoceptors are present in corpus cavernosum, little is known of their physiological significance. Intra-cavernosal injection of propranolol does not prevent erection in normal subjects, making it unlikely that the effect is on erectile tissue.

Alpha-blockers lower blood pressure without interfering with erectile function. Indeed, as discussed previously, injected intracavernosally they induce relaxation of penile smooth muscle leading to tumescence. Alpha-blockade can, however, cause failure of ejaculation. Clonidine is an $alpha_2$-agonist reported to cause erectile failure, probably by a central effect.

There are reports of the calcium channel blocker, verapamil, causing erectile failure. Yet intracavernosal injection of verapamil induces erection. But in contrast to the effect of calcium channel blockers on erectile tissue, they have been shown to prevent apomorphine and oxytocin-induced penile erection in rats. This suggests that calcium channel blockers may interfere with the central processes mediating erection. Other antihypertensive vasodilators, including hydralazine and prazosin, have been reported to cause priapism.

Pinacidil is an antihypertensive vasodilator which opens potassium channels. In isolated human corpus cavernosum it abolishes spontaneous contractile activity and relaxes smooth muscle preparations precontracted by noradrenaline. It is yet to be tested clinically in humans, but tests on monkeys have shown that it induces erection.

Alcohol

Surveys have shown that alcohol may enhance sexual enjoyment, presumably by disinhibiting feelings and behaviour, particularly in women. However, many men report the converse. Acute intoxication is frequently described as a cause of erectile failure, but it is not clear by what mechanism. It is generally assumed that alcohol has a direct pharmaco-logical inhibitory effect on genital responses. But experiments in man and animals fail to show inhibition of spinal mechanisms. Thus, alcohol's adverse effect may be on perceptual or cognitive processes during sex.

Examining apomorphine-induced erections in rats shows that alcohol inhibits erection in a dose-dependent manner. This suggests alcohol may interfere with dopaminergic receptor mechanisms, or a second neurotransmitter/neuropeptide mediating apomorphine-induced erection, possibly oxytocin.

Sustained heavy drinking can affect erectile function through effects on several different organ systems, including the nervous system, endocrine system and the liver. In addition the psychosocial consequences of alcohol dependence, such as depression, low self-esteem and marital conflict, create sexual problems. Peripheral neuropathy occurs in alcoholism and may involve the sensory fibres of the dorsal nerve of the penis, resulting in diminished tactile sensation.

Nicotine

Cigarette smoking has been associated epidemiologically with erectile failure. This may be via its link to vascular disease. But there is evidence of a more direct relationship to sexual dysfunction, including case reports of sexual function returning rapidly in men who stop smoking. Experimental studies suggest that nicotine's vasoconstrictory effect plays a causal role, but only at high doses (heavy smoking of cigarettes high in nicotine). Cigarette smoke extracts inhibit methacholine-stimulated prostacycline secretion in a dose-dependent way. As previously discussed, prostacycline is a vasodilator and thought to be a local mediator of erection.

Smoking has also been shown to inhibit papaverine-induced erection. The smoking of two cigarettes shortly before testing by men who previously obtained a full erection with papaverine prevented a second erection in over half the sample. The average drop in intracavernous pressure was more than 30 mmHg ($P<0.01$). Cigarette smoking may thus give a negative result when papaverine is used diagnostically to establish arterial sufficiency.

Drugs with anti-androgenic effects

There are different types of anti-androgenic agent. Some are used for their anti-androgenic effect, as for example in the treatment of carcinoma of the prostate. Others are not used as anti-androgens, and their effect on the endocrine system is a side-effect. Drugs in the latter group include cimetidine, digoxin and metclopramide. It is quite likely that these drugs cause sexual problems by alternative mechanisms.

Cyproterone acetate is an anti-androgen used in the treatment of sex offenders and occasionally in severe acne. It reduces sexual interest and activity, but does not impair the erectile response to erotic films. Medroxyprogesterone acetate (MPA) has also been used in sex offenders. In a laboratory study of MPA there was a significant reduction in reported levels of subjective arousal to erotic stimuli, but genital arousal decreased only slightly (Bancroft, 1989). Nocturnal penile tumescence was significantly decreased during MPA administration and appeared to be related to decreases in total testosterone. The effects of both these drugs resemble the effects of hypogonadism.

Buserelin is a synthetic gonadotropin-releasing hormone (GnRH) analogue which produces a short phase of stimulation followed by a selective inhibition of secretion of pituitary gonadotropins, resulting in 'medical castration'. It is used in the palliative treatment of advanced prostatic cancer and advanced male breast cancer. It can cause loss of sexual appetite and impair erection.

Hypolipidaemic agents

The isobutyric acid derivatives gemfibrozil and fenofibrate are used to reduce serum triglyceride and cholesterol levels in patients with hyperliperdaemia unresponsive to dietary restriction. They are indicated in men under 55 years to reduce the risk of coronary artery disease. They cause erectile failure in a minority by an unknown mechanism.

Medical and surgical causes of sexual dysfunction

Sexual dysfunction can be a specific symptom of neurological, endocrine or vascular disease. It can also be a non-specific consequence of ill health or a psychological complication of organic disease through anxiety, depression, effects on body image or other cognitive processes. Only the first group of conditions will be described (abnormalities of sex steroid production have already been discussed above).

Neurological causes of sexual dysfunction

An integrated pattern of sexual desire, arousal, consummatory behaviour and experience depends on the orchestrated activity of neurones at all levels of the central and peripheral nervous system. It seems reasonable to predict that a wide variety of neurological lesions and diseases would cause sexual dysfunction. The little attention given to sex in the neurological literature suggests that this may be the case, but detail is scant.

The diagnosis of a neurogenic sexual problem in psychiatric practice is invariably suggested by the medical history followed by a selective neurological examination, for example for signs of peripheral neuropathy in a patient with diabetes. Faced with a sexual problem of possible neurological origin, further assessment should be based on the neuro-scientific principles as outlined above, and not on statistical associations. Again using the example of diabetic neuropathy: it is bad practice to assume automatically that a diabetic patient with erectile dysfunction has an organic problem, as the rushed or unskilled clinician often does. Psychological factors must be explored, and evidence of neuropathy, vascular disease and poor glycaemic control actively sought. In many cases the cause is multifactorial (see below).

Epilepsy

There has been wide variation in the reported rate of sexual dysfunction in subjects with epilepsy. Several studies have highlighted the high frequency of global hyposexuality (lower sex drive with less frequent sexual intercourse and problems with arousal) and erectile dysfunction in temporal lobe epilepsy (TLE) specifically. Shukla *et al* (1979), for example, reported hyposexuality in 63% of men with TLE compared with 12% in those with generalised seizures. Similar figures on hyposexuality have been reported in women.

There have been other studies challenging these high rates and suggesting that sexual dysfunction in TLE is related to poor social adjustment. Other potential aetiological factors that have been examined are anticonvulsants and their effects on sex steroids. Free testosterone levels may be low in patients on anticonvulsants, suggesting the high rate of sexual dysfunction (see Toone, 1986, for review). However, the evidence for this is conflicting and unconvincing.

The role of the amygdala in sexual appetitive behaviour discussed above is consistent with low sex drive in TLE. Animals with medial amygdala lesions differ from sham-lesioned controls with respect to precoital sexual arousal. Behavioural analysis suggests that lesioned animals are deficient in processing information on sexually exciting stimuli. Several lines of neuroscientific evidence suggest that hippocampal lesions might also be expected to cause sexual dysfunction.

Hypothalamo-pituitary disease

Numerous clinical case reports identify loss of sexual appetite and failure of arousal with structural lesions of the hypothalamus. These include sexual problems not explained by endocrine changes nor corrected by hormone replacement. A recent clinical study of women with well-defined hypothalamo-pituitary disease found that 45 of 46 previously sexually active women reported significant sexual dysfunction (Hulter & Lundberg, 1994). Lack of sexual appetite (79%), problems with lubrication (65%) and problems with orgasm (69%) were documented and were unrelated to changes in pituitary hormone release or sex steroid levels. Raised prolactin, for example, was present in only seven women and did not correlate with symptoms. These findings are again consistent with the animal research already presented.

Multiple sclerosis

A questionnaire study of 217 patients with multiple sclerosis found that sexual dysfunction was reported by 56% of the women and 75% of the men (Valleroy & Kraft, 1984). Among the women, the most commonly occurring sexual symptoms (in decreasing order of frequency) were decreased sensation, decreased sexual appetite, decreased frequency or loss of orgasm, and difficulty with arousal. Men reported erectile dysfunction most frequently, followed by decreased sensation, decreased sexual appetite, and orgasmic dysfunction. Although fatigue affected sexual performance, loss of mobility, weakness and depression were not significantly associated with sexual dysfunction. Localised areas of demyelination in the spinal cord and brain presumably account for the specific sexual deficits. There was an association with spasticity and bladder dysfunction, but in their absence sexual dysfunction still affected 50% of patients (see Dupont, 1995, for review).

Spinal cord injury

As already mentioned, reflex erection continues to occur in some men with complete transaction of the spinal cord above the sacral segments despite the absence of penile sensation. Erection in response to sexual thoughts have been called psychogenic to differentiate them from reflex erections. Although this response is psychogenic in the first instance, once an erection is developing, receptors in the penis are stimulated by the tumescence and the reflex mechanism is also activated.

If the sacral cord is damaged, reflex erections are lost, but it is claimed that psychogenic erections can still occur. Psychogenic erections have been reported in men with complete lesions of the cord as high as T12, suggesting that they are mediated by the sympathetic pathway. We have already seen that the sympathetic system tonically inhibits erection, but the above observations suggest that there is also a sympathetic erectile pathway. However, the clinical data on which this claim is based have been disputed.

Psychogenic erections in paraplegic men are usually short-lived, only partial and lack the rigidity needed for coitus; they involve swelling of the corpora cavernosa, but not the corpus spongiosum (Chapelle *et al,* 1980). Reflex erections are characterised by greater rigidity and involve the corpus spongiosum.

There are few data on women with spinal cord injuries. A questionnaire study of 23 women (18 paraplegic and five quadriplegic) with an average age of 38.5 years found that 30% had ceased intercourse after the injury, and 20% continued at decreased frequency. Of the 16 sexually active subjects, about half had become anorgasmic during intercourse. A careful detailed neurological study of both male and female patients with anorgasmia has indicated a role for the spinothalamic system in orgasm. These patient showed dissociated sensory loss due to anterior spinal cord lesions, while dorsal column functions at the lumbosacral level were preserved (for review see Berard, 1989).

Peripheral nerve lesions

The pelvic nerves carry the parasympathetic fibres from S3 and one other nerve root (either S2 or S3 depending on the individual). They join fibres from the hypogastric nerves (sympathetic) to form the pelvic plexus (sometimes called the inferior hypogastric plexus) in the pelvic fascia on the lateral side of the rectum, seminal vesicles, prostate and posterior bladder (see Fig.4).

Damage to the pelvic plexus causes erectile dysfunction after pelvic surgery. Its efferent fibres (the cavernous nerves) supply the corpora cavernosa and are damaged during radical retropubic prostatectomy, radical cystectomy, and abdominoperineal resection of the rectum. They may also be damaged during transurethral resection of the prostate, external sphincterotomy, internal urethrotomy and drainage of prostate abscess. Rupture of the membranous urethra with pelvic fracture may be followed by neurogenic dysfunction, but this may also be the result of surgery at a time when anatomical landmarks are obscured by oedema and haemorrhage.

Radical prostatectomy is the most effective treatment for localised prostastic adenocarcinoma, but it has been eschewed in favour of less effective treatments because of the complication of erectile failure. Recently, however, anatomical studies have precisely localised the microscopic cavernosal nerves and demonstrated their relations to other structures. This has led to modifications of surgical technique which spare these nerves and preserve erectile function.

Vasculogenic erectile dysfunction and diabetes mellitus

Masters & Johnson (1966) claimed that erectile dysfunction was psychogenic in 95% of cases. Subsequent research has shown that potential organic causes are present in 50% and that 25% of men may have a vascular lesion compromising erectile function. Evidence of peripheral vascular disease, a history of ischaemic heart disease or CVA, hypertension, smoking, obesity and diabetes mellitus should alert the clinician to this possibility, which increases with age.

Vascular occlusion at the bifurcation of the aorta may cause erectile dysfunction accompanied by claudication (Leriche syndrome). Arteriosclerotic changes and thrombi in the common and internal iliac, internal pudendal and penile arteries are associated with an insidious onset and progressive loss of erectile ability. Morning erections may be maintained while coitus becomes more difficult, but these become weaker and eventually cease. The time between the initial difficulty in maintaining an erection throughout intercourse and complete global loss varies considerably. It may be months, when secondary performance anxiety may have intervened, or take five years. There is no entirely reliable way of establishing that arterial insufficiency, rather than psychological factors, is the main cause, and often both are implicated. Loss of nocturnal penile tumescence (NPT) strongly favours an organic explanation, but there are still methodological problems associated with monitoring NPT. The persistence of NPT does not rule out a vascular cause; consider the external iliac steal syndrome in which erection is lost after the initiation of pelvic thrusting. In this condition the blood supply to erectile tissue is sufficient for erection at rest, but muscular activity causes dilatation of the arteries supplying the buttocks and legs and blood is shunted away from the penis. Some patients report gluteal pain after loss of erection, but others are indistinguishable from patients with performance anxiety on history alone.

The arterial supply of the erectile tissue can be evaluated most simply by the intracavernosal injection of a vasoactive drug, such as papaverine or prostaglandin E1. A complete sustained erection rules out arterial insufficiency, but a negative result can still occur as a result of anxiety. A non-invasive alternative is penile blood pressure measurement using the Doppler technique. Other methods used for evaluating the penile vasculature are Doppler pulse wave analysis, NPT monitoring using a device which measures rigidity as well as tumescence (the RigiScan), radio-isotope washout studies, duplex sonography and, if vascular surgery is being considered, phalloarteriography (see Gregoire & Pryor, 1993)

The competence of the venous drainage system can also be assessed. Venous leaks of various kinds cause erectile failure in men of all ages, becoming more prevalent with age. The site of leakage may be detected by injecting contrast material into the cavernous bodies (cavernosography) after an intracavernosal injection of a smooth muscle relaxant. Diagnostic confirmation depends on demonstrating decreased cavernosal pressure after the injection (cavernometry) in the presence of an adequate arterial supply as shown by Doppler ultrasound. The outcome of surgery for this pathologically heterogenous group is disappointing – 30% will show improvement maintained at one year. The term veno-occlusive dysfunction has been introduced to acknowledge the possibility that leakage may occur from failure of cavernous muscle to expand sufficiently to occlude the outflow of blood through the emissary veins.

Diabetes mellitus

Erectile dysfunction has been reported in 34–75% of diabetic men, the figure varying according to the characteristics of the sample and methodology. Most reports suggest that sexual appetite and ejaculation are unaffected. Attempted analyses of the relative contributions of organic and psychological factors have proven difficult, but there is wide agreement that the illness has profound psychological effects which play a role in the development of sexual dysfunction.

A minority of patients have erectile dysfunction at the initial clinical presentation of hyperglycaemia. In many of these men erectile function recovers with insulin treatment. This observation is thought to reflect reversal of neuronal biochemical abnormalities as blood sugar is lowered by insulin.

Despite adequate control of blood sugar, however, erectile dysfunction is a common complication of diabetes in the early years of the disease and increases with age. The two most important organic mechanisms are thought to be arterial insufficiency, particularly of the cavernosal artery, and peripheral neuropathy. Veno-occlusive dysfunction may also contribute, and there have been a few poorly substantiated reports of hypothalamo-pituitary-gonadal axis abnormalities.

A significant correlation between peripheral sensorimotor impairment and erectile dysfunction is clearly established. Clinically this is demonstrated by increased threshold for vibration and loss of ankle tendon reflexes. Impaired sensory conduction in the dorsal nerve of the penis has been demonstrated in diabetic men with erectile dysfunction and such measurement may become part of the clinical assessment of this group of patients in the future.

It is more difficult to demonstrate the significance of autonomic neuropathy. There is no way of clinically testing the integrity of the parasympathetic fibres to the penis. Clinical tests, such as pulse beat-to-beat variation, considered to reflect parasympathetic function, show little correlation with erectile function. Yet it is the parasympathetic supply to erectile tissue that activates the vascular changes which initiate and maintain erection. Post-mortem studies, however, have revealed damaged autonomic fibres in diabetic men with erectile failure.

Biochemical studies have shown abnormalities in all three autonomic neuroeffector systems (see Fig. 3) in cavernosal nerves in diabetes, including decreased VIP and acetylcholinesterase-positive fibres. Clinically, a patient with autonomic neuropathy but adequate arterial supply shows a complete erectile response to intracavernosal injection of a vasoactive drug.

Hyperprolactinaemia

The physiological role of prolactin in sexual behaviour is unclear. It is secreted by the anterior pituitary gland under the inhibitory control of the hypothalamic tuberoinfundibular dopamine system acting on dopamine D2 receptors. Thus, antipsychotic drugs cause hyperprolactinaemia and this has been implicated as a cause of sexual dysfunction in patients on these drugs.

The role of prolactin in sexual dysfunction is suggested by clinical observations in patients with hyperprolactinaemia due to prolactinomas. Erectile failure is almost always present and recovers rapidly when the hyperprolactinaemia is treated.

Hyperprolactinaemia impairs gonadal function and is also associated with reduced sexual appetite, making it difficult to ascertain the mechanism for erectile dysfunction. Animal experiments indicate that hyperprolactinaemia affects erectile function independently of sexual appetite and gonadal function, and that it exerts this effect on brain mechanisms. There is also pharmacological evidence that prolactin inhibits central dopaminergic control of erection. In women, hyperprolactinaemia has been associated with mild depression and a decrease in orgasmic frequency, but it is not clear to what extent reduced frequency of orgasm is related to failure of arousal.

Conclusions

Understanding the biology of mammalian sexual activity forms the basis of the clinical approach to organic sexual dysfunction. Social attitudes, culture, beliefs and emotions have unique salience in human sexual activity, but organic research and the poor results of psychological treatment outcome studies indicate that their causal significance in sexual dysfunction has been overestimated. Sexual consummation depends on hypothalamic integration in humans as it does in rodents, and remarkable instances of evolutionary conservation have been discovered, such as the integrative role of ancient polypeptides like oxytocin. We must, however, remain wary of biological reductionism and anthropomorphism. Experimental findings from animal models should be generalised to humans only with caution and when there are no alternative data on which to base intervention.

Only the psychiatrist working in the sexual and marital therapy clinic is equipped to recognise the possible contribution of organic factors. On occasions this amounts to making a diagnosis of previously unrecognised disease, such as a pituitary microadenoma. More often it will be the psychiatrist who will assess the relative contribution of organic disease to the problem and identify the need for appropriate physical tests. With the recent emergence of uroandrology, the psychiatrist with an interest in sex therapy needs to keep abreast of a rapidly developing field of biomedical technology in order to liaise effectively with surgical colleagues.

Finally, organic sexual dysfunction secondary to psychotropic medication is one of the commonest problems in psychiatry. Many clinicians will choose to ignore it, often in the mistaken belief that it is unavoidable. Many will avoid even asking patients about their sexual function for a host of other misguided reasons. We know that sexual dysfunction was the most frequently cited side-effect leading to non-compliance with antihypertensives in a large primary care project. Psychotropic drugs have considerably more deleterious effects on sexual function than antihypertensives. But as Monteiro *et al* (1987) demonstrated, patients rarely report these effects unless questioned directly. It remains to be systematically studied, but it should come as no surprise if sexual dysfunction emerged as the commonest reason for not continuing with prescribed psychotropic medication.

References

American Psychiatric Association (1994) *Diagnostic and Statistical Manual of Mental Disorders* (4th edn) (DSM–IV). Washington, DC: APA.

Balon, R., Yeragani, V. K., Pohl, R., *et al* (1993) Sexual dysfunction during antidepressant treatment. *Journal of Clinical Psychiatry*, 54, 209–212.

Bancroft, J. (1989) *Human Sexuality and its Problems.* Edinburgh: Churchill Livingstone.

Berard, E. J. (1989) The sexuality of spinal cord injured women: physiology and pathophysiology. A review. *Paraplegia*, 27, 99–112.

Bulpitt, C. J., Dollery, C. T. & Carne, S. (1976) Changes in the symptoms of hypertensive patients after referral to hospital clinic. *British Heart Journal*, 38, 121–128.

Chapelle, P. A., Durand, J. & Lacert, P. (1980) Penile erection following complete spinal cord injury in man. *British Journal of Urology*, 52, 216–219.

Dupont, S. (1995) Multiple sclerosis and sexual function – a review. *Clinical Rehabilitation*, 9, 135–141.

Everitt, B. J. (1990) Sexual motivation: A neural and behavioural analysis of the mechanisms underlying appetitive and copulatory responses of male rats. *Neuroscience and Biobehavioural Reviews*, 14, 217–232.

Gregoire, A. & Pryor, J. P. (1993) *Impotence: An Integrated Approach to Clinical Practice.* Edinburgh: Churchill Livingstone.

Harrison, W. M., Rabkin, J. G., Ehrhardt, A. A., *et al* (1986) Effects of antidepressant medication on sexual function: a controlled study. *Journal of Clinical Psychopharmacology*, 6, 144–149.

Heath, R. (1964) *The Role of Pleasure in Behavior.* New York: Harper & Row.

Hulter, B. & Lundberg, P. O. (1994) Sexual function in women with hypothalamo-pituitary disease. *Archives of Sexual Behaviour*, 23, 171–183.

Jacobsen, F. M. (1992) Fluoxetine-induced sexual dysfunction and an open trial of yohimbine. *Journal of Clinical Psychiatry*, 53, 119–122.

LeVay, S. (1993) *The Sexual Brain.* Cambridge, MA: MIT Press.

Masters, W. H. & Johnson, V. E. (1966) *Human Sexual Response.* London: Churchill.

Medical Research Council (1981) Adverse reaction to bendrofluazide and propanolol for the treatment of mild hypertension. *Lancet*, ii, 539–543.

Monteiro, W. O., Noshirvani, H. F., Marks, I. M., *et al* (1987) Anorgasmia from clomipramine in obsessive–compulsive disorder: a controlled trial. *British Journal of Psychiatry*, 151, 107–112.

Murphy, M. R. (1993*a*) The neuroanatomy and neurophysiology of erection. In *Impotence – An Integrated Approach to Clinical Practice* (eds A. Gregoire & J. Pryor), pp. 29–48. Edinburgh: Churchill Livingstone.

—— (1993*b*) The pharmacology of erection and erectile dysfunction. In *Impotence – An Integrated Approach to Clinical Practice* (eds A. Gregoire & J. Pryor), pp. 55–77. Edinburgh: Churchill Livingstone.

——, Seckl, J. R., Burton, S., *et al* (1987) Changes in oxytocin and vasopressin secretion during sexual activity in men. *Journal of Clinical Endocrinology and Metabolism*, 65, 738–741.

——, ——, Checkley, S. A., *et al* (1990) Naloxone inhibits oxytocin release at orgasm in man. *Journal of Clinical Endocrinology and Metabolism*, 71, 1056–1058.

Oomura, Y., Aou, S., Koyama, Y., *et al* (1988) Central control of sexual behavior. *Brain Research Bulletin*, 20, 863–870.

Saenz de Tejada, I., Goldstein, I., Azadzoi, K., *et al* (1989) Impaired neurogenic and endothelium-mediated relaxation of penile smooth muscle from diabetic men with impotence. *New England Journal of Medicine*, 320, 1025–1030.

Segraves, R. T. (1989) Effects of psychotropic drugs on human erection and ejaculation. *Archives of General Psychiatry*, 46, 275–284.

Sherwin, B. B. & Gelfand, M. M. (1987) The role of androgen in the maintenance of sexual functioning in oophorectomized women. *Psychosomatic Medicine,* 49, 397–409.

Shukla, G. D., Srivastava, O. N. & Katiyar, B. C. (1979) Sexual disturbances in temporal lobe epilepsy: a controlled study. *British Journal of Psychiatry*, 134, 288–292.

Toone, B. (1986) Sexual disorders in epilepsy. In *Recent Advances in Epilepsy* (vol. 3) (eds T. A. Tedley & B. S. Meldrum), pp. 233–261. Edinburgh: Churchill Livingstone.
Valleroy, M. L. & Kraft, G. H. (1984) Sexual dysfunction in multiple sclerosis. *Archives of Rehabilitation and Physical Medicine*, 65, 125–128.

Additional reading

Bancroft, J. (ed.) (1995) *The Pharmacology of Sexual Function and Dysfunction.* Amsterdam: Elsevier Science.
Riley, A. J., Peet, M. & Wilson, C. (1993) *Sexual Pharmacology.* Oxford: Clarendon Press.

2 Gender development

Susan Golombok and Robyn Fivush

The development of gender identity and role ● *Puberty and the development of sexual relationships* ● *Conclusions*

Gender development originates from the moment of conception. When a female egg unites with a male sperm to form either an XX or an XY chromosome pair, males and females embark upon different developmental pathways. This chapter will explore the various theoretical explanations of the processes involved in the development of gender identity (a person's concept of him- or herself as male or female) and gender role (the behaviours and attitudes considered appropriate for males and females in a particular culture). The development of male and female sexual relationships will then be examined.

The development of gender identity and role

Prenatal influences

Is the function of genes and of the hormones which are present in the developing foetus simply to determine our physical characteristics as male or female? Or does our biological makeup also influence the development of gender identity and role? This issue has been addressed by studying individuals with biological anomalies to discover whether, for example, an atypical genetic pattern or an excess or deficiency of prenatal sex hormones has an effect on these aspects of gender development. If so, the variation in sex-typed behaviour can, at least in part, be attributed to the biological anomaly under investigation, and can help us to understand the role of specific biological factors on normal gender development. For example, if children exposed prenatally to unusually high levels of male sex hormones are found to be extremely masculine and those exposed to unusually low levels are much less so, then male hormones would appear to be influential in the development of male gender role behaviour.

But first, it is important to point out that the categorisation of hormones as either male or female can be misleading. Androgens are commonly referred to as male hormones because of their role in male sexual differentiation, whereas progesterone and oestrogens are often described as female hormones because they control the female reproductive cycle. In fact, both sexes produce all three hormones, but in different relative amounts. Moreover, the so-called female hormones can act like androgens; both oestrogen and some synthetic forms of progesterone can have a masculinising effect on behaviour (Hines & Green, 1990).

Exposure in the womb to abnormally high or low levels of male or female sex hormones can occur in two ways. Firstly, there are certain genetic conditions which cause an overdose or a deficit of specific sex hormones in the developing foetus. These infants are born with genital malformation, either masculinisation of the genitals of genetic females or feminisation of the genitals of genetic males, depending upon the effect of the condition on sex hormone production. The extent of the masculinisation or feminisation varies from one child to another so that in some cases the genitals are ambiguous in appearance, while in others a genetic female appears to be male, and vice versa. These individuals are called pseudohermaphrodites, meaning that they possess both male and female sexual structures. Secondly, synthetic hormones have been prescribed to women experiencing a difficult pregnancy. This practice began in the 1940s and continued until the 1970s when it became clear not only that this treatment was largely ineffective but also that women who had been prescribed the hormone diethylstilbestrol (DES) were at risk for vaginal and cervical cancer.

Gender identity

The role of androgens in gender identity has been examined by studying girls with congenital adrenal hyperplasia. This is a genetically transmitted disorder in which malfunctioning adrenal glands produce high levels of androgens from the prenatal period onwards. Girls with this syndrome are genetically female and have female internal reproductive organs but are born with masculinised external genitals. When assigned and raised as boys, these genetic girls adopt a male gender identity and role. The condition is usually treated by surgically feminising the genitals during infancy, and by administering corticosteroids thereafter, which reduces the level of androgen production.

Studies of the effects of prenatal androgenisation on gender identity have examined girls who were treated early in life to avoid the confounding effects of increased levels of male sex hormones postnatally. If genetic females with congenital adrenal hyperplasia are raised as girls from birth, they develop a female gender identity in spite of their prenatal androgenisation. They are quite sure that they are girls and have no desire to change sex (Money & Ehrhardt, 1972). Thus prenatal androgenisation does not appear to affect the formation of gender identity.

Investigations of genetic males with complete androgen insensitivity syndrome tell us what happens when the body cannot respond to male sex hormones. This is a condition in which the tissues of a genetic male are insensitive to androgen, causing the genitals to be female in appearance. These infants are raised as girls. When they reach puberty they develop breasts and look just like other adult women. They do not menstruate, however, and are infertile. The syndrome is often not detected until puberty, when menstruation fails to occur. Individuals with complete androgen insensitivity syndrome develop a female gender identity and role in spite of the presence of a Y chromosome (Money & Ehrhardt, 1972).

Studies of pseudohermaphrodites provide strong evidence that gender identity is determined by psychological rather than biological factors. Biological males with complete androgen insensitivity syndrome who look female at birth and who are raised as girls can develop a female gender identity, and biological females with congenital adrenal hyperplasia who look like boys and who are treated as boys can develop a male gender identity – in spite of incongruent sex chromosomes, gonads, hormones and internal reproductive organs! The most important factor in determining gender identity seems to be the sex to which the infant is assigned and reared.

However, findings reported by Imperato-McGinley *et al* (1979) challenge the view that biology has no role to play in the development of gender identity. These researchers investigated a group of boys in the Dominican Republic who, due to a rare genetic disorder, were born with under-developed male genitals which made them look like girls. The children were reared as girls until the raised levels of male hormones produced at puberty caused them to develop a penis and male secondary characteristics. These genetic males then turned into men, adopting a male gender identity and male sex role behaviour. This research suggests that male hormones may be important in gender identity formation. But social factors cannot be ruled out as an explanation. The parents may have been aware of the condition because the children's genitals were not identical to those of normal females. In fact, the children were nicknamed 'guevodoces', meaning 'testicles at 12'. Because fertile men hold a much higher status in the Dominican Republic than infertile women (the alternative had they remained female), both the children and their families would have benefited from the change.

So what can we learn from research on pseudohermaphrodites? It seems that gender identity is largely determined by psychological rather than biological factors, and that the sex to which an infant is assigned at birth is the first crucial step in this process. We cannot, however, definitively conclude that biological factors play no part in the development of gender identity.

Gender roles

Although prenatal androgens are not a major influence on gender identity, they do appear to play a part in the development of gender roles, predisposing us towards masculine gender role behaviour. Comparisons between girls with congenital adrenal hyperplasia who were treated early in life and control groups of girls unaffected by this disorder found the androgenised girls to be more interested in active outdoor play, to prefer boys as playmates, to spend more time playing with masculine toys, and to see themselves and be seen by others as tomboys. They were less interested in traditionally female activities such as doll play, baby-care and fantasy games involving role-play as a wife or mother (Ehrhardt *et al*, 1968; Berenbaum & Hines, 1992). Boys with congenital adrenal hyperplasia also showed higher levels of energy expenditure in play and sports than did a control group of their unaffected brothers (Ehrhardt, 1975).

Progesterones can have either a masculinising or a feminising influence on sex role behaviour. Natural progesterone and some synthetic progesterones are feminising because they interfere with the action of androgens. Other synthetic progesterones mimic androgens and thus have a masculinising effect (Goy & McEwen, 1980; Hines, 1982). Girls prenatally exposed to synthetic progesterones with androgenic properties show a similar pattern of tomboyish behaviour to girls with congenital adrenal hyperplasia (Money & Ehrhardt, 1972). Also, higher scores on a projective test of aggression have been obtained by both females and males exposed to androgenic progesterones. These studies provide further evidence that prenatal androgenisation causes a predisposition towards male sex role behaviour.

In contrast, the outcome of prenatal exposure to non-androgenic progesterones is a tendency towards female sex role behaviour, particularly for girls. Prenatally exposed girls show more interest in doll play, child care, feminine clothing, and less physically active play, and less interest in tomboyish behaviour than unexposed controls (Ehrhardt *et al*, 1984). The consequence for boys is less conclusive. There are some reports of less energetic, assertive, aggressive and athletic behaviour, but other studies have failed to demonstrate a clear effect for boys (Ehrhardt *et al*, 1984). One explanation is that sufficient androgens are present in the male foetus to override the effect of the natural or synthetic progesterone. Because boys are under pressure to conform to stereotypically masculine behaviour, any tendency towards less typically male behaviour that may arise from an elevated level of natural or non-androgenic synthetic progesterone may be counteracted by cultural influences.

Although it seems that the development of sex role behaviour may be influenced to some extent by sex hormones, with androgens masculinising behaviour and non-androgenic progesterones having a feminising effect, a number of methodological problems are associated with this research (Bleier, 1984). The samples studied were small and often included children across a wide age range; furthermore, the interviewers were sometimes aware of the nature of the child's condition, which may have biased the results. It is also conceivable that knowledge of the unusual hormonal condition may affect the behaviour of parents or the children themselves, so that tomboyish behaviour in girls prenatally exposed to an excess of male hormones may be noticed more by parents, and their daughters may be under less pressure to conform to the female role. In the past, many girls with congenital adrenal hyperplasia did not receive surgery until after they had become aware of their masculinised genitals which may well have affected their behaviour. Nowadays, however, the majority of these girls are feminised in infancy, and yet continue to be less feminine than their peers. Interestingly, the findings of more recent studies of prenatal androgenisation that have corrected for the methodological problems summarised by Bleier are similar to those of the original investigations. Although the methodological difficulties prevent us from drawing any firm conclusions, the research findings are relatively consistent in suggesting that there might be a link between sex hormones and sex role behaviour, with androgens predisposing towards masculinity and non-androgenic progesterones towards femininity.

How might prenatal sex hormones influence gender role behaviour? It is thought that sex differences in prenatal hormone levels produce sex differences in the organisation of neural substrates of the brain, causing the threshold for some behaviours to be lower for girls and for others to be lower for boys. According to this theory, a high level of prenatal androgens masculinises the brain so that it takes a weaker stimulus to evoke male sex typed behaviour such as play with cars and trucks, and a stronger stimulus to evoke female sex role behaviour such as doll play, whereas a low level of androgens has the opposite effect. These prenatally determined differences in sensitivity to stimuli are thought to help explain why boys and girls differ in patterns of play, in levels of activity and in aggressive behaviour (Money & Ehrhardt, 1972; Hines & Green, 1990).

The theory that prenatal sex hormones produce sex differences in brain structure and behaviour has aroused a great deal of controversy, particularly because it derives from animal research which is often criticised as irrelevant to human behaviour, and because the mechanisms involved in the link between sex hormones, sex differences in brain structure and sex differences in behaviour in humans have not been clearly determined. The theory has also been criticised for failing to take account of psychological and social influences on sex-typing. It is to these social and psychological processes that we turn next.

Psychoanalytic theory

According to traditional psychoanalytic theory, gender development is rooted in the phallic stage of psychosexual development which occurs at about five years of age (Freud, 1905, 1920, 1933). Until this time, both boys and girls are believed to identify with the mother. On entering the phallic stage, the identification process in boys and girls begins to diverge.

A boy is thought to experience sexual desire for his mother and to see his father as a rival. But because he fears retaliation by his father, specifically that his father will castrate him, he develops castration anxiety. This conflict, between his sexual desire for his mother and his fear of castration by his father, is known as the Oedipal conflict. Freud believed that it is in order to resolve the conflict that boys shift their identification from the mother to the father and take on his male characteristics. In this way he avoids castration which he fears so much, and comes to realise that the possession of a penis will allow him to have sexual relationships with women when he grows up.

The mechanisms involved in female identification are rather different, and less clearly described by Freud. For girls it is penis envy, rather than castration anxiety, which is considered to form the basis for gender development. At first a girl, like a boy, is thought to view her mother as a love object and her father as a rival. But when she discovers that she does not possess a penis she experiences penis envy, believing that she has already been castrated and blaming her mother to whom she develops a deep hostility. The father then replaces the mother as a love object. Eventually, she comes to understand that her desire for a penis is unattainable. In order to overcome her penis envy she substitutes her wish for a penis for a wish for a baby. The resolution of the Oedipal conflict in girls involves transferring identification back to the mother and adopting a female identity and role.

Many of Freud's critics have questioned his ideas about penis envy, arguing that although this may be a real phenomenon, it is based more on culture than on biology. Thus, even psychoanalysts trained under Freud, such as Helene Deutsch (1933), Karen Horney (1933) and Clara Thompson (1943), believed that females come to envy the penis because the penis represents power and control in society. What little girls come to realise early in development is not that a penis *per se* is important, but that having a penis means having power and control over one's life, and not having a penis means being denied opportunities and autonomy. While this reformulation of Freudian theory may make a great deal of sense, it does not change any of the basic ideas about sexual development. These theorists still assume that penis envy is a major factor in female sexual development. Further, being male is still seen as better than being female, although for cultural rather than biological reasons.

More radical reinterpretations of traditional psychoanalytic theory have involved questioning the assumption of male superiority. From this approach, females are examined in their own right rather than in comparison to males. Eric Erikson (1968) argued that the female experience of body was fundamentally different than the male experience of body. Whereas the male sense of bodily self involves protrusion and projection into external space, the female sense of bodily self is directed toward inner space, a sense of containment and surround. Females do not have penis envy; rather they have a different but very positive sense of their own body. In fact, Erikson argues that males may envy females because females have the ability to create life. To overcome this "womb envy", males feel the need to accomplish things in the world, leading to their being more outer-directed. Females are more secure because of their creative powers, and develop caring and nurturing relationships.

Nancy Chodorow (1978) has also reinterpreted some of Freud's basic ideas about early development. Instead of focusing exclusively on the phallic stage of psychosexual development, Chodorow argues that gender identity begins in infancy. At this early point in development, Chodorow agrees with Freud that the breast, and by extension the mother, is the most important object in the infant's world. Both boys and girls are assumed to begin with a female gender identity. As they grow older, females continue to identify with the mother and their self-concept develops from this interpersonal relationship. Males, in contrast, begin to differentiate more and more from the mother, and in the process of forming a male gender identity, turn away from all that is female. Males define themselves as separate and individuated; moreover, they repress all feminine tendencies in themselves and begin to denigrate femininity in others.

It is important to point out that there is virtually no empirical support for Freud's theory, or for the various reformulations and reinterpretations. Nevertheless, Freud has had a major impact on our thinking about gender development. He was the first theorist to focus on developmental issues, and his ideas have had a profound influence on more recent social–cognitive explanations of gender development.

Social learning theory

From the perspective of classic social learning theory, the two processes which are important for children's gender development are differential reinforcement and modelling. The process of reinforcement is based on the principle that behaviour is modified by its consequences. Behaviour which has favourable consequences (reinforcement) is more likely to be repeated, while behaviour which is not rewarded or is punished is less likely to be performed again. Sex-typed behaviour is thought to result from the differential reinforcement of boys and girls; for example, girls will generally receive a much more favourable response than boys for playing with dolls, and boys are more likely than girls to be reinforced for playing with cars and trucks, so these behaviours come to be performed with different frequency by girls and boys.

There is much evidence to suggest that parents of preschool children do treat their sons and daughters differently, although the extent to which they are producing sex-typed behaviour, rather that simply responding to pre-existing differences between boys and girls, remains unknown (Maccoby & Jacklin, 1974). Right from birth, parents interact with their infants differently according to whether they are baby boys or baby girls. They dress their girls in pink, decorative clothes and their boys in blue, functional ones, and surround them with sex-typed toys and furnishings. From as early as 12 months, infants are encouraged to play with sex-typed toys and to avoid play activities which are considered more appropriate for children of the other sex. The differential encouragement of sex-typed activities in boys and girls becomes even more apparent as infants grow into toddlers (Fagot, 1978).

However, differential reinforcement by parents seems to decline once children reach school age. At this stage of a child's development, friends take on a more important role. Peers consistently and strongly reinforce sex-typed toy choice and play, and punish cross-gender activities.

The observation and imitation of models is the other mechanism that is considered by social learning theorists to be operative in gender development. According to classic social learning theorists, boys and girls learn sex-typed behaviour by imitating models of the same sex as themselves, particularly the same sex parent. However, the idea that children acquire sex-typed behaviour by directly imitating same sex parents is now thought to be rather simplistic, and a modified version of social learning theory has been proposed to explain the contribution of modelling to gender development (Perry & Bussey, 1979). It seems that children do not simply imitate the behaviour of individual models of the same sex as themselves. Instead, they learn which behaviours are considered to be appropriate for males and which for females by observing many men and women and boys and girls, and by noticing which behaviours are performed frequently by females and rarely by males, and vice versa. Children then use these abstractions of sex-appropriate behaviour as models for their own imitative performance.

Thus contemporary social learning theorists no longer consider the modelling of same sex parents to be a primary mechanism in gender development. Instead, children observe a wide variety of role models in their daily life and tend to imitate those whom they consider to be typical of their sex. Friends, in particular, appear to be important role models; school-age boys and girls show a strong preference for same sex peers. But it is gender stereotypes, rather than specific individuals, that seem to be most influential in the acquisition of sex-typed behaviour. Gender stereotypes are pervasive in our society, and children are aware of these stereotypes from as early as two years of age. Not only do children learn about gender stereotypes from interactions with others, but they are also exposed from an early age to sex-stereotyped characters in books and on television.

Cognitive developmental theory

Cognitive developmental theories constitute the third major psychological approach to the understanding of gender development. A central tenet of cognitive developmental theory is that children play an active part in their own development; they seek out for themselves information about gender and socialise themselves as male or female.

Early studies focused on children's developing understanding of the concept of gender (Stagnor & Ruble, 1987). Basic gender identity is established at about 2–3 years. By this age, children know that they are male or female, and can correctly label other people as male or female as well. It is not until they reach the stage of gender stability a year or two later that they realise that gender is stable across time; that a male friend used to be a baby boy and will be a man when he grows up. At this stage, children still believe that gender can change; if a girl puts on boy's clothes, has a boy's haircut and plays with boy's toys, she will become a boy. Gender constancy is the final stage in the development of the gender concept. When this stage is reached, at about 5 or 6 years, children understand that gender is a characteristic which does not change; even if a girl dresses and behaves like a boy she will still be a girl.

According to Kohlberg, it is when children reach the stage of gender constancy that they begin to identify with their own gender, seek out information associated with their own gender, come to value the characteristics and behaviours associated with their own gender, and engage in gender-related activities. Gender knowledge increases in content and complexity throughout childhood and children are more likely to imitate models of their own sex once they have reached gender constancy (Slaby & Frey, 1976). Children know a great deal about gender and consistently show a preference for toys and activities associated with their own gender by the time they achieve basic gender identity at about 2–3 years (Maccoby & Jacklin, 1974; Martin & Little, 1990).

Gender schema theorists have examined the way in which children organise knowledge about gender. The term schema is used in psychology to refer to an organised body of knowledge. Gender schemas refer to organised bodies of knowledge about gender, and are functionally similar to gender stereotypes. From as early as 2–3 years, soon after they begin to label themselves and others consistently as male or female, children organise information according to gender. If told that a person is male or female, children will make gender-related predictions about that person's behaviour, even in the face of opposing information. So preschool children will predict that a boy will like to play with cars and guns, even if told that he likes to play with dolls. As children grow older, not only do they learn more about gender-related behaviours and characteristics, but they also begin to organise their knowledge in more complex ways. They do not simply assume that because a child is male, he will necessarily like to play with cars and guns; if told that the boy likes to play with dolls, they are able to predict that he may like other stereotypically female activities as well (Martin *et al*, 1990). Children know more about behaviours and characteristics associated with their own gender than the other gender, and this seems to occur from as early as two years of age.

Gender schemas influence the way in which we perceive and remember information about the world around us, so that we pay greater attention to, and are more likely to remember, information that is in line with our gender schemas than opposing information. Children as young as five years have been shown to have a better memory for events which fit with gender stereotypes than those which do not. For example, they are more likely to remember a picture of a woman, than of a man, cooking a meal (Liben & Signorella, 1980).

Puberty and the development of sexual relationships

The onset of puberty is associated with an increase in bursts of gonadotrophin-releasing hormone from the hypothalamus, causing an upsurge in the production of follicle stimulating hormone (FSH) and luteinizing hormone (LH) by the pituitary (Hopwood *et al*, 1990). The age at which puberty begins is influenced by both genetic and environmental factors, including geographic location, ethnicity, emotional state and nutrition (Hopwood *et al*, 1990). In boys, these hormones cause the testes to produce testosterone, which is largely responsible for the development of male physical characteristics and reproductive function. In girls, increased levels of FSH and LH cause the ovaries to produce oestrogen, which stimulates the development of a female body shape and the reproductive organs. Girls have male as well as female sex hormones, although at much lower levels than boys. It is the androgens produced at puberty that are responsible in girls for the growth of pubic and body hair. Just as girls have male sex hormones, boys have low levels of female sex hormones.

Girls usually enter puberty between the ages of 8 and 14. The development of breasts and a female body shape results from an increase in fatty tissue. This is followed by the growth of pubic and underarm hair. Puberty is also characterised by a growth spurt, development of the reproductive organs and the start of menstruation. It is thought that girls need to attain a critical percentage of body fat before menstruation will begin (Frisch & McArthur, 1974). In boys, puberty begins two years later, on average, than in girls. Physical changes include growth of the penis and testes, as well as of pubic, body and facial hair. During the growth spurt there is a rapid increase in height and in muscle tissue resulting in a male body shape. Boys also begin to ejaculate, and their voice deepens.

The beginning of sexual activity in adolescents is influenced by social factors as well as by hormones. The way in which biological and social factors interact to influence the development of sexuality has been examined by following up more than 1000 adolescents over a two-year period (Udry, 1990). Whereas the onset of interest in sex was associated with an increase in androgen levels in both boys and girls, the antecedents of sexual behaviour differed between the sexes. For boys, initial involvement in sexual activity was highly dependent on hormones and not much affected by social influences. In contrast, girls' first involvement in sexual activity was much more influenced by social factors, such as whether or not their best friend had had sex, than by hormones.

In western society, sexual activity has always been more acceptable for boys than for girls, and adolescent boys have been much more likely than adolescent girls to engage in sexual relationships. But the gap between the sexes has narrowed in recent years as more adolescent girls have become sexually active. For most young people today, sexual intercourse first takes place during the teenage years. In a survey of 16–25-year-olds in Los Angeles, the average age of first sexual intercourse was 14.9 years for boys and 15.9 years for girls (Moore & Erickson, 1985). Adolescents in Europe are slightly older when they first have sex. Recent surveys in the Netherlands and West Germany showed that about 50% of 17-year-olds have experienced sexual intercourse. In the UK, a survey of 16–24 year olds similarly showed that the median age at first intercourse was 17 years (Johnson *et al*, 1994). Sexual activity with a partner of the same sex has been reported to be experienced by about 10% of adolescents in the US (DeLamater & MacCorquodale, 1979) and by about 6% of 16–24-year-olds in the UK (Johnson *et al*, 1994).

It is often assumed that male and female sexuality are qualitatively different, and that men are much more interested in sex than are women. But just how different are the sexual experiences of men and women? The studies of Masters & Johnson (1966) did much to increase our understanding of the physiological changes which take place during sexual arousal, and demonstrated that in spite of differences in anatomy and reproductive function, men and women experience a similar pattern of sexual response. In addition, Heiman (1975) demonstrated that women become just as aroused by erotic material as men, although they are not always aware of their sexually aroused state. However, women are less likely than men to reach orgasm during sexual intercourse. In the first large-scale survey of sexual behaviour, it was found that 30% of married women had never experienced an orgasm. Two decades later, it was still the case that a substantial minority (10–15%) of married women never or seldom reached orgasm; and Hite (1976) found that only around 30% of women in her sample regularly had an orgasm during sexual intercourse without additional clitoral stimulation. Gender differences also exist for masturbation. Only 58% of women compared with 98% of men had masturbated at least once.

These surveys suffer from a number of methodological problems, particularly the use of samples which are unrepresentative of the general population, which make it difficult to draw general conclusions from the findings. But they do provide information about sexual activity that cannot be obtained by other types of investigation. Such surveys are thought to give reasonably accurate estimates of sexual behaviour, although the subjects were probably more sexually active than average. *The Hite Report* obtained a response rate of only 3% from a sample that was unrepresentative in the first place. The value of this survey lies in the detailed accounts of female sexuality, which provided new insight into women's sexual experiences.

Conclusions

This chapter has examined various aspects of what it means to grow up male or female. We have seen that gender development constitutes a complex interaction between biological, psychological and social factors. Although we have focused on the ways in which females and males differ, it should be borne in mind that there are also great similarities between the sexes. Just as importantly, not all girls are alike nor are all boys alike. The differences we have discussed are group differences. It must be remembered that each individual is unique and will display a unique developmental pathway.

References

Berenbaum, S. A. & Hines, M. (1992) Early androgens are related to sex-typed toy preferences. *Psychological Science*, 3, 202–206.

Bleier, R. (1984) *Science and Gender: A Critique of Biology and its Theories of Women*. Oxford: Pergamon.

Chodorow, N. J. (1978) *The Reproduction of Mothering: Psychoanalysis and the Socialisation of Gender*. Berkeley: University of California Press.

DeLamater, J. & MacCorquodale, P. (1979) *Premarital Sexuality: Attitudes, Relationships, Behaviour*. Madison: University of Wisconsin Press.

Deutsch, H. (1933) On female homosexuality. Reprinted in *Psychoanalysis and Female Sexuality* (ed. H. M. Ruitenbeek), 1967, pp. 106–129. New Haven: College and University Press.

Ehrhardt, A. (1975) Prenatal hormone exposure and psychosexual differentiation. In *Topics in Psychoneuroendocrinology* (ed. E. J. Sachar). New York: Grune & Stratton.

——, Epstein, R. & Money, J. (1968) Fetal androgens and female gender identity in the early treated adrenogenital syndrome. *John Hopkins Medical Journal*, 122, 160–176.

——, Meyer-Bhalburg, H. F., Feldman, J. F., *et al* (1984) Sex-dimorphic behaviour in childhood subsequent to prenatal exposure to exogenous progestogens and estrogens. *Archives of Sexual Behaviour,* 13, 457–477.

Erikson, E. (1968) Womanhood and the inner space. In *Women and Analysis* (ed. J. Strouse), 1974, pp. 291–319. New York: Grossman.

Fagot, B. I. (1978) The influence of sex of child on parental reactions to toddler children. *Child Development,* 49, 459–465.

Freud, S. (1905) Three essays on the theory of sexuality. In *The Standard Edition of the Complete Works of Sigmund Freud, Vol. 7* (ed. J. Strachey), 1953. London: Hogarth Press.

—— (1920) Beyond the pleasure principle. In *The Standard Edition of the Complete Works of Sigmund Freud, Vol. 18* (ed. J. Strachey), 1953. London: Hogarth Press.

—— (1933) Psychology of women. In *New Introductory Lectures on Psychoanalysis.* London: Hogarth Press.

Frisch, R. E. & McArthur, J. W. (1974) Menstrual cycles: fatness as a determinant of minimum weight for height necessary for their maintenance and onset. *Science,* 185, 949–951.

Goy, R. W. & McEwen, B. S. (1980) *Sexual Differentiation in the Brain.* Cambridge, MA: MIT Press.

Heiman, J. R. (1975) The psychology of erotica: women's sexual arousal. *Psychology Today,* 8, 90–94.

Hines, M. (1982) Prenatal gonadal hormones and sex differences in human behaviour. *Psychological Bulletin,* 92, 56–80.

—— & Green, R. (1990) Human hormonal and neural correlates of sex-typed behaviours. *Review of Psychiatry,* 10, 536–555.

Hite, S. (1976) *The Hite Report.* New York: Macmillan.

Horney, K. (1933) The denial of the vagina. In *Psychoanalysis and Female Sexuality* (ed. H. M. Ruitenbeek), 1967, pp. 73–87. New Haven, CT: College and University Press.

Hopwood, N., Kelch, R., Hale, P., *et al* (1990) The onset of human puberty: Biological and environmental factors. In Adolescence and Puberty (eds J. Bancroft & J Reinisch). New York: Oxford University Press.

Imperato-McGinley, J., Peterson, R., Gautier, T., *et al* (1979) Androgens and the evolution of male gender identity among male pseudohermaphrodites with 5a reductase deficiency. *New England Journal of Medicine,* 300, 1233–1237.

Johnson, A. M., Wadsworth, J., Wellings, K., *et al* (1994) *Sexual Attitudes and Lifestyles.* Oxford: Blackwell Scientific Publications.

Liben, L. S. & Signorella, M. L. (1980) Gender related schema and constructive memory in children. *Child Development,* 51, 111–118.

Maccoby, E. & Jacklin, C. (1974) *The Psychology of Sex Differences.* Stanford, CA: Stanford University Press.

Martin, C. L. & Little, J. K. (1990) The relation of gender understanding in the children's sex-typed preferences and gender stereotypes. *Child Development,* 61, 1427–1439.

——, Wood, C. H. & Little, J. K. (1990) The development of gender stereotype components. *Child Development,* 61, 1891–1904.

Masters, W. & Johnson, V. (1966) *Human Sexual Response.* Boston: Little & Brown.

Money, J. & Ehrhardt, A. (1972) *Man and Woman, Boy and Girl: The Differentiation and Diamorphism of Gender Identity from Conception to Maturity*. Baltimore: John Hopkins University Press.

Moore, D. & Erikson, P. (1985) Age, gender and ethnic differences in sexual and contraceptive knowledge attitudes and behaviour. *Family and Community Health*, 8, 38–51.

Perry, D. & Bussey, K. (1979) The social learning theory of sex difference: imitation is alive and well. *Journal of Personality and Social Psychology*, 37, 1699–1712.

Slaby, R. G. & Frey, K. S. (1975) Development of gender constancy and selective attention to same sex models. *Child Development*, 46, 849–856.

Stagnor, C. & Ruble, D. N. (1987) Development of gender role knowledge and gender constancy. In *Children's Gender Schemata: New Directions for Child Development* no. 38 (eds L. S. Liben & M. L. Signorella), pp. 5–22. San Francisco: Jossey Bass.

Thompson, C. (1943) 'Penis envy' in women. In *Psycholanalysis and Female Sexuality* (ed. H. M. Ruitenbeek), 1967, pp. 246–251. New Haven, CT: College and University Press.

Udry, J. (1990) Hormonal and social determinants of adolescent sexual initiation. In *Adolescence and Puberty* (eds J. Bancroft & J. Reinisch). New York: Oxford University Press.

Further reading

Golombok, S. & Fivush, R. (1994) *Gender Development*. Cambridge: Cambridge University Press.

3 Sexology and male sexuality: a history of socio-medical attitudes towards sexual behaviour

Sue Collinson

Myth, magic and rejuvenation • *Moral hygiene and 'lost manhood'* • *Spermaticidal anxiety* • *Control and continence* • *Hype, hyperidrosis and hypersexuality* • *Sexual pathology* • *Sexual psychology* • *The third sex* • *From disease to desire: variety is the spice of life*

Sexology, by which human sexuality became the object of a specific science, originates in Britain from around the middle of the 19th century. This was at a time when medicine itself was undergoing a transformation into a science which appeared to promise an unprecedented technical potential to conquer and control ill-health and disease. There is, however, a rich history and wide pre-scientific literature on the subject of sex and sexuality which still today informs many of our beliefs and attitudes. Indeed, we justify our interest in sex-related behaviour on the grounds that it offers us an explanation of social organisation, although as Freud observed, the focus of interest has changed, during its long history, from the instinct itself to its object (Freud, 1977). Interpretations of the nature of sexuality and its relationship with love and reproduction range from the ancient Greek perception which linked sexuality to appetite, thus categorising it as one of the lower functions of humankind, to the Christian suspicion of sexuality, with its separation of the biological function of sex from the spiritual nature of love. This is the legacy which has influenced European attitudes towards sex for generations, and which persists even today in the omission of ideas of love from discussions of the biology of reproduction.

The extensive pre-scientific literature dealing with human sexuality is dominated by concerns with male potency. By the late 19th century, Freud may have pathologised perceptions of phallic symbolism and iconography, but phallism has been celebrated, venerated and recorded for as far back as there are records of human behaviour. The central image of the male generative organ has for centuries been used to symbolise the regenerative power of nature, and the loss of that potency, as well as the desire for its enhancement, has been responsible for generating a long tradition of therapies for the rejuvenation of male sexuality. Even when sex becomes a subject of serious scientific investigation, the literature shows us that the central concern is with male sexuality. It is against this context, of the idea of the social and psychological primacy of masculine sexual behaviour, that the prehistory of sexology can be understood. The history of the importance of male sexuality also contributes to an understanding of the long and enduringly uneasy relationship between medicine and sexuality. It can also be used to illustrate the confusion that existed between concepts of sexual instinct and sexual force; the issue of sexuality as the motive force for reproduction; and the eventual emergence of the idea that sexual variations represented 'degenerate' forms of the 'natural' norm. This in turn increasingly informed a powerful public morality during the 19th and 20th centuries, which was founded upon exacting definitions of personal, social and racial hygiene.

Finally, the professionalisation of doctors and the medicalisation of those aspects of social behaviour represented by an individual's sexuality was eventually to invite medical intervention in the sexual lives of healthy individuals to an unprecedented extent. Sex, like other 'diseases', was endowed with its own taxonomy of deviance, and then responded to with a range of interventions, which could include institutionalisation. A complex situation arose whereby, in an increasingly secular world, the doctor became the arbiter of appropriate moral and social sexual behaviour. Concern over public morality, the extent of prostitution and the spread of venereal disease during the 19th century was taken as justification for attempts to classify and construct forms of social control over certain types of sexual behaviour, particularly those which were judged to be related to criminality, deviance and insanity. The emergence of eugenics in the wake of post-Darwinian biology appeared to give scientific validation to the development of social strategies which were designed to intercede in the sexual life of the nation.

As sexuality and sexual behaviour were drawn into the domain of scientific investigation during the second half of the 19th century, sex researchers began to develop a taxonomic account of the aetiology and range of sexual variety. By the end of the century, the work of Richard von Krafft-Ebing, Havelock Ellis and Sigmund Freud among others had helped to establish classificatory and analytical descriptions of human sexual behaviour, aligning studies of sexuality with the pathological descriptions of psychiatry and criminology, rather than with biology. While their work laid the foundations for the removal of the moral dimension within both medical and social attitudes towards sexuality, in order to understand fully the complex relationship between sexual variety and sexual morality, we need to have some knowledge of the cultural factors which historically have determined our attitudes towards the meaning and significance of sex.

Myth, magic and rejuvenation

Examples abound in the myths and legends of early literature which confirm the importance of male sexuality, and its close relationship with power and regeneration. The rejuvenation of sexual power was an art, often practised by women using a combination of magic, ritual and physical intervention, and its ultimate, mystical ideal was to cheat ageing and death. When Medea was given the task of rejuvenating Aeson, she made her potion from "pebbles from the furthest Orient, hoarfrost gathered under the moon, wings and flesh from the infamous horned owl, entrails of a werewolf, the skin of the Cynyphian watersnake, liver of a very long lived stag, the head of a crow nine centuries old, and a thousand other things". After boiling these ingredients together, Medea cut Aeson's throat to bleed him, made him drink the potion, and also infused it into his wound. The effects were immediate: his beard and hair turned from grey to black, and his limbs filled out into the form of youth.

The ancient Greek understanding of sex as an appetite has persisted until the present day, in the form of the belief in the existence and efficacy of the aphrodisiac qualities of certain foods and other substances. The widespread use of the rhino horn as unicorn horn; the concept of the oyster as amorous, the lobster as lecherous; the secret recipes of the various elixirs of youth; and the later patenting of pills and potions under such names as Orvieta, Elixir Vitae and Elixir Renovans have always found a market. The recipes from classical to modern times, collected by Norman Douglas in his cookbook *Venus in the Kitchen or Love's Cookery Book*, are all designed to enhance male arousal. They include a pie of bull's testicles garnished with sparrows' and pigeons' brains; a pig's vulva marinated in white wine (to be served hot); marmalade of carnations "for people of cold temperament"; and, "for the timid", leopard's marrow cooked in goat's milk and abundant white pepper, and eaten on toast.

The spring or fountain of youth is another enduring and potent symbol of rejuvenation. One of the many fantastic legends which adorned the life of Prester John, the mythical king of the Orient, was the existence in his kingdom of the Fountain of Youth, which lay "less than three days journey from the river of Paradise" (the Ganges). Drunk from three times a day on a fasting stomach for three years, three months and three hours, a man would live and remain youthful for three hundred years, three months, three weeks, three days and three hours. Belief in the restorative powers of water has persisted. The waters of Tonbridge Wells were described by A. Veteran in his 1847 *Hints to the Sick* as effective for enlivening "the nobler parts of the body and spirits", producing a "sweet balsamick, spirituous and sanguineous temperament: which naturally incites men and women to amorous emotions and titillations" and enables them "to procreate". The waters at Bath, Buxton and the spas of central Europe are enjoyed to this day.

There was also a widely held belief that the consumption of the sexual parts, and their products, of young male animals promoted sexual rejuvenation. A well-established practice was to eat the testes of young lambs when they were castrated. There was, and perhaps still is, a powerful belief that semen, when ingested, also possesses valuable stimulant qualities. Havelock Ellis recommended it as a "physiological aphrodisiac" which acted as a general and sexual rejuvenator (Ellis, 1948). Ellis pointed out that John Hunter had observed that when semen is "held in the mouth for some time it produces a warmth similar to spices which lasts some time". Ellis discovered that Australian aboriginals customarily administered a potion of semen to dying or feeble members of the tribe. The Marquis de Sade, too, insisted that ingestion of semen was part of the attraction of fellatio, while W. L. Howard, in his article on 'Sexual perversion' for the *Alienist and Neurologist* in January 1896, recorded a case in which the stimulant action of semen had created as irresistible a desire for it in one of his patients as that of the dipsomaniac for alcohol.

The business, and enjoyment, of sex experienced a golden age during the 18th century. James Graham, perhaps the Hugh Heffner of his times, opened a Temple of Health in 1780 in an elegant, ten-roomed Adam house in Adelphi Terrace, London. Clients were attended by scantily-clad 'Goddesses of Health'. At first Graham gave lectures and simple electrical demonstrations, and sold a range of potent, rejuvenating medicines. However, by 1781, he had installed in the Temple the 'Grand Celestial Bed'. For £50, clients could pass the night in this extraordinary and exotic rejuvenation apparatus, which was twelve feet long by nine feet wide, supported by 40 pillars of brilliant glass and overhung by a super-celestial dome surmounted by Cupid, Psyche and other figures playing musical instruments. The legend over the bed read "Be Fruitful, Multiply and Replenish the Earth". Other features included silk sheets, golden musical pipes, satin curtains, perfumed pillows, and mattresses stuffed with the tails of English stallions. Artificial lodestones continually poured forth an everflowing circle of magnetic attraction, to create the "superior ecstasy which the parties enjoy in the Celestial Bed".

Moral hygiene and 'lost manhood'

This pre-Victorian enjoyment, in an age of romanticism and revolution, of an apparently liberalised sexual code may in fact be responsible for the subsequent reappraisal, during the 19th century, of sexual moralism. Both the social and scientific context of 19th century culture, which is much nearer to our own than that of the apparently more liberal 18th century, meant that the conventions of courtship and marriage, as well as the sexual practices and attitudes which existed outside these conventions, needed to be redefined. During the late 18th and early 19th centuries, rapid industrialisation encouraged the movement of a significant proportion of the population into dense and unregulated urban areas. For the first time, extremely large numbers of people were living in very close proximity. The simultaneous decline in the authority of religion, especially in the new cities, raised important issues concerning morality and the regulation of social behaviour. By the second half of the 19th century, the complex issue of the 'social question' had become inextricably linked to the idea that the prosperity of the nation was dependent upon the health, hygiene (both physical and moral) and composition of the population. Sexuality and sexual behaviour thus had a dual significance, for both the individual and the race.

The consequences of urban change led to the conceptualisation of the process of 'degeneracy', which proposed that there was a falling away of type, accompanied by the unchecked multiplication of large numbers of 'unfit' urban dwellers, whose degeneracy was manifest in different forms of individual behaviour which included criminality, lunacy, alcoholism and perverse sexual behaviour. Thus, attitudes towards sexual behaviour changed during this century, partly in response to the increasingly scientific nature of the theory and practice of medicine, but also because of the social significance which was now attached to sexually irregular behaviour. The body of serious medical literature concerned with sexual behaviour grew. Prominent among its concerns was an anxiety, informed by a background belief in the fertility of the unfit, urban working classes, that there was a decline in middle-class masculinity and sexual vitality. Theories of the importance of male sexuality became concerned with the idea of 'lost manhood'. This concept began to gain credibility at the same time as the theory of 'degeneration', and both have a significance for the history of sexology because of the way in which they informed the growing 'moral hygiene' movement of the second half of the 19th century.

The theory of degeneration originates with the work of B.-A. Morel (1809–1873), a medical doctor who was strongly influenced by religion and anthropology. His degeneration hypothesis is both psychiatric and socio-anthropological, with its description of degenerations as "deviations from the normal type which are transmissible by heredity and which deteriorate progressively towards extinction". Degenerates possessed a hereditary predisposition, and degeneration could be caused by a range of factors, including intoxication, the social milieu, and moral sickness. Morel's theory influenced a great number of medical and non-medical social theorists during the course of the 19th century, including Cesare Lombroso (1836–1909), who proposed that sexual deviates were on a lower rung of the evolutionary ladder, Max Nordau (1849–1923) and Richard von Krafft-Ebing (1840–1902). It was also taken up by neo-Darwinists who interpreted degeneration as regression in the Darwinian sense.

Spermaticidal anxiety

Central to this idea of lost manhood, which has underpinned attitudes towards adolescent male sexuality from the first half of the 19th century until quite recent times, was a belief in the dangers of masturbation, those "sickly joys" and "nightly pollutions" which were believed prematurely to drain and exhaust the practitioner, and to lead to an untimely enfeeblement, sterility, impotency and ageing. This physical deterioration, engendered by an excessive loss of sperm, led also to warnings against the marriage of older men to young wives, although a judicial amount of "connexion was absolutely necessary to prevent atrophy of the testicles". During this period, huge sums were paid for quack remedies by young men suffering from 'spermatorrhoea'. By the middle of the 19th century, spermatorrhoea had become absorbed into medical theory and practice as a male sexual disorder, and was regarded as part of the 'aetiology of impotence'. Young men submitted to cauterisation, blistering, applications of camphor, and infibulation. A range of metal and leather fasteners were available commercially, as well as devices such as strait waistcoats, hand 'mufflers', and the "armed bougie", with which to cauterise the internal surface of the urethra with nitrate of silver. Occasionally men underwent castration.

Although there is a wide body of evidence which shows us that the Victorian era was not a time of universal sexual repression and prudery, the perception of the 19th century as an era of inflexible morality and punitive religious values is still widespread. The role of the medical profession towards the sexual problems of patients was, however, a vexed one, for most practitioners either possessed only a very limited knowledge of such matters, or felt a distaste towards having to deal with them. Generally speaking, formal medical advice to men on sexual matters during the first decades of the century was based upon ideas of continence. Sexual activity should be limited to the purposes of reproduction within marriage. The gratuitous expenditure of semen, in the form of onanism, was regarded as a primary cause of physical and moral degeneration. Each male had a bank of precious semen, on which he should not go overdrawn.

The concept of 'spermatorrhoea' was developed by a Swiss doctor, Samuel Auguste Andre Tissot (1728–1797), who published *Onanism* (1760) which described the dangers of wilful masturbation, and by Claude Francois l'Allemand (1790–1853), who wrote of wet dreams as a foul and pernicious disease in *Des Partes Seminales Involuntaires*, published in three volumes between 1836 and 1842. L'Allemand described spermatorrhoea as a progressive disease, during which the semen became "less rich", leading to infertility. At the same time the patient became physically weak and debilitated, leading to atrophy of the testicles and eventual death. This doctrine was picked up and disseminated in England by William Acton (1813–1875), a urologist who proposed, in *Functions and Disorders of the Reproductive Organs* (1857), that masturbation led to blindness and insanity. Acton's book was, in fact, entirely about male sexuality, and addressed the issue of male sexual anxiety by examining fears of impotence and masturbation. He attempted to combine information about male sexual physiology with social and moral opinion within the broader thesis of abstinence and restraint. On the other hand, another 19th century physician, Charles Drysdale (1829–1907), was an advocate of regular sex, with contraception, as a cure for spermatorrhoea. His book, *Natural, Sexual and Physical Religion* (later *The Elements of Social Science*), advocated regular use of the sex organs from puberty onwards by both sexes in free, non-marital unions. While Drysdale was obviously not a typical Victorian physician, there is now evidence that many doctors did privately advise young men to engage in premarital sexual activity rather than sexual abstinence, as a way of dealing with the dangers of masturbation. An enormous amount of the medico-psychological literature from this time was concerned with masturbation, and there is a wide and well-researched body of literature on the relationship between masturbation and insanity and nervous disorders. The work of the British psychiatrist, Henry Maudsley, typifies the development of the theories dealing with this relationship. He initially believed that masturbation caused insanity, but eventually modified this position to a belief that insanity was one of the causes of masturbation. Observation appeared to bear this out: as Hare remarked, "acuteness of observation" led to the identification of hebephrenia, which was typically attributed to masturbation (Hare, 1962).

Control and continence

The publication of Darwin's *Origin of Species* (1859) and *The Descent of Man* (1871) also had a significant impact upon the interpretation of sexual behaviour, not least because it was followed by a misinterpretation of what Darwin was attempting to say about sexual selection. Many of Darwin's followers interpreted his work as claiming that sex existed for the good of the species, and this in fact became the dominant view by the mid-20th century, inspiring studies in sexuality as well as helping to de-stigmatise the study of sex. However, it also helped Darwin's cousin, Francis Galton, to propose that sexual selection could be used to improve race. By 1885 he had founded the 'science' of eugenics, which promoted the principle of judicious marriages between the clever and the wealthy (more or less synonymous definitions for Galton), as well as birth control. For eugenicists, the essential problem was how to encourage a sense of 'sexual responsibility' in order to ensure that sexual selection fostered racial progress. Implicit within the doctrine was the notion that the planning of sexual behaviour could bring about a society of good citizens. One of the most important founding figures in the history of British sexology, Havelock Ellis, was also a eugenist.

The prevailing belief in the importance of sexual health inevitably produced a rich seam of theories and doctrines which were concerned with the regulation of sexual behaviour and which, prefiguring many of the vogues of the late 20th century, offered a variety of routes to sexual well-being. The new science of nutrition, and the realisation of its importance to the health and well-being of the individual, was drawn into the domain of sexual behaviour, encouraging the development of a range of food products as cures for concupiscence. Farinaceous foods such as Graham's Crackers and Kellogg's Cornflakes were invented at this time, and marketed to be eaten as remedies for the disease of lust. John Harvey Kellogg, a Seventh-Day Adventist, also advocated vegetarianism, the water cure and clothing reform as the keys to abstinent living. A sufferer from klismaphilia, Kellogg had an enema every day after breakfast as a substitute for erotic functioning. He also believed that 'sex activity' was not necessary to health, declaring that the "reproductive act is the most exhausting of all vital acts. Its effect upon the undeveloped person is to retard growth, weaken the constitution and dwarf the intellect". He maintained that it was important for sperm to be reabsorbed internally, as it played an important part in the development of the nervous system. While the sperm reabsorption nourished the nervous system, masturbation starved it, undermining an interior balance and consensus, with the result that, unreplenished, the nervous system entered into a state of exhaustion and debilitation.

Hype, hyperidrosis and hypersexuality

The development of endocrinology during the second half of the 19th century increased interest in the function of the 'ductless' glands. Charles Brown-Sequard, who succeeded Claude Bernard to the Chair of Experimental Medicine at the College de France in Paris, spent years investigating the role played by the male sex gland, and came to the conclusion that, as well as their external secretion, testicles possessed an internal secretion which went directly into the blood stream traversing the glands, and which not only inspired the male's sex instinct, but was also the "true motive power behind the activities of the male brain and nervous system generally". While in France this was happily interpreted to mean that sexual excitement aided and enhanced mental activity, and inspired a range of bizarre therapies involving the surgical grafting of the testes, and intravenous injections of the testicular extracts, of young, male animals onto and into elderly and anxious men, British physiologists were more sceptical about this 'organotherapy', preferring to remain within the biological tradition as represented by Patrick Geddes and J. Arthur Thomson in *The Evolution of Sex* (1889). These biologists drew on examples from observation of non-human behaviour to describe the "divergent evolution of the sexes". The female was 'anabolic', the male 'katabolic', and all species were characterised by the dominance of the energetic male over the passive female.

The old idea of sexual desire as an appetite was given a new veneer during the late 19th century, by the work of Frank G. Lydston (1857–1923) on the relationship between hunger and sexual psychopathy. Not unlike the ancient Greeks, he proposed that sexual instinct was given to man not for pleasure but for procreation, and was therefore, "in effect, a species of hunger". He was concerned to shift the discussion of sexual psychopathy away from the moral standpoint towards a physical explanation. His interest was in the sexual function of the cerebellum, which, he maintained, determined the fundamental sexual differences between men and women. "Men have a greater cerebellar development than women, consequently more powerful sexual impulses. It has been noted that men whose cerebellar development is extreme – a mark of atavism – are likely to be the victims of inordinate sexual desire." Lydston's biogenetic and evolutionary thesis presented sexual perversion as a congenital abnormality.

The decline, during the 19th century *fin de siècle*, of mid-Victorian optimism and confidence brought to the fore the social consequences of the darker side of urbanisation. The drain of imperial demands upon the nation, the reconstruction of the world according to the demands of capitalism and technology, and the sense of impending war, created a new set of dilemmas for European civilisation. Urban man, the 'brain worker', was envisaged as undergoing a physical debilitation as a result of his unnatural lifestyle; concern was expressed that the sexual organs of the brain worker, the intellectual, were shrinking in size and potency. Max Nordau, the German psychiatrist, had claimed in *Degeneration* (1895) that "great minds...cannot simultaneously create ideas and children", while George M. Beard, the American neurologist, conducted research into this form of neurasthenia as a product of modernisation, and found that its exacerbatory features included the necessity for punctuality, the disorderly city, tobacco and railway travel. In *Sexual Neurasthenia* (1881) Beard noted with concern that the "functional nervous diseases of men are now in the same condition as the diseases of women half a century ago. Symptoms of mental depression, morbid fear in all its types and phases, hyperidrosis, nervous dyspepsia, palpitation, deficient mental control...". While civilisation was unmanning civilised men, however, the muscle worker, who was regarded as nearer in kind to both the primitive and the deviant forms of humankind, was also thought to possess a sort of hyperpotency, or *furor sexualis*. This belief in the hypersexuality of the lower class male, and which included the black and the socially deviant, constituted a potent threat to the white male's sense of his racial and social superiority. While the capacity for sexual restraint was indicative of the superior individual, the sexual incontinence of the working classes threatened the quality of the national stock.

Sexual pathology

Once matters of human sexuality fell within the medical domain, it was inevitable that the doctor's surgery in some sense replaced the confessional, reflecting the conversion of sexual 'sin' into sexual 'sickness'. The medical literature on sex expanded as doctors, and in particular psychiatrists, began to transform their observations and case notes into theoretical explanations of the nature and variety of human sexual behaviour. Richard von Krafft-Ebing (1840–1902) published an extensive collection of his cases in *Psychopathia Sexualis* (1886), in which he described in great detail examples of fetishism, homosexuality, sadism and masochism. These main categories were supplemented by cases of zoophilia, satyriasis, exhibitionism and voyeurism. Krafft-Ebing believed that these variants in sexual behaviour represented "hereditary taint" and "moral degeneration". He also warned of the "danger of the sex drive" and that sexual pathology posed a threat to society. All of Krafft-Ebing's fetishists were men, although he described homosexuality as an "antipathetic sexual instinct" in both men and women. Transvestism, transsexuality and homosexuality all represented stages in this disease of antipathetic sexual instinct. His *Textbook of Insanity* (1876) describes masturbation as the greatest source of sexual evil, and a critical factor in the development of sexual deviations. Krafft-Ebing's significance is that he described for the first time many of the variants of sexual behaviour. He is often judged harshly today as having a repressive and punitive attitude towards sexual behaviour; in fact, his intention in drawing up a comprehensive map of the variants of sexuality was to construct an account of diversity which would help fellow physicians to cope with the sexual problems of patients. Public readership was not his intention. When *Psychopathia Sexualis* became a well-known source for sexual titillation, he amended it by translating many of the accounts of sexual deviance into Latin.

It was also at about this time that a partial shift occurred, away from an emphasis on male sexual functioning, towards 'maternalism' and the sexual and reproductive responsibility of women. Although the maternalist movement was primarily and almost exclusively concerned with the creation of a healthy population, the wider context, in which a growing number of women were working in the professions, and the increasingly influential women's suffrage movement, contributed to a re-evaluation of women's place in society, as well as an examination of the broader question of the nature of sex itself and the way in which it influenced and informed social behaviour. Marie Stopes (1880–1958) advocated the unity of love and sex. Her book, *Married Love: A New Contribution to the Solution of Sex Difficulties* (1918), promoted the use of birth control in order that women could enjoy sex without constraint or fear of inevitable pregnancy and childbirth. Karl Pearson (1857–1936) attempted to create a new "science of sexualogy" (sic) to determine the status of women. Writing about sex also ceased to be almost exclusively medical, as social scientists began to claim sex as an object of study for their discipline, while even those such as Ellis, Freud and Hirshfeld, whose original discipline was medicine, incorporated the social sciences into their methodology.

Sexual psychology

Henry Havelock Ellis (1859–1939) challenged the prevailing notions of sexual normality through concepts of individual and cultural relativism. He developed the extremely influential idea of a continuum of sexual behaviour, between 'normal' and 'abnormal' sexual phenomena, mainly through studying the sexual lives and habits of friends and contemporaries. He published his vast *Studies in the Psychology of Sex* between 1896–1928, in which he described the great range of sexual experiences, practices, customs and cultural variations, drawing upon the different disciplines of anthropology, cultural history and zoology, as well as medicine. In his biography, *My Life* (1939), he called for sexual freedom and for the reform of social attitudes and legal curbs. Havelock Ellis was one of the first people to introduce the work of Freud (1856–1939) into the British discussion. Ellis and Freud shared points of similarity which included an emphasis on the importance of infant sexuality, and agreement on elements of intersexuality, but also diverged significantly. Ellis was interested in the social significance of sex, while Freud was more interested in studying the dynamic unconscious. However, Ellis gave support to both Freud and Ernest Jones in the early days of psychoanalysis in England, at a time when the medical profession on the whole was dismissive of psychoanalytic writing.

The development by Freud of psychical analysis, later psychoanalysis, which relied upon the interpretation or analysis of what the patient says, or omits to say, brought together in Vienna a group who shared his views on psychoanalytic practice. There were later to be some notable defections from this group, including Alfred Adler, Carl Jung and Wilhelm Stekel (1868–1940). In *Three Essays on Sexuality* (1905), Freud proposed that the aims of pleasure and procreation do not coincide completely, and that from a very early age sexual energy was directed towards self-discovery, reality and knowledge. Adult sexual behaviour had infantile origins which contributed to the development of the adult sexual instinct and personality as a whole. Thus, repression of natural, human, sexual curiosity could lead to the development of obsessional neuroses and hysterical debilitation in both women and men.

Stekel diverged in thinking from Freud because he claimed that neuroses and sexual disorders derived from mental conflict, and were therefore potentially curable; if the analyst could uncover the source, this would lead to the cure of the patient. Stekel had a deep interest in interpreting symbolism in human behaviour. He saw sexual motive or sexual sublimation in almost every human action: the woman dithering over a choice of hats cannot make up her mind because she has made a poor choice in her husband; a collector of ephemera is an off-course Don Juan; those late for appointments are younger children resentful at their position in the family. In *Disorders of the Instincts and Emotions*, first published in the 1930s, Stekel wrote that every person was influenced from head to foot by his (sic) sexuality. No gesture, word or movement was exempt from sexual influence. Furthermore, "a man is like his penis. The penis is an image of the entire man – a thing that in many cases may be demonstrated through practical experience" (Stekel, 1953). According to Stekel, this intimate synonymy between being and sex led to parapathiacal behaviour, and the close correlation in most men's lives between vocation and sexuality. Choice of vocation was actually an attempt to solve mental conflicts through the displacement of them into the mechanical: that is to say, their vocation. At its crudest, the shoe fetishist became a cobbler; while members of the medical profession were "voyeurs who have transferred their original sexual curiosity into the art of diagnosis".

Wilhelm Reich (1897–1957) had an even more thoroughgoing belief in the interdependence of the social and sexual. He maintained that the eventual failure of the Russian Revolution was attributable to the disregard for sexual as well as social liberation. Reich advocated sex between adults and children, as well as believing that the sexual repression of adolescents led to juvenile delinquency, neuroses, perversion and political apathy. He was convinced that regular orgasms were necessary for the mental health of both men and women. Because the orgasm was the key to psychological health, if an individual's sexual energy became bottled up, the resulting sexual tension led to neurosis. Similarly, if there was a revolution in attitudes leading to non-repressive sex, all forms of perversion would disappear. In 1924 he published *The Function of the Orgasm: Sex-Economic Problems of Biological Energy*; by 1936 he had founded the International Institute for Sex-Economy, in Norway. In 1939 he set up the Orgone Institute in Maine, US, where he developed the orgone box, a device for collecting sexual energy, which was then stored in an accumulator and used to strengthen the body against disease and to increase the potential for orgasm. Reich's attempt to synthesise Marxism and psychoanalysis in America in the 1950s led to an inevitable confrontation with authority. He died in prison in 1956.

The third sex

The idea of a sexual continuum was taken up by Ellis's friend Edward Carpenter, a homosexual. Throughout history, attitudes towards homosexuality have depended entirely upon the nature of culture and society. In Britain, certainly during the 19th and most of the 20th century, homosexuality has been viewed legally and socially as a deviance. The development during the 19th century of a medical model of homosexuality meant that as well as experiencing moral censure, homosexuals have also been regarded as mentally ill. Edward Carpenter advanced the concept of an intermediate sex, building upon a theory of congenital homosexuality developed by Karl Ulrichs, a German lawyer. This third sex, the 'urning', was the product of the anomalous development of the originally undifferentiated human embryo, resulting in the female mind in a male body, and vice versa. The idea of the third sex was further developed by the sexologist Magnus Hirschfeld (1868–1935), who was also homosexual, and the founder of the Institute for Sexual Science in Berlin. He proposed that most people were originally bisexual but during their natural development lost the desire for the same sex, and became heterosexuals. 'Psychohermaphrodites' were men and women with normal development of the sexual organs, but who could love people of either sex because their 'feeling centres' for one sex or the other were imperfect. The third category, of homosexuals, had normal sexual organs but the early desire for same sex individuals in the feeling centre had failed to recede, leading to men loving men and women loving women. The inclusion of the significance of hormones in the development of sexual differentiation contributed to a gradual reduction in punitive attitudes towards homosexuals, although it did not diminish the power of medicine to produce authoritative theories about homosexuality. The idea of homosexuality as a crippling disease eventually gained wide acceptance, and from the 1930s onwards this was especially so, as evidenced by the wide range of 'cures' being offered, from hypnotism to chemical experimentation and, by the 1960s, electric shock treatment and aversion therapy, which had first been applied to fetishism in the 1950s. These various attempts to offer sexual adjustment were motivated by the belief that individuals who were unable to conform to the prevailing social and cultural norms would on the one hand never achieve satisfaction, while on the other they would also operate as a subversive social subgroup.

From disease to desire: variety is the spice of life

The first major statistical survey of sexual behaviour was carried out by an American, Alfred Charles Kinsey (1894–1956), who was not medically qualified. He used standardised interviews to study the sexual life of American people in the 1930s and 1940s, and the results of his huge study were published as *Sexual Behaviour in the Human Male* (1948) and *Sexual Behaviour in the Human Female* (1953). Using a taxonomical methodology, Kinsey identified areas of congruence between a range of subgroups within the US population, and one of the results of his work was to replace ideas of normal and abnormal with natural and unnatural. He did not create a greater tolerance towards homosexuals, although he did show that a great number of people were involved in homosexual behaviour and that not all were necessarily homosexual, but rather that homosexuality exists potentially in all persons. He also described the sexual needs of the young. Perhaps Kinsey's great achievement was a demystification of sexual activity, showing it as a commonplace and banal part of human activity.

While it is still difficult to establish Kinsey's motivation for his work, William E. Masters and Virginia E. Johnson had an implicit therapeutic intent behind theirs. *Human Sexual Response* (1966) was a biological description of sexual response during the human life cycle, while *Human Sexual Inadequacy* (1970) examined the psychological aspects of sexual behaviour, as well as giving impetus to the clinical study of sexual problems in marriage. *Human Sexual Inadequacy* was essentially an account of an 11-year period of clinical work and research carried out by Masters and Johnson, which involved the treatment of a group of 790 examples, in over 500 marital partnerships, of sexual difficulties which the authors classed together as sexual dysfunctions. The work of Masters and Johnson helped to move the consideration of sexual problems away from the framework of psychopathology to those of learning, and failure to establish effective learning. They also initiated a more general separation of sexual difficulties from sexual problems, and they helped to develop the idea of couple-based rather than individual therapy, as well as the rather more controversial idea of 'surrogates' to provide psychological and physical input during therapy. Perhaps most importantly of all, they helped create the distinction between sexual dysfunction and disorders of sexual desire.

There are continuing attempts to explore and explain the aetiology of certain sexual conditions, especially homosexuality, but the idea of a continuum between the extremes of 'normal' and 'abnormal' has persisted, and indeed has contributed substantially to an understanding that, once decriminalised and stripped of moral interpretation, many of the varieties of sexual behaviour once classified according to the great case-book medicine of the late 19th century as a collection of loathsome diseases, are a reflection of the diversity of social forces in general. Just as Freud broadened the concept of sexuality to include all pleasurable bodily functions, sexology has become a multidisciplinary study with contributors from a wide variety of disciplines. It is not, however, except in a narrower medical formulation, a 'science', and this leaves the historians, sociologists and anthropologists who have contributed to the body of literature on human sexuality on uneasy ground. All the evidence tends to show us that our sexual definitions are socially and historically derived, and that our attitudes towards sex have been enriched and enlivened, circumscribed and impaired by the endless variety and change in cultural patterns which describe the history of humankind. Human sexuality is one of the fundamental forces which shape personal and social life, either through expression or repression, and is often expressed in the form of a power struggle between sexual drive and social structure. As Freud suggested, "perhaps we must make up our minds to the idea that altogether it is not possible for the claims of the sexual instincts to be reconciled with the demands of culture". Even this, however, presents us with an implicit, biological mandate and it is possible that the fact that we treat biological research with more respect than the social sciences reveals the true nature of our debt to the Victorian age, when ideological issues were embedded in and won through scientific argument. It is necessary to remember, as Padgug (1979) has written, that "biological sexuality is the necessary precondition for human sexuality. But biological sexuality is only a precondition, a set of potentialities, which is never unmediated by human reality".

References

By a veteran (1847) *Hints to the Sick, the Lame, and the Lazy; or, Passages in the Life of a Hydrotherapist*. London: J. Ollivier.

Douglas, N. (ed.) (1952) *Venus in the Kitchen; or, Love's Cookery Book*. London: William Heinemann.

Ellis, H. H. (1939) *My Life*. London: William Heinemann.

Freud, S. (1977) Three essays on the theory of sexuality. In *On Sexuality* (Vol. 7), p. 82. Harmondsworth: Pelican Freud Library.

Hare, E. H. (1962) Masturbatory insanity: The history of an idea. *Journal of Mental Science*, 108, 1–25.

Kinsey, A. C., Pomeroy, W. B. & Martin, C. E. (1948) *Sexual Behaviour in the Human Male*. Philadelphia: W. B. Saunders.

—, — & — (1953) *Sexual Behaviour in the Human Female*. Philadelphia: W. B. Saunders.

Masters, W. H. & Johnson, V. E. (1966) *Human Sexual Response*. London: Churchill.

— & — (1970) *Human Sexual Inadequacy*. London: Churchill.

Padgug, R. A. (1979) Sexual matters: on conceptualising sexuality in history. *Radical History Review*, 20, 9.

Stekel, W. (1953) *Disorders of the Instincts and the Emotions. Impotence in the Male. The Psychic Disorders of the Sexual Function in the Male.* London: Vision Press.

4 Sexual therapy and the couple

Michael Crowe

Classification of sexual problems • Causal factors • Treatment of sexual problems in couples • General therapeutic principles • Relationship therapy • Incompatible sexual drives • Management of erectile problems • Management of early ejaculation • Management of delayed ejaculation • Management of vaginismus • Female lack of arousal and anorgasmia • Conclusions

---

The treatment of sexual dysfunctions is perhaps in a greater state of flux than at any time since the publication of Masters & Johnson's *Human Sexual Inadequacy* (1970). There are more numerous and varied approaches than ever before, both those that apply psychotherapeutic methods and those that use a very straightforward organic solution for this complicated series of problems. There is, especially among men with erectile dysfunctions, a high demand for quick and easy treatment methods in this field, and there is a risk that the more psychotherapeutic methods are being passed over in many clinics in favour of the more direct urological or pharmacological forms of treatment. It is my belief that this is unfortunate, since it means that the relationship in which the sexual dysfunction exists is being ignored in favour of a rather unthinking reliance on mechanistic solutions, and many of these solutions may end up creating more problems than they solve.

Masters & Johnson (1970), in their pioneering work on human sexual inadequacy, were the first to describe the couple as the unit for therapy. They used a then quite novel method which involved taking the couple to a hotel where they stayed for a two-week period and attended the therapists every day to report on the progress of their 'homework exercises'. In the current climate of the National Health Service such a procedure would be impossibly expensive, but many of the more practicable techniques of these pioneers have been adopted by present-day therapists. In particular the focus on the couple as the unit of therapy has been followed by many, although not all, of the sexual dysfunction clinics in this country.

In spite of this, the concept of the couple as the focus for therapy is far from being universally accepted. In the most widely used diagnostic manuals (ICD–10 and DSM–IV) there is still an implicit assumption that a sexual problem 'belongs' to only one person. This may be appropriate for many problems, such as the loss of erection in someone who is not in a relationship, or who has several relationships in all of which it occurs.

However, for many problems it is simply inappropriate, and one problem in particular which is highly unsuitable for classification in this way is that of 'low sexual desire' occurring in an ongoing relationship. Here the problem is one of definition, in that the partner with the 'low desire' is only experiencing a problem in relation to the higher sexual desire of the other, and it may equally well be that the other partner has unacceptably high demands. In such cases it would seem that to treat the problem without reference to the couple and their relationship would be to ignore at least half the problem. Other sexual problems would appear to be intermediate in this respect. For example, a couple with an unconsummated relationship in which the wife has vaginismus and the husband suffers from primary impotence may reasonably be treated as two separate individuals, but a more satisfactory approach would certainly be to treat them together as a couple.

The psychosexual approach, originated by Masters & Johnson (1970) and extended by Kaplan (1974), is still the most influential in the field. The way in which it is used varies greatly from one centre to another, although there are many factors in common between the different approaches. There are some units that rely more on the psychodynamic understanding of the problem in treating it, while others have a more behavioural approach. Others, such as my own unit at the Maudsley Hospital, take an eclectic view of the therapy of couples, which includes both behavioural and systemic techniques, along with a more traditional Masters & Johnson approach to the sexual problems themselves. The possible advantages of the various approaches have yet to be put to the test in terms of a controlled trial of different therapeutic methods.

As a postscript to this introduction it should be added that, in discussing couples, I am including a number of different combinations. Heterosexual couples may be married or unmarried, and some these days will be in relationships in which they are living separately and meet only at intervals. Homosexual couples, both male and female, have most of the same kinds of problems as heterosexuals, and are just as entitled to be treated in a psychosexual clinic, but many of these have added difficulties over issues of discrimination and dilemmas about 'coming out' with family and friends. In this chapter I will be describing mainly heterosexual couples and individuals, but most of what is said would apply equally well to homosexuals.

Classification of sexual problems

In treating a couple or individual with a sexual dysfunction, it is useful to think in terms of a classification that can embrace all the various types of problems which are presented. The classification in Table 4.1 (from Hawton, 1985) is a useful one which distinguishes between those cases

Table 4.1 Classification of sexual problems

Aspect of sexuality affected	Women	Men
Interest	Impaired sexual interest	Impaired sexual interest
Arousal	Impaired sexual arousal	Erectile dysfunction
Orgasm	Orgasmic dysfunction	Premature ejaculation Delayed ejaculation Ejaculatory pain
Other dysfunctions	Dyspareunia Sexual phobias Vaginismus	Dyspareunia Sexual phobias

with a disturbance of sexual interest and those with a dysfunction as such, although in other ways it is less satisfactory, especially as it does not take account of the relationship involved in the sexual problem. This I will cover in a later section, but it should be emphasised at this point that there are many different possible factors contributing to a sexual problem, both in the individual and in the relationship.

Sexual problems may be divided into those that involve motivation, interest or desire on the one hand, and those that involve a failure of sexual function on the other. The phobias and interest problems in the above table fall into the former category, while all the others are problems of function. In many of the problems of function it is possible (although less desirable) to treat the individual alone, but in the great majority of problems of desire I would maintain that to treat the individual alone would be to leave out a most important source both of causation and of information.

Causal factors

The great majority of sexual problems are multifactorial (Crowe & Jones, 1992). In the average case presenting at the clinic it is possible to discern aetiological factors deriving from organic illnesses or medication, from current anxiety and stress, from earlier life experiences, and from problems in the relationship. Perhaps the most researched condition in the field, and the one in which it is easiest to make a diagnosis as to the cause of the problem, is erectile dysfunction. However, even in this condition it is usually impossible to pinpoint one unique cause of the problem, and it is usually necessary to make a formulation that involves at least three possible causes (for example ageing, alcohol and relationship difficulties). In almost all the other conditions, both those involving motivation and those involving function, the problem of disentangling the various causative factors is even more difficult.

Causative factors in sexual problems may be divided into those of organic origin, those of individual psychological origin, and those deriving from the relationship. There are a great many possible organic factors in sexual, and especially erectile, dysfunctions which may contribute to the problem, and some of these are listed in Table 4.2.

Table 4.2 Organic factors leading to sexual dysfunctions

Neurological	Spinal injuries and cord compression Multiple sclerosis Brain disorders including tumours and cerebrovascular accidents Peripheral neuropathy Autonomic neuropathy (e.g. in diabetes mellitus)
Hormonal	Pituitary tumours Loss of testicles (e.g. by accident or in the treatment of cancer; more likely to cause loss of libido than erectile dysfunction) Post-menopausal problems in the vaginal walls
Vascular	Blockage of the larger vessels Atheroma and 'pelvic steal' syndrome Damage to arterioles (e.g. in diabetes mellitus) Leakage from the penile veins
Pharmacological	Antipsychotics and benzodiazepines Some antihypertensives Thiazide diuretics Antidepressants (tricyclics more likely to cause erectile problems, MAOIs and SSRIs to lead to delayed ejaculation and anorgasmia) Alcohol and other substances of misuse
Pelvic problems	Vaginitis Fibroids, cysts, tumours and sometimes constipation Salpingitis and other pelvic inflammations Pelvic injuries
Ageing	Reduction of interest Delay in arousal – need for more stimulation Retarded ejaculation and delayed female orgasm

Some of the individual psychological factors are shown in Table 4.3. It should be remembered that in most cases these factors remain somewhat speculative, even at the end of therapy, and in our work it is usual to use the discussion of these factors not as a definitive explanation of the sexual problem but more as a means of involving the couple or individual in thinking about possible alternative reasons for the problem, to extend their flexibility of conceptualisation, and thus their commitment to therapy.

In addition to these individual factors, it is possible in most cases where there is an ongoing relationship to perceive aspects of that relationship that might be contributing to the sexual problem. As with the psychological factors above, it is always a matter of uncertainty as to whether a particular aspect of a relationship is making a significant impact on the sexual interaction.

In thinking about relationships and their impact on other issues, it is always helpful to think systemically. This is a conceptualisation often used in family therapy, in which the individual is considered as part of a wider system including other family members and society. One particularly useful concept in systems theory is that of 'circular causation' in which, for example, when two people are interacting, the actions of one may become the 'cause' of the other's actions, in a continuous cycle, but neither is considered responsible for the development of the situation as a whole. Who has 'caused' the problem is a matter of arbitrary

Table 4.3 Individual factors contributing to sexual problems

Psychiatric difficulties	General anxiety Depression and other neurotic problems General emotional inhibition Low self-esteem
Problems deriving from the past	Previous traumas (e.g. sexual abuse and rape) Ignorance or negative attitudes Cultural factors and beliefs
Current life stresses	Work difficulties (e.g. overwork, threat of redundancy, unemployment) Recent retirement Physical illness or handicap Worry about children or elderly relatives Recent childbirth
Performance anxiety	Common in almost all dysfunctions, and consists of anxiety when the sexual act is contemplated or attempted

punctuation, and it would be just as right to punctuate the sequence before the woman's action as to do so before the man's. This 'systems thinking' (Crowe & Ridley, 1990) helps the therapist to avoid taking sides in a conflict, but instead to help the couple to understand that there are other ways to solve conflicts than to appoint a judge and deliver a verdict as to who was to blame.

Table 4.4 gives some of the relationship factors which are hypothesised to contribute to sexual problems in couples.

In our present multicultural society it is also important to remember that there is a wide variety of sexual practices, rules, taboos and myths which cannot be taken for granted. For example, the Muslim community looks very sternly on any form of masturbation, and it may cause unbearable conflict in a Muslim man who has premature ejaculation for the therapist to suggest the stop–start or squeeze technique to be practised alone. The therapist must be alert to such complications of therapy, and it is useful in training courses to emphasise the variability of cultural and ethnic differences in sexual practice.

Within the typical Western culture, too, there are myths and beliefs which are quite pervasive and powerful. Zilbergeld (1980) has usefully discussed these myths, and Baker & de Silva (1988) found them to be held fairly frequently by the clients attending a London sexual dysfunction clinic, and to be relevant to the management of these clients in psychosexual therapy. Typical of these myths is that "the man in a sexual relationship is responsible for orchestrating the experience of both partners" and that "men are always willing and ready for sex".

Table 4.4 Relationship factors contributing to sexual problems

Equal or symmetrical relationship	Resentment and anger
	Constant hostility
	Excessive politeness (as seen in some cases of non-consummation)
	Difficulty in communicating about sex
	Lack of trust
	Problems with confidentiality (with friends or family)
	Difficulty in 'closing the bedroom door'
Unequal or complementary relationship	'Patient and therapist' style relationship
	Perpetrator and victim relationship
	Unequal levels of assertiveness
	The aftermath of an affair
	The partner with an alternative sexual need (e.g. fetishism)

Given the wide variety of possible causes for sexual dysfunctions, and the impact that sexual therapy may have on both the individual and his/her relationship, any comprehensive approach to treatment should take account of organic, psychological and relationship factors. The remainder of this chapter will be concerned with how to do this, bearing in mind the most recent developments in physical treatment as well as individual and couple psychotherapy.

Treatment of sexual problems in couples

Although Masters & Johnson's break with the past involved the definition of the couple as the focus of therapy, there is still today some ambivalence on the part of the therapeutic world to the treatment of the couple together. In her influential book *The New Sex Therapy*, Kaplan (1974) advised taking the dysfunctional partner out of sex therapy when there was a 'block' to progress, and giving him/her some intensive individual psychotherapy before getting the couple together again for sex therapy. It is also of interest that the chapter on marital therapy in her book was written by another author, suggesting perhaps that she saw it as being an optional extra. In their 'multidimensional model' for the treatment of desire disorders, however, Rosen & Leiblum (1989) used biological, psychological and interpersonal elements, and described a number of cases in which resentment and power struggles seemed to be perpetuating the desire disorder in the less interested partner.

My own preference, especially in the context of problems of sexual interest, is to stay as far as possible with the couple as the focus of therapy, and to do most of the necessary individual work with the partner present. In some situations it may be preferable to work with the individual, especially if the female partner has a history of sexual abuse as a child. But even this may be linked to the couple therapy through her sharing with the male partner some of the experiences she has been discussing in her own sessions (Douglas *et al*, 1989), if only to explain to him why some of the 'normal' sexual activities in their relationship are causing her problems.

It is true that in an increasing number of cases at present there is no regular partner to be brought to therapy, and in these circumstances it is obviously better to treat the person attending the clinic alone than to refuse treatment altogether. However, I would maintain that it is preferable, if there is a relationship, to treat the couple together wherever possible.

General therapeutic principles

In treating sexual dysfunctions and sexual motivation problems it is important not to appear to promise too much. I very rarely use the word 'cure' in relation to sexual therapy. It is much better to speak of adjustment, or of coping with a problem, rather than offering the hope of cure. In only one area can one safely refer to a cure with a minimal risk of relapse; this is the treatment of vaginismus in which, if the couple have been able to have pain-free penetration, they will fairly predictably go on to have successful intercourse thereafter. In most other areas (e.g. erectile problems, premature ejaculation, delayed ejaculation, anorgasmia and dyspareunia, as well as motivational problems) any improvement may well be succeeded by a later relapse. Watson & Brockman (1982) found that only 55% of 29 couples who had improved their sexual adjustment in treatment had maintained that improvement at follow-up.

The general principles of therapy are quite similar in most clinics where the modified Masters & Johnson approach is practised. There is an emphasis on homework exercises involving the 'sensate focus' approach, and in addition it is useful to increase communication especially about sex and related issues. The techniques of sensate focus are well known, and consist essentially of a prolonged kind of foreplay, with the addition of body oil and, in the early stages, a ban on intercourse and on touching genitals or erogenous zones. There is then a gradual inclusion of genital contact, of other specific techniques for specific problems (see below), and eventually of intercourse. Sensate focus is designed originally to reduce pressure to perform, and the related performance anxiety. It also has the potential to release inhibited urges, and in some couples it has the paradoxical effect of making them wish to break the ban on intercourse. Sometimes this is successful in terms of their presenting problem, but the therapist should be cautious in welcoming the improvement because it may be short-lived, especially if they seem to be taking future success for granted.

Another principle of this approach to therapy is what has been called 'permission-giving' (Annon, 1974). In many couples there are cultural or individual inhibitions on sex, and it is very useful in the early stages of sexual therapy to make it clear to them that whatever seems right to both partners is acceptable to the therapist. It may also be necessary to help some couples with quite simple educational input about sexual function. For example, a couple attended with infertility and a complaint that the wife was 'ejaculating' post-coitally. It transpired that they were only achieving very minimal penetration due to her vaginismus, and it then became quite easy to treat them for this problem, following which they were able to achieve a pregnancy. However, their ignorance of sexual functioning could have led to prolonged investigation and physical treatment if the right questions had not been asked.

In many cases there is a relationship difficulty in addition to the sexual dysfunction, and it is always helpful to deal with this so as to facilitate compliance with the homework exercises. Such difficulties may include unspoken resentment, hostility, tension, poor communication, inhibitions, or negative attitudes to the expression of emotion. The management of these difficulties will be described later in the chapter, and for greater detail the reader is referred to Crowe & Ridley (1990).

In some clinics, including our own at the Maudsley Hospital, relaxation exercises are taught, and in the process of deep breathing and muscle relaxation we also instruct the couple in the exercises devised by Kegel (1952) which contract and relax the muscles of the pelvis and vaginal wall. The exercises are also thought to be useful in the management of erectile disorder, and have been shown to achieve as good results as venous ligation in male clients with erectile disorder and demonstrated venous leakage (Claes & Baert, 1993).

Following the sensate focus stage, the couple will usually be encouraged to attempt intercourse, often in the 'woman above' position, which has a number of advantages. Firstly, it gets away from the conditioned anxiety that usually occurs in the traditional position; secondly, in the case of a dysfunctional male, it makes it easier for him to penetrate without excessive manoeuvring; and in a dysfunctional woman it gives her more freedom of movement.

Relationship therapy

Couples often express negative feelings and attitudes to therapy and (more often) towards each other, and it can be hypothesised that in many cases the communication problems are a major factor in keeping the sexual problem alive. It is in these circumstances that couple therapy can be used to overcome blocks to progress. The many difficulties in communication and problems of resentment between the partners make it helpful to see the couple, if possible, together for the majority of the therapeutic time, and to have at the therapist's disposal a means of assessing and modifying the relationship at the same time as carrying out the sexual therapy.

There are many forms of couple therapy that may help to overcome the communication blocks and resentments which exist in a couple with a sexual problem. Perhaps the longest established is psychodynamic couple therapy (Daniell, 1985), but this is a rather long and drawn-out way of helping couples and less suitable for incorporation into sexual therapy. Rational–emotive (Dryden, 1985) and cognitive (Beck, 1988) approaches to couple therapy also have considerable promise, and may prove useful and be fairly compatible with sexual therapy. Behavioural couple therapy (BCT) has been practised for over 20 years (Jacobson & Margolin, 1979; Stuart, 1980) and is very compatible with sexual therapy, as it includes homework exercises and other tasks, and is orientated towards positive change.

In our clinic we employ a mixed approach known as behavioural-systems couple therapy (BSCT) which includes most of the techniques of

BCT but also some systemic interventions. We have found it both compatible with sexual therapy and relatively easy to teach, as well as offering more help than BCT in those couples who show ambivalence and relative lack of cooperation with therapy. The approach is described in much greater detail in Crowe & Ridley (1990).

In BSCT the general approach is one of problem-solving, and in contrast to other forms of couple therapy there is little emphasis on finding the 'cause' of a particular problem, but instead a focus on factors which may have contributed to the initiation or maintenance of the problem, and factors which have modified the problem at different times (e.g. a relaxed holiday or having sexual relations in the early morning). The question is always 'how' rather than 'why'.

A good general tactic for a therapist doing BSCT is to 'de-centre' as soon as practicable in the session. This entails asking the partners to talk to each other without addressing the therapist directly. They may find this rather strange at first, but in due course it becomes easy and natural, and it is very helpful to the therapist, because he/she can observe the interaction between them in the session instead of relying on their accounts of what happens at home. It is also very necessary with many couples for the therapist to keep the momentum going, and to ensure that each partner is heard by the other as well as by the therapist. A good principle at this stage is to make it clear that they should take each other seriously, both in understanding feelings and in respecting wishes.

Another principle is to concentrate as much as possible on the relationship as the focus of attention, rather than trying to solve the individual's presenting problem without reference to the relationship. If two people can each make a small modification in their behaviour, it seems intrinsically likely that the resulting change will be more long-lasting than if only one changes.

The two elements in BSCT (behavioural and systemic) can be conceptualised as forming a hierarchy of alternative levels of intervention (ALI). This hierarchy is shown diagrammatically in Fig. 4.1. The behavioural levels include reciprocity negotiation and communication training, and these form the basic foundation of therapy, or the lower level of the hierarchy. Above these are two 'structural' interventions (Minuchin, 1974; Haley, 1976), namely arguments/role-play in the session, and tasks (often timetabled) to be carried out between the sessions. Above these again is the use of paradoxical injunctions (Selvini Palazzoli *et al*, 1978), and above paradox is another alternative, namely to accept the problem or seek other forms of therapy (e.g. individual psychotherapy or, in the case of erectile disorder, pharmacological treatment). Reasons for moving up the hierarchy are the existence of blocks to progress in the lower level approaches, the presence of too much individual focus in the couple's self-appraisal, or too much rigidity in the system (preventing change with the more straightforward approaches). The progress is not all one-way;

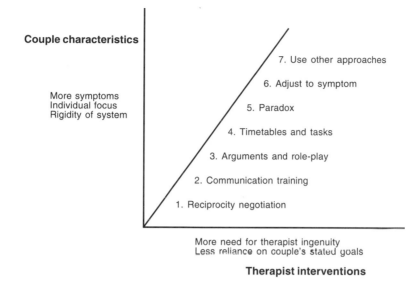

Fig. 4.1 The heirarchy of alternate levels of intervention (ALI).

thus it is quite possible to move down the hierarchy, if in response to an intervention at the 'upper levels' the couple become more amenable to straightforward behavioural suggestions. The behavioural levels form the mainstay of treatment, with the more systemic levels used only as it becomes necessary. It is also quite possible to use different types of intervention in the same session depending on the exact type of problem the couple is presenting at the time. I will now give more detail about some of the individual approaches that make up BSCT. The numbers refer to those in Fig. 4.1.

(1) Reciprocity negotiation

The first resort in BSCT is reciprocity negotiation (RN). In this basic approach the couple is encouraged to take specific issues on which they disagree and negotiate more positive ways of solving the problems. The resentments may be dealt with by translating past into future, negative into positive, general into specific, and overambitious tasks to more practicable ones. Thus, a couple in which the wife was continually complaining about her husband's critical comments were asked to think of an alternative approach. The husband agreed to mention only the things he approved of in her behaviour, as long as the wife tried to do some of the things that would answer his criticisms. In another similar case the husband continually returned home late from work, and his wife expressed her criticism very bitterly. The compromise they reached was that he would try to be in by a certain time, and if delayed would telephone to explain the delay. In return his wife would be careful to talk in a friendly and encouraging way in the first half-hour after his arrival.

(2) Communication training

At a similar level on the hierarchy is communication training. This approach is primarily behavioural, in that it assumes that the couple have good motivation, and that the problems in communication are due primarily to lack of knowledge or experience rather than deliberate or unconsciously motivated misunderstanding or miscommunication. However, it also has things in common with the work of Satir (1964) and other systemic therapists, who have postulated that "all behaviour is communication". The whole concept of communication thus has many wider connotations than a simple improvement in the giving and understanding of messages between partners.

In the present instance, however, we are mainly concerned with communication as a technique, and certain simple principles should be observed. The partners should speak in brief sentences, and acknowledge what they have heard from their partner (Jacobson & Margolin, 1979). They should avoid 'mind reading', and should try to begin all statements with the pronoun 'I' rather than trying to speak for the other person. They should be encouraged to show empathy for the partner's feelings, and should as far as possible use positive and constructive comments rather than negative or critical ones.

For example, a wife was complaining that her husband kept "groping" her when she was at the kitchen sink. Instead of simply telling him to stop it, she was encouraged to suggest an alternative way to approach her, and opted for him to kiss her on the cheek if he wished to make contact when she was busy in the kitchen.

In another instance a wife was in the habit of going into monologues about the insensitivity of her husband's mother and the fact that he always seemed to defend his mother when the wife mentioned her. The therapist was able to reduce the monologues by persuading the wife to leave 'gaps', bringing the husband into the discussion, and the wife was pleased that he began to understand her point of view when the therapist insisted that he should say what he really thought about his mother and her rudeness. It became easier for him to do this when she was not being so vehement in her complaints about the mother, because he was not having to correct her 'overstatements', and therefore not appearing so defensive to his wife.

Communication training is thus primarily a means of ensuring the kind of positive, constructive and forward-looking interaction which is required for reciprocity negotiation, and can be seen as being in the same area of therapeutic activity. It is, however, probably more suited to those couples who are able to think abstractly.

(3) Arguments and role-play

The next stage up in the hierarchy is that of 'structural' interventions in the session. Here we are entering a different dimension in which the therapist begins to decide what is needed by the couple and intervenes in session to change their experiences of each other there and then. Thus, in a couple where neither of them shows their feelings, but acts in an overpolite way, the therapist might ask them to argue in the session about something very trivial. Such a subject is chosen because it is innocuous, and if the argument becomes heated the partners do not envisage much harm coming to the relationship. One such couple had a lively argument about whether the toilet roll should be hung with the paper hanging down next to the wall or away from it. The important thing is not the rights or wrongs of the argument, but that they should argue openly and feel confident about expressing their feelings. If one partner is more inhibited the therapist should encourage him/her to speak up more loudly or not to give in so easily; however, this does not mean siding with that person in the argument itself, but simply to modify the process of argument. Often it is more appropriate for the couple to 'agree to differ' on the topic than for one or the other to win the argument.

In a related area it is sometimes useful, when the partners are finding difficulty in empathising with each other, for the therapist to suggest that they should use 'reversed role-play' in the session, in which each takes the part of the other in a discussion of an issue which has caused distress. At the end of about five minutes they are asked to 'de-role' and to feed back what they have learnt about the other's point of view and feelings.

(4) Timetables and tasks

These are usually given as homework exercises at the end of the session. The therapist returns to the session after some discussion with colleagues (if available) and gives a kind of formulation of the couple's current situation, along with some tasks to be carried out before the next meeting. Such tasks may be very simple ones, such as to arrange for a joint outing (perhaps linked with the instruction to keep it a secret so as to strengthen the boundary around the couple relationship), or simply to have a ten-minute talk together once a day at a set time and with no interruptions.

More complicated tasks can be set, and may be timetabled. For example, a couple in which the male partner is morbidly jealous may be asked to have a half-hour talk at a set time of day about the man's jealous obsessions and the woman's response to them. If, however, the topic is raised at any other time the woman is to say "That's fine, but we can't discuss it now: we will give it our full attention at 8 pm this evening". Such timetables are quite useful in another way, in that they 'legitimise' the jealousy or other such behaviour, rather than labelling it as sick or psychiatrically disturbed.

Timetables can also be used for sexual drive incompatibility in couples (see below), but using days rather than times of day as the basic unit for the timetable.

(5) Paradox

When faced with a situation in which the couple seem to be stuck in an unhelpful sequence of interaction, or seem to be fixed in their view that it is entirely one partner who is to blame for the problem, or when all other interventions lower down in the hierarchy have proved ineffective, the therapist has the option of using a paradoxical intervention (Selvini Palazzoli *et al*, 1978). The paradox is a method that relies on circular causation, and aims at a kind of reshuffling of the forces working within the relationship to make it difficult to maintain the *status quo*.

In framing a paradox it is necessary to think in terms of the behaviour complained of in the 'patient', the reciprocal behaviour in the partner, and the apparent benefit which these could be providing for the couple (or, to put it the opposite way round, the feared consequences of giving up this particular interaction). The paradoxical message, which combines all these elements, usually begins with a 'positive connotation' of their relationship, then prescribes the behaviour complained of and the reciprocal behaviour, and gives the systemic reason (or benefit to the couple) of continuing to do both things. Sometimes they respond by anger when such a message is given, and may deny that there could be any benefit to them: in other cases there is an immediate understanding of the meaning of the message and a humorous response. It does not matter in the short term whether the couple obey or disobey the implied instructions in the message; what helps is for them to realise that there are several ways of looking at the problem and they are liberated from their previous sense of hopelessness because there is in the last analysis another way out of the painful dilemma of therapeutic failure.

An example of a paradox is given by the case of a professional couple who had had continual power struggles over trivial issues, and a more serious struggle over the recent emancipation of the wife from domestic duties to being a college lecturer. After many attempts by the therapist to help them to use negotiation and communication training to improve their daily interaction, he came to them at the end of the sixth session with this message. "My colleagues have been giving me a hard time in discussion of your problems. They think I have been hopelessly ambitious in expecting you to have a peaceful relationship and feel that I have been misleading you. The suggestion now is that you should have regular rows about your domestic arrangements; that you, David, should pick on Barbara's shortcomings and you, Barbara, should do your best to be rebellious and difficult, because this way you will avoid the bigger issue of how to adapt to the new circumstances you are in, and how to learn to respect each other as separate individuals." This message went down surprisingly well, and they both reassured the therapist that he had not misled them, but thanked him for the insight he had given them. They did much better in the subsequent sessions, and were soon able to be discharged from the clinic.

Paradox is not something we use regularly, but when it is used it may have the effect of unblocking an unhelpful series of interactions and leading to better functioning within the relationship. It may be given in some cases in the form of a 'split team message': this involves the giving of a paradoxical message, but accompanied by an alternative behavioural task, with part of the team 'supporting' the paradox and the other part on the side of the straightforward task. At times this seems less radical than a full paradox, and at the same time gives the couple the option of accepting either the paradoxical or the straight task, putting greater responsibility on them for making the choice.

(6) Adjust to symptom

In couple therapy generally, and in couple work in relation to sexual problems, it is necessary to remember that not all such difficulties are amenable to this type of therapy. In some cases it is important to remember that the symptom may have to be accepted and lived with. This is particularly the case in, for example, erectile disorder in the elderly, and if both partners are philosophical about not having a sex life it may be that too much emphasis on therapy will simply make them more unhappy, and it is best to resign themselves to the absence of sex. However, in these kinds of cases it is often very useful for them to develop different ways of showing physical affection, and in some this can form an effective substitute for sex itself. Also, their communication can often be greatly improved by communication training, and a much freer and more open discussion of sex-related topics can make a big difference to their general satisfaction.

(7) Use other approaches

In other cases it may be best to move away from the psychosexual approach to a different form of treatment. In the case of erectile disorder this is likely to be a more physical treatment, such as intracavernosal injections or vacuum devices. In anorgasmia it may involve the woman having individual psychotherapy to explore some of the past traumas which are contributing to the current problems. In either case it is useful at times to revisit the couple therapy to monitor how these other forms of therapy are impacting on the relationship.

Therapy in couples with incompatible sexual drives

This section is carefully titled to emphasise the point made above that disorders of desire should be defined not only in terms of the partner with the lower desire, but also in respect of the other partner in the context of the relationship. The possibility remains that the problem is with the 'high desire' partner or with the interaction between the two, rather than with the 'low desire' partner. There is an unfortunate tendency to label people as having 'conditions', of which low or inhibited sexual desire is one (see the discussion above on DSM–IV and ICD–10), and this has certainly led to undesirable and probably unnecessary treatment for those whose sexual interest is lower than that of their partner but not in any other sense abnormal.

There is a different dynamic in the relationship depending on whether the man or the woman has the higher sexual drive. If it is the man (which is the more common situation in younger couples) there is either a continual pressure on the woman for sex or a resentful acceptance by the man of the relative infrequency of its occurrence. If it is the woman with the higher drive the conflict is rather more subtle, with veiled and coded criticisms of the man and much tension and anxiety. In both cases the reluctant partner is likely to use emotional withdrawal as a frequent tactic, and this will often be accompanied by avoidance of the partner at bedtime (e.g. by watching late television or staying up to do chores). In addition to being withdrawn the more reluctant partner is likely to be less assertive than the enthusiastic one, and to take a quiet and diplomatic line in arguments.

There are three components of sexual desire as proposed by Levine (1984). These are (a) a biological urge, (b) a cognitive and culturally determined 'sex wish', and (c) an affective and interpersonal aspect that is seen as the most important part of the equation and which is closely involved in the relationship. It may be that the low sexual drive in a particular individual is the result of illness (for example, the loss of testosterone due to a pituitary tumour) and it is very necessary to exclude such factors by careful history-taking and investigation. Other factors contributing to the problem could be clinical depression or a previous history (usually in the female) of rape or sexual abuse. But it is also important to be sure that the sexual drive in the less enthusiastic partner is indeed reduced, and that it is not that the other partner has an excessive need for sex. In a couple with a disparity in sexual motivation, it is vital to look for the two relationship factors that are most likely to be contributing to the problem, namely inequality and withdrawal.

Therapy for these couples includes the modified Masters & Johnson approach, with an additional aspect of encouraging playfulness in the couple's sexual life. It is also helpful to encourage a reduction of inhibitions in both partners, and to ensure that the partner with the 'high' drive is not therapeutically neglected or treated as the completely normal one, since they may be contributing quite markedly to the problem by their sexual approach or attitudes (Rosen & Leiblum, 1989). In the interactional sphere it is also important to elucidate the ways in which the reluctant partner may feel that sex is an unwelcome imposition because of other non-sexual aspects of the relationship.

The therapeutic approach should in addition be able to take account of the individual as well as the interactional aspects of the problem, and it may often be necessary to see both partners separately as well as together for part of the therapy time. Having said that, there are almost no cases in which the relationship is so good that there is no need for work on it, and even if that were the case it would be useful to have the assistance of the partner in helping the reluctant individual to resolve the problem.

Two particular interventions deriving from BSCT are helpful in resolving this type of conflict. The first is the encouragement of arguments (level 3) and the second is the use of a sexual timetable (level 4). In cases with male reluctance, the use of arguments on trivial issues can be extremely helpful in raising assertiveness in the male partner. He is often a man who prefers to swallow his anger and acts as a diplomat rather than a fighter. If his partner is lively and volatile this can lead to a great inequality in assertiveness, and the unspoken resentments can lead him to be reluctant to initiate the sexual interaction that his partner greatly desires. The couple may find that many of their periods of tension are associated with a lack of sex, which the woman complains about and the man excuses. The in-session arguments that the therapist encourages need to be on an unimportant subject, or such a man will not tolerate them, but having begun to argue and to become comfortable with the assertiveness involved, the couple may find it an enjoyable experience and laugh at themselves and each other.

In due course this may be associated with sexual success, and in one case of the successful use of this technique the husband said that he had eventually realised that his sexual life was "too serious to be taken seriously". He and his wife were both in their 50s and widowed, and had moved in to her house after their marriage. He was the typical diplomat in the relationship and she was volatile and temperamental. They had had very little sexual activity in the marriage, and she blamed him heavily for this, as he "never approached her". Physically thay were both healthy, but sometimes when he attempted sex he was unable to have an erection. The therapy looked at many aspects of their relationship, but the key intervention was the encouragement of trivial arguments. He took to this quite readily, but she had some problems, not only with his unusual assertiveness but also with the implication that she might be partly responsible with him for the sexual problem. She eventually dropped out of the joint sessions, but he continued with therapy alone, and the couple resumed a quite active sexual relationship, with his potency more reliable than before.

The second type of intervention in this situation is the sexual timetable. This is more useful where there is a reluctant female partner (Crowe & Ridley, 1986). The couple are usually in a state of fairly constant conflict over sexual relations, with the male partner very demanding and the female either resisting or giving in without much enjoyment. There is a fairly frequent assumption by both partners that it is the reluctant partner who has something wrong with her, and that "any normal woman would want sex as much as her partner does". The first step in therapy may be to challenge this assumption, by questioning both of them on their perceptions and preconceptions on the issue. It is better not to impose the therapist's own views, but if the woman says anything to challenge the apparently mutual beliefs about sex the therapist should make the most of the disagreement and build on it.

The timetable is usually raised at quite an early stage, by asking how often each partner would like sex to occur. They will usually come up with quite different wishes in this respect, and if, for example, the man suggests every night and the woman once in two weeks the therapist then asks them to suggest a compromise frequency. This may be once or twice per week, and if they can agree on this, the next step is to agree that, for the present, sex will take place at that frequency. It is vital, however, that they agree not only how often, but also on which night(s) or day(s) it should take place. Then, on those nights on which sex is forbidden, the woman can relax in the knowledge that she will not be pressurised, and can even (as she often wants to do) be physically affectionate without the fear that it will inevitably lead to sexual intercourse. On the 'sex' nights, in contrast, the man can relax in the knowledge that he will receive sexual satisfaction, and the woman can prepare herself for it because the pressure is off on the other nights. The arrangement can continue for as long as the couple feel it is helpful, but in most cases they decide to give up the timetable after a few weeks, when they can talk more freely and without tension about the sexual issue, because the timetable has released them from their tension and opposition.

In one such case the couple had been married for about five years and had two small children. The husband put pressure on the wife for sex almost every night, and she objected strongly to this. When sex happened, however, she would often enjoy it and was orgasmic. They failed to respond to the conventional sensate focus approach, partly because of the wife's extreme slowness of response and partly owing to the husband's impatience. She then suggested that, if she knew that sex would be happening on a particular occasion, she could prepare for it and be a willing participant. The timetable was suggested and she opted for two nights per week. They specified the nights, and the husband agreed to the scheme, saying that although he preferred sex to be "spontaneous" he would be happy to know that it was going to happen in a reliable way rather than accept the pressure and uncertainty every night. They managed very well with this arrangement, and when last seen she had changed her wish to sex three times per week, and they were insisting on continuing the timetable indefinitely, because it had transformed their general relationship as well as the sexual problem.

Couple therapy in the management of erectile problems

This is now probably the most common problem presenting in sexual dysfunction clinics (Tiefer & Melman, 1989). It is very tempting, especially in urology-based clinics, to assume that the erectile problem is simply a physical one. Bancroft (1989), however, has argued cogently for therapists not to ignore the man attached to the dysfunctional penis. I would take this further and maintain that the partner, if there is an ongoing relationship, is of almost equal importance.

It is clearly necessary (as argued in other chapters of this book) to investigate thoroughly the possible physical causes of the problem, and according to one's speciality and training, one will use more or less of the relevant but invasive investigations such as nocturnal penile tumescence studies, cavernosograms, hormone levels and penile-brachial blood pressure measurement. In our clinic we move to these measures usually as a second stage, only if psychosexual therapy (including the partner if available) is unsuccessful and if an intracavernosal injection of papaverine or prostaglandin at higher doses is ineffective. Thus, as with the ALI hierarchy above, we tend to work in a progressive manner, moving in this case from the less invasive to the more invasive interventions as the case demands.

Thus in a case of erectile dysfunction where there is a partner available and willing to be involved in therapy, it is usual to begin with a Masters & Johnson approach. This means, in most cases, sensate focus (SF) with a ban on intercourse and on the genital or erogenous areas being touched. The couple then move to genital SF, and in successful cases to intercourse, often with a recommendation for the 'woman on top' position at first. In many couples who respond quite well to SF, there is still, even at the end of treatment, some uncertainty as to whether the erection will be strong enough to achieve penetration. The couple may then be instructed to use genital sensate focus as the main type of sexual interaction, and to proceed to sexual intercourse only when they feel confident enough to do so, perhaps on only about one in three occasions on which sexual play takes place.

In many cases there is also a relationship problem, and if this is the case it is appropriate, and indeed necessary, to address this at the same time as the sexual one. The behavioural-systems approaches outlined above will be useful, including the use of the ALI hierarchy to decide in which mode to treat the problem presenting at the particular stage of therapy.

One typical relationship aspect of erectile dysfunction is where the partner is herself rather uninterested in sex. She may also be suffering from the same kind of performance anxiety as her partner, and this may inhibit the erection as much as his anxiety does. If she can be encouraged to increase her commitment to the sexual aspect of the relationship, for example by realising that she may obtain some increased gratification from a successful outcome of therapy, and feel more relaxed about the whole area, the man may improve his erectile response simply from her increased enthusiasm. This emphasis on the interactional aspects of the problem can increase their success rate in a very simple way and may obviate the necessity for more physical approaches.

It should be understood that only about one couple in three with erectile dysfunction will respond to psychosexual therapy with a reasonable result; the others need some additional physical treatment to succeed in reversing their dysfunction. Of these the first resort would normally be to use a drug such as yohimbine by mouth. This has been shown by Riley *et al* (1989) to be better than placebo in a controlled trial in men with erectile problems. It seems to be more effective in those men with preserved morning erections than those without, but it only works in about 50% even of these. There are other problems with the use of this drug, in that it is not fully approved for use, and it appears to raise blood pressure in some men (by about 10 mm Hg). However, there are a number of men who have returned to a full sex life with the aid of yohimbine, and who relapse whenever they stop taking the medication.

The next resort in men with erectile dysfunction is the use of intra-cavernosal injections to produce penile tumescence. Even in men with absent morning erections, this approach is successful in about 90% of patients. However, the treatment is not acceptable to all such men (or their partners) and many who achieve technical success do not continue to use the treatment to achieve intercourse. There appears to be a differ-ence between men with functional impotence (often an older age group) and those with diabetes, spinal injuries or other organic reasons for their problems: the latter are much more enthusiastic and assiduous in their use of intracavernosal injections (Crowe & Qureshi, 1991). The compounds used in intracavernosal injections are phentolamine, papaverine, prosta-glandin E or vasoactive intestinal polypeptide. Papaverine is the compound with which sex therapists have the greatest amount of experience, and despite its lack of full approval from the Committee on the Safety of Medicines, it has proved satisfactory in a large number of patients. The most serious, but extremely rare, side-effects are prolonged erections (which require emergency decompression by withdrawal of blood and the injection of an antidote, usually metaraminol) and Peyronie-type deformity of the penis. It is said that prostaglandin E is less likely to produce priapism, and it is fully approved, but it is more liable to cause penile discomfort than papaverine after injection. The jury is still out as to which preparation it is better to use in the long term.

In some men who are either unwilling to use intracavernosal injections or in whom they are ineffective, it is possible to recommend the use of vacuum devices. These consist of a glass tube that fits over the penis and produces a passive enlargement when the air is extracted from the tube. The 'erection' is maintained by the use of a band round the base of the penis (Witherington, 1988). The results are not always satisfactory, and some men complain of numbness and discomfort: however, they seem to be an acceptable alternative in many cases, particularly elderly men.

The use of teflon implants, although popular with some surgeons and their patients, should be seen as a last resort, particularly as there is no possibility of normal function if the implants fail and have to be removed. They are indicated after severe Peyronie's disease with deformity of the penis. They are of two types, inflatable and semi-rigid, and a follow-up by Melman *et al* (1988) has shown that the majority of such patients are satisfied with the results.

Arterial surgery to improve the blood supply of the penis has had mixed results, and unless there is a clearly demonstrated single blockage in the vessels should probably not be recommended. Surgery to reduce venous drainage is sometimes successful, but in one series (Lewis, 1988) there was only a 24% success rate, and in view of the technical difficulty of the operations many surgeons are now not recommending them.

Management of early ejaculation

This is a very common problem in the general population, affecting perhaps 25% of men (Sanders, 1987). However, it is not as commonly seen in sexual dysfunction clinics as erectile dysfunction. The partner may be the main 'complainant' because the problem interferes with her enjoyment. It is important, as before, to include the partner in the assessment and treatment of the problem, and in many cases the reduction of anxiety produced by sensate focus, relaxation and improved communication can have the effect of delaying ejaculation sufficiently to enable satisfactory intercourse.

The 'stop–start' technique of Semans (1956) is useful. It is similar in essence to the 'squeeze' technique recommended by Masters & Johnson, but easier to teach and easier to use. In the stop–start technique the man learns, in homework exercises, to delay ejaculation in self-stimulation by approaching the 'point of inevitability' and then ceasing the stimulation until the urge abates. The penis becomes quite refractory after a successful trial of this, and the man finds that he can, by successively stopping and starting, delay ejaculation for up to 15 minutes. He is then asked to repeat the homework using body oil or a similar lubricant on his hand, until he can again last for 15 minutes. His partner then stimulates him in a similar way, with a dry and then a lubricated hand, and they again do this on several occasions until he can last for 15 minutes. The technique can then be used in oral sex, and eventually in intercourse, the couple stopping their movements as the point of inevitability is reached and then resuming when the urge has worn off.

Some antidepressants, especially clomipramine and the SSRI preparations (e.g. fluoxetine and sertraline) have a side-effect of delaying ejaculation (and incidentally also orgasm in women). This can be used in severe cases of early ejaculation, although it is not something that works in every case, and in many men the effect may be minimal or absent. The drug may be taken 30 minutes or so before intercourse, but is not dramatically effective if used alone, and is best used along with the stop–start technique and good couple therapy in addition.

Management of delayed ejaculation

Delayed ejaculation is a much rarer condition than the previous two, and comparatively difficult to treat. It often presents as infertility, although in other cases the presenting issue can be the man's lack of sexual fulfilment, his sense of being 'used' as a kind of stud by his partner, or her guilt that he is not getting the kind of pleasure that she obtains. The management of the problem again is easier if both partners are involved in therapy. Masters & Johnson prescribe 'superstimulation', which involves the penis being rubbed very vigorously with the hand lubricated with body oil until ejaculation occurs. This is easier in those cases where the man can already ejaculate in masturbation, but even where this cannot be achieved before therapy it can sometimes happen during superstimulation. Some men with this problem can only masturbate to ejaculation using unusual techniques such as rubbing the penis against the sheets, or stimulating the base of the penis and the scrotum. For them, when intercourse is attempted, it may be necessary to include these activities in some way in order to help ejaculation to occur. For others, ejaculation may only be brought about by the use of a vibrator held at the head of the penis, and in others the additional use of yohimbine 30 mg by mouth an hour before sex is attempted may assist ejaculation. In yet other cases it seems that they can only succeed if they deliberately try not to ejaculate. When, by whatever means, ejaculation occurs intravaginally, men with delayed ejaculation may suddenly feel liberated and be able to do so more easily in future. However, as in much sexual therapy, it is usually more a case of achieving control of the problem rather than a 'cure'.

Management of vaginismus

In the treatment of this problem the main emphasis is on gradual retraining of the muscles surrounding the vagina to relax. This is achieved by the use of graded dilators (smooth tapered tubes of different sizes) or by the use of fingers. It is always possible for the woman with this problem to be examined internally using one finger, and she, and later her partner, can then be encouraged to insert a finger in the same way. Eventually, after a variable period of homework, they will be able to use a larger dilator or three fingers to penetrate, and it is at this stage that intercourse is usually permitted, preferably at first in the 'woman on top' position.

Some couples have great difficulty progressing with this therapy, and this is as much due to the husband's reluctance to cause any discomfort as the wife's fears of penetration. Patient work by the therapist and at times the use of a paradoxical approach can unblock the system and achieve progress, but the overall results, although better than for any other dysfunction, are not quite the 100% reported by Masters & Johnson.

Female lack of arousal and anorgasmia

The general approach to these problems follows the usual sensate focus pattern, with prolonged mutual stimulation and communication about sexual matters. Two particular aspects of the relationship are important. The first is to check whether the man's sexual technique is being unhelpful to the woman in either inhibiting arousal or in failing to arouse her in the way she prefers, and therefore reducing her satisfaction. The second is whether the man is expecting too much sexual pleasure or satisfaction in his partner, almost as an obsessive task in which he has to succeed and gain her approval and gratitude. In this latter situation it may help them to read Zilbergeld's (1980) "myths of male sexuality", which help to dispel some of the prevalent beliefs about male responsibility for the whole sexual experience, and about male readiness for sex under all circumstances.

It is useful for the woman to be able to share with her partner some of the techniques which she has found helpful in achieving an orgasm alone. In some women this may involve the use of the vibrator, in others the use of a water spray or jacuzzi, and in yet others specific manual stimulation which the man may not be aware of. Communication and the sharing of responsibility for sexual arousal are important aspects of this stage of therapy in anorgasmia.

Another area which may need exploration is the possibility that the woman may have experienced, either in childhood or later, sexual traumas such as abuse or rape. If this is found it may be necessary to see her individually for a number of sessions (see Douglas *et al*, 1989), in order to help her with her disturbing memories and distorted ideas of guilt following the sexual trauma. It is usually much easier to proceed with joint sessions with the partner after such an individual series, and the treatment of the dysfunction will be facilitated by the sexual abuse work.

Conclusions

The treatment of sexual dysfunctions and motivation problems is in my view best carried out by seeing the couple together, at least for the major part of the therapy. This enables the therapist to take account of the non-sexual aspects of the relationship, and to reverse some of the misunderstandings, communication problems and resentments that may be contributing to the dysfunction. Even where there is no serious relationship difficulty, it is helpful to see both partners in order to allow the non-dysfunctional partner to help the other with therapy and homework exercises. The use of the behavioural-systems approach to couple therapy provides a highly compatible adjunct to Masters & Johnson type therapy, and can help to improve communication, negotiation and rigidity in the system and enhance the outcome of sexual therapy.

Given the fact that most sexual problems involve the participation of two individuals, each with his or her own insecurities, stresses and sexual histories, it would be very surprising if the interaction between these two people was irrelevant to their sexual relationship. Whether one is dealing with desire disorders, erectile problems, vaginismus or problems of orgasm and ejaculation, it would seem that the therapist is losing many opportunities for effective intervention by ignoring the relationship.

References

Annon, J. S. (1974) *The Behavioural Treatment of Sexual Problems, Vol. 1, Brief Therapy*. Honolulu: Enabling Systems.

Baker, C. D. & de Silva, P. (1988) The relationship between male sexual dysfunction and belief in Zilbergeld's myths. *Sexual and Marital Therapy*, 3, 229–238.

Bancroft, J. (1989) *Human Sexuality and its Problems*. Edinburgh: Churchill Livingstone.

Beck, A. T. (1988) *Love is Never Enough*. New York: Harper and Row.

Claes, H. & Baert, L. (1993) Pelvic floor exercise versus surgery in the treatment of impotence. *British Journal of Urology*, 71, 52–57.

Crowe, M. & Ridley, J. (1986) The negotiated timetable: a new approach to marital conflicts involving male demands and female reluctance for sex. *Sexual and Marital Therapy*, 1, 157–173.

—— & —— (1990) *Therapy with Couples: a Behavioural-Systems Approach to Marital and Sexual Problems*. Oxford: Blackwell.

—— & Qureshi, M. J. H. (1991) Pharmacologically induced penile erection (PIPE) as a maintenance treatment for erectile impotence. *Sexual and Marital Therapy*, 6, 273–285.

—— & Jones, M. (1992) Sex therapy: the successes, the failures, the future. *British Journal of Hospital Medicine*, 48, 474–482.

Daniell, D. (1985) Marital therapy: the psychodynamic approach. In *Marital Therapy in Britain* (ed. W. Dryden), pp. 169–194. London: Harper and Row.

Douglas, A., Matson, I. C. & Hunter, S. (1989) Sex therapy for women incestuously abused as children. *Sexual and Marital Therapy*, 4, 143–160.

Dryden, W. (1985) Marital therapy: the rational emotive approach. In *Marital Therapy in Britain* (ed. W. Dryden), pp. 195–221. London: Harper and Row.

Haley, J. (1976) *Problem Solving Therapy*. New York: Harper and Row.

Hawton, K. (1985) *Sex Therapy: a Practical Guide*. Oxford: Oxford Medical Publications.

Jacobson, N. S. & Margolin, G. (1979) *Marital Therapy: Strategies based on Social Learning and Behavioural Exchange Principles*. New York: Brunner/Mazel.

Kaplan, H. S. (1974) *The New Sex Therapy: Active Treatment of Sexual Dysfunction*. New York: Brunner/Mazel.

Kegel, A. H. (1952) Sexual function of the pubococcygeus muscle. *Western Journal of Surgery, Obstetrics and Gynaecology*, 60, 521–524.

Levine, S. B. (1984) An essay on the nature of sexual desire. *Journal of Sex and Marital Therapy*, 10, 83–96.

Lewis, R. W. (1988) Venous surgery for impotence. *Urologic Clinics of North America*, 15, 115–121.

Masters, W. H. & Johnson, V. E. (1970) *Human Sexual Inadequacy*. Boston: Little, Brown and Co.

Melman, A., Tiefer, L. & Pedersen, R. (1988) Evaluation of the first 406 patients in a urology department based centre for male sexual dysfunction. *Urology*, 32, 6–10.

Minuchin, S. (1974) *Families and Family Therapy*. London: Tavistock Publications.

Riley, A. J., Goodman, R. E., Kellett, J. M., *et al* (1989) Double-blind trial of yohimbine hydrochloride in the treatment of erectile inadequacy. *Sexual and Marital Therapy*, 4, 17–26.

Rosen, R. C. & Leiblum, S. R. (1989) Assessment and treatment of desire disorders. In *Principles and Practice of Sex Therapy*, 2nd edn (eds S. R. Leiblum & R. C. Rosen), pp. 19–47. New York: Guilford Press.

Sanders, D. (1987) *The Woman Report on Men*. London: Sphere Books.

Satir, V. (1964) *Conjoint Family Therapy*. Palo Alto, CA: Science and Behaviour Books.

Selvini Palazzoli, M., Boscolo, L., Cecchin, G., *et al* (1978) *Paradox and Counterparadox*. New York: Jason Aronson.

Semans, J. H. (1956) Premature ejaculation, a new approach. *Southern Medical Journal*, 49, 353–357.

Stuart, R. B. (1980) *Helping Couples Change*. New York: Guilford Press.

Tiefer, L. & Melman, A. (1989) Comprehensive evaluation of erectile dysfunction and medical treatments. In *Principles and Practice of Sex Therapy*, 2nd edn (eds S. R. Leiblum & R. C. Rosen), pp. 207–236. New York: Guilford Press.

Watson, J. P. & Brockman, B. (1982) A follow-up of couples attending a sexual dysfunction clinic. *British Journal of Clinical Psychology*, 21, 143–144.

Witherington, R. (1988) Suction device therapy in the management of erectile impotence. *Urologic Clinics of North America*, 15, 123–128.

Zilbergeld, B. (1980) *Men and Sex*. London: Fontana.

5 Physical treatments for sexual dysfunctions

Kevan R. Wylie

---

*Male erectile disorder • Ejaculatory and orgasmic problems • Libido
and desire disorders • Other sexual problems*

This chapter summarises some of the non-psychological treatment options available for patients with sexual dysfunction. While this should primarily be considered for patients with an organic cause for their problem, there will be many patients who will insist on some kind of treatment other than psychological interventions. It should be stressed that in many cases a willingness to offer a physical treatment can serve as a useful in-road to discussing psychological issues with the patient.

Male erectile disorder (MED)

This is not the most common sexual dysfunction in men, but it is the problem that doctors are most likely to see in clinical practice. While it is important to ensure that as accurate a diagnosis as possible is made regarding aetiology, in practical terms there are often at least two options that can be made available to any individual patient, depending upon the aetiology. It is often worthwhile describing in detail to the patient the various options available, providing, of course, that the doctor is willing to make available the treatment chosen, or at least provide referral to a colleague where necessary. I usually present the range of treatment options as along a spectrum. At the most 'natural' level there is counselling and sex therapy, either alone or in conjunction with couple/relationship work where indicated. Next along the spectrum are various medications (topical and oral), intracavernosal injections (ICIs), vacuum constriction devices (VCDs), a group of miscellaneous treatments, and at the end of the spectrum, surgical intervention which is usually reserved for those patients where other solutions have been unsuccessful.

Topical medications

One of the simplest options for men who have difficulty achieving an erection is to suggest the application of transdermal nitrate patches to the shaft of the penis. These may result in local vasodilation of penile arteries.

However, the success rate is highly variable and many men complain of systemic side-effects, particularly headache. It is often necessary to apply one 5 mg patch up to an hour before the desired effect. Transvaginal absorption by the partner and subsequent partner headache can be overcome by the use of condoms, but this in itself may affect the man's already unstable erection.

Other agents under investigation include Minoxidil paste, nitric oxide, various polypeptides, and evaluation of traditional Chinese herbal preparations including ginseng, which have a high reported response.

Oral medication

At present there are no licensed medications available in the UK. The most widely known of the oral agents is yohimbine hydrochloride. This is an indole alkaloid which is chemically similar to reserpine. It is a presynaptic alpha-2 adrenergic receptor blocker. It increases parasympathetic (cholinergic) and decreases sympathetic (adrenergic) activity. Yohimbine is believed to aid in erectile functioning because it may increase noradrenergic activity in the penile corpora carvernosal tissue, which has a high density of alpha adrenoceptors. It has a product licence in the US where it is indicated as maybe having "activity as an aphrodisiac". Most of the studies that have looked at the efficacy of this drug can be criticised from a methodological point of view. The response rate appears to be around 40%, and is of most benefit in cases of psychogenic aetiology or where a good genital vascular supply exists. The most common side-effects are anxiety (and so is best avoided in patients with anxiety disorder and panic attacks) including sweating, restlessness, agitation, diarrhoea and symptoms resembling that of influenza. It is contraindicated in patients with renal disease and in those patients receiving antihypertensive medication. The tablets can be prescribed on a named-patient basis, with improvement reported at a dose of 5.4 mg tds which can be doubled if success does not occur. There are reports that the drug may have some value taken on an 'as required' basis one hour before desired activity.

Other drugs under investigation include specific alpha-2 adrenoreceptor antagonists, phosphodiesterose inhibitors, opiate antagonists and dopamine agonists. Antidepressants, especially trazadone and amitriptyline, may offer some advantage. The latter is useful in diabetic patients with concomitant pain. Over-the-counter agents advocated include various amino acids, ginseng, Royal Jelly, zinc and pyroxidine and vitamin E.

Testosterone

Many patients believe that their erectile problem is a result of testosterone deficiency or receptor insensitivity. In patients with evidence of hypogonadal states, testosterone replacement will result in an improvement in sexual interest and activity alongside mood elevation and restoration of ejaculation. Androgen-dependent spontaneous erections will also be restored by replacement (i.e. nocturnal and diurnal erections). Erections in response to an external erotic stimuli are not affected.

In normal men only 2% of testosterone is unbound (free levels) with the rest being bound to albumen, globulin and other proteins. It is the non-protein bound, free testosterone that is physiologically active. The interested reader is referred to McClure (1988).

Factors that can affect the steroid binding globulin or increase resistance of the body to testosterone (e.g. obesity, alcohol, stress) must be carefully considered and appropriate counselling offered. Laboratory investigations include establishing the free androgen index (total testosterone divided by sex hormone binding globulin) and gonadotrophin estimations. Before any prescription is issued prostatic cancer should be excluded (by digital rectal examination, prostate-specific antigen estimation and, in older men, transrectal ultrasound scans of the prostate and/or urinary flow rates). Testosterone is usually given as Restandol 40 mg tds, and if this offers clinical improvement can be converted to three-weekly intramuscular injections (e.g. Sustanon 250 mg) or six-monthly subcutaneous implants. A new transdermal delivery system is now available where two 12.2 mg patches are applied every night to achieve replacement.

Patients receiving testosterone supplements should be warned about the risk of baldness and suppression of spermatogenesis. The incidence of prostatic cancer is not increased, but in those patients with pre-existing carcinoma the rate of growth is exacerbated. Hence yearly prostate monitoring as described is essential on all patients over the age of 40 receiving this treatment. The prevention of osteoporosis should be considered when assessing the risk/benefit ratio in an individual.

Intracavernosal injection (ICI)

Injection of vasoactive drugs directly into the penis is highly effective. Originally this mode of treatment allowed patients with organic erectile dysfunction restoration of their erections. However, it is now an established treatment for patients with psychological MED, as the resulting response reduces the anxiety that comes to be associated with attempts at sexual intercourse, with an improvement in the patient's general confidence. Traditionally papaverine and phentolamine have been the agents used and they still have a place in diagnostic centres. These drugs have the effect of inducing smooth muscle relaxation. In the UK, alprostadil now has a product licence and has become the main agent used in ICI. Alprostadil, a prostaglandin E1, is presented in a box complete with syringe pre-filled with distilled water, needles, swabs, drug and dilatant, and a patient information leaflet. It costs approximately ten times more than papaverine, currently retailing at around £10 per box, but is prescribable on the NHS. Each box offers a single-use facility. Three dose options are available.

The main side-effects of intracavernosal injections are: local haematomas and bruising, which is particularly the case when superficial veins are damaged by the injection process; transient light-headedness and dizziness due to systemic absorption of the vasodilator (or perhaps the injection *per se*); fibrosis at the site of repeated injection; introduction of infection and priapism. Pain at the time of injection is discomfort from needle entry and as a consequence of the agent. Pain caused by the injection of the agent is more marked with prostaglandin E1, but again this tends to be only transient. For those patients who have difficulty with self-injection or who have manual dexterity problems, the use of auto-injector pens which sell at approximately £20 can be recommended.

Attention to technique and attainment of the correct dosage of the drug are of paramount importance. When a patient decides on this form of treatment there is often benefit from talking the patient through the technique and injecting the patient directly on the first occasion. The makers of Caverject (alprostadil, Upjohn Pharmaceuticals) provide a patient information video which can be viewed in the clinic or taken home. It is wise to watch the patient self-inject on at least one occasion to ensure that the correct angle of injection is being made. This should usually be at 2 to 3 o'clock alternating with 9 to 10 o'clock to the full depth of a 30 gauge needle. Patients should be advised against injecting against resistance. Patient instruction is described further by Gregoire (1993).

The usual starting dose for prostaglandin is 2.5 µg increasing in similar increments. Patients with neurogenic or psychogenic MED may have prolonged responses to even small doses. Each vial contains the equivalent of 20 µg in a 1 ml syringe. Higher doses can be used for diagnostic and resistant cases. The equivalent for papaverine would be starting at 12.5 mg and increasing at similar increments. Non-response to papaverine at 75 mg usually necessitates reducing the dose of papaverine and adding phentolamine (up to 4 mg in titrated doses). This is probably best carried out in specialist clinics.

The side-effect all patients must be warned about is of prolonged erection (priapism). This complication is seen more often with papaverine compared with prostaglandin E1. This can become painful for the patient and the risk of tissue hypoxia and necrosis should not be underestimated. The consequence can be worsening of the patient's ability to have an erection in the future. My advice to patients is that if an erection is sustained for four hours, action must be taken immediately to ensure detumescence. Practical advice to the patient includes exercising (walking or running up and down the stairs) to encourage arterial shunting, and topical application of ice packs. This has no value in stasis priapism. Patients must return to the prescribing doctor or to any casualty department for treatment.

Caverject packs contain instructions to advise doctors how to manage the priapism. For doctors dispensing papaverine or other agents, patients should have a telephone number for contact or an instruction sheet to give to other doctors to act upon.

Treatment involves aspiration of blood from the corpora cavernosum, and a 23 gauge butterfly needle is used to remove up to 60 ml of blood. If this is unsuccessful then a vasoconstrictive agent can be administered through the same butterfly needle. It is recommended that phenylephrine is used. The strength of injection needed is 200 µg/ml, i.e. 0.1 ml (1 mg of a 10 mg in 1 ml vial) diluted to 5 ml with water for injection. Care should be taken regarding the hypertensive effects this agent may have if absorbed systemically. If priapism persists then urgent urological assistance will be required to consider shunting procedures. It is usually considered that ICI is contraindicated in patients with sickle-cell anaemia due to the increased risk of priapism in this group.

Patient partner acceptability is an important consideration for this treatment, and the drop-out rate after a year may be as high as 60%. These patients may opt to try another treatment such as vacuum constriction devices. Others may report an increase in spontaneous erections. In patients where the agents are absolutely crucial to attaining erections (i.e. in organic disease such as diabetes) there may be a role in seeing both partners to ensure that the rest of their 'sexual script' allows for variety and acceptability of the injections. Partners often wish to be involved in the technique. The role of massaging the corpora needs to be emphasised, and has the dual effect of increased physical stimulation which is often important for older patients, as well as ensuring good distribution of the drug between the cavernosa. When patients return to the clinic complaining that the drug has lost its effect or is not working at home, it is often necessary to ask the patient to inject themselves again in clinic to ensure that correct technique and dosage is being used. With alprostadil, injections can take place up to three times a week, but with papaverine it is usually restricted to once a week.

Vacuum constriction devices (VCDs)

The concept of a VCD was first described in 1917 in the US. A cylindrical tube is placed over the penis and a vacuum created using a hand-held or electrical pump. This creates a negative pressure around the shaft of the penis sufficient to draw blood into the erectile tissue and thereby causes an artificial erection. This erection is maintained by placing a constriction ring around the base of the penis to prevent escape of blood. These devices allow up to 87% of patients with MED to achieve an erection (Turner *et al*, 1991). They are most effective in patients with venoocclusive disease (constriction of proximal penile veins may enhance penile rigidity) and least effective in those with cavernosal fibrosis (e.g. post-priapism).

Patients are advised not to use the ring for greater than 30 minutes at any one time because of the danger of ischaemia and necrosis. They are relatively contraindicated in patients with clotting abnormalities and may be difficult for patients to use where there is Peyronie's disease or poor dexterity. Additionally, patients should be warned that the ring might prevent or cause painful ejaculation.

To maximise uptake of the VCD, potential patients should be encouraged to practise with the device at home with their partner. With several VCDs available in the UK, and with prices ranging from £120–£420, the choice of the VCD is often a personal decision. Options include manual or battery-driven pumps. Choice may also be influenced by sales brochures and videos, easy payment options, and the return of sale facility offered by some companies. Demonstration in the clinic room may also be valuable. VAT exemption is possible in patients with chronic MED.

Despite this only 50–60% of those choosing this treatment will opt to use it regularly. Reasons for lack of initial uptake include unsatisfactory quality of erection due to pivoting of the penis (which can be alleviated by double constriction rings and/or generous use of lubricating gel to ensure the ring is adjacent to the abdominal wall), a shorter erection with reduced girth, the high initial purchase price, or a belief that the device is cumbersome.

Seventy to ninety per cent of regular users and partners report satisfaction, and there is evidence that satisfaction increases with continual use. However, a significant number will discontinue use of their VCD for the following reasons: ineffective erections; pain, discomfort and bruising; recovery of spontaneous erections; too time-consuming; and lack of partner acceptance (Vrijhof & Delaere, 1994).

Choice of ICI or VCD?

Patient preference will play a part in this decision, but the physician can guide the patient in making his decision. Both methods produce satisfactory erections, with up to 90% of patients achieving success with either method. The drop-out rate is greater for ICI. In a large follow-up study of predominantly organic aetiologies, the drop-out rate at 12–96 months was reported as 11.25% (Virag *et al*, 1991) whereas in a psychogenic aetiology prospective study the drop-out rate at six months was 60% (Turner *et al*, 1989). Reasons for dropping out include lack of spontaneity, aesthetic obstacles, limitations on sexual frequency, cost, worry about side-effects, and the emergence of underlying psychopathology. This latter point emphasises the need for careful assessment and consideration of attempting some form of sex therapy, particularly in those men with predominantly psychogenic MED. Some patients have a fear of injecting themselves, especially into the penis. Where there is fear of needles, appropriate management can include referral to a behavioural nurse or psychologist for desensitisation therapy, or use of topical anaesthetic to reduce the discomfort of needle entry.

The erections that occur with ICI tend to be superior, particularly with regard to penile girth, which may increase by 100% with papaverine but only 60% with VCDs (Chancellor *et al*, 1994). The VCD may result in floppy penis syndrome or pivoting proximal to the constriction ring. Use of ICI tends to be restricted to two or three times a week (less with papaverine) but prolonged intercourse can occur. In contrast, with VCDs, several lovemaking sessions can occur daily, with the proviso that the ring is released after 30 minutes for a period of time. ICI tends to be a more easily concealed option.

VCDs do not have the serious side-effects of priapism and fibrotic plaques seen with ICI. However, failure to release the constriction ring after 30 minutes can have devastating effects for patients who fall asleep. The VCD has a higher initial cost to the patient unless assistance is provided. Hospital-based services might find it more economical in the long term to provide the VCD for free, so reducing clinic returns and prescription charges.

A treatment 'resistance' to papaverine may occur in severe cases of vasculogenic MED and in these cases VCD may be a more useful option. Both ICIs and VCDs can be helpful in those patients with concurrent premature ejaculation, should this require treatment.

Surgical interventions

The role of surgery can be considered according to aetiology. Firstly, arteriogenic MED, alone or combined with venoocclusive disease, accounts for 80% of all cases of vasculogenic MED. In the majority of these patients there is widespread atherosclerosis which is rarely helped by surgical intervention. However, patients with a localised arterial occlusion or stenosis (comprising less than 5% of cases in a urological impotence clinic) are often amenable to surgical repair. Typically, these are younger males who have suffered pelvic trauma, and in such cases surgical repair results in up to 80% of patients regaining and retaining their potency (Goldstein, 1986). Operative success depends upon the aetiology, surgical technical skill, and accurate preoperative imaging to identify the location of the damaged vessel. Duplex colour doppler ultrasonography following ICI of papaverine or alprosotadil has established itself as the imaging technique of choice. This minimally invasive investigation identifies abnormalities of flow within penile arteries. Surgery involves either arterialisation of a major penile vein (usually the deep dorsal vein), and hence formation of an artificial arterio-venous fistula, or revascularisation of the damaged artery . The revascularisation of the penile arteries involves bypassing the damaged segment by anastomosing the inferior epigastric artery to the dorsal or cavernous arteries. Complications are usually transient and are due to the formation of a 'high flow' state within the penile vessels. They include priapism, oedema especially of the glans, pain and paraesthesia around the site of incision.

Secondly venogenic MED is considered. There remains controversy as to whether venous MED is due to a primary venous abnormality, which results in an inability of the corpora to retain sufficient blood to maintain an erection, or whether this venous leakage arises secondary to disease of corporal smooth muscle – the so-called venoocclusive disease. It has been shown that SPACE (single potential analysis of cavernosal electrical activity), a measure of the 'healthiness' of the corporal tissue, is an important prognostic factor in the outcome of penile venous surgery (Steif *et al*, 1994). For diagnostic purposes cavernosometry and cavernosography remain the most useful investigations. However, these are uncomfortable invasive procedures which should not be undertaken in patients unwilling to consider surgery. Whatever the cause of the condition, cavernosography will demonstrate any excessive leakage of the contrast medium through abnormal venous channels. The aim of the surgical treatment is to ligate these abnormal veins, although a number of surgical techniques have been described which vary enormously as to the extent of the ligation. Overall the results of surgery for venous disease are disappointing. Although some good short-term results have been reported, the number of patients who retain potency decreases markedly with time. This may be due to failure to obstruct the anatomical channels, development of new venous leaks, undiagnosed arterial insufficiency, or to other poorly understood factors.

A summary of published data shows that immediately after surgery anything between 30–80% of patients are able to achieve full erection (without ICI augmentation). However, by 12 months this figure drops to around 24% (Freedman *et al*, 1993). Many patients will remain partial responders and be dependent upon ICI for full erections even after surgery. Better than average longer-term results are achieved in patients with mild cavernosal leakage with no arterial component. Patients with the worst outcome following venous surgery are usually elderly, have coexisting arterial disease, and have widespread venoocclusive disease.

Thirdly, in Peyronie's disease, where potency remains but intercourse is significantly impaired due to the curvature of the penis, the best treatment is Nesbit's procedure, whereby the penis is straightened. Patients should be informed about concomitant penile shortening of about 1 cm. Where potency is impaired, ICI or a penile prosthesis should be used, with or without excision of the plaques. There are reports that long-term treatment with Potaba (potassium para-amine benzoate, an antifibrosis agent) may be beneficial.

Penile prostheses

Penile prostheses are rarely used as a first-line treatment for patients with MED. Nevertheless, when other forms of therapy (VCD or ICI) have failed or are no longer considered satisfactory by the patient or his physician, consideration should be give to the insertion of a penile prosthesis. This is especially true in younger men with vasculogenic MED (e.g. due to longstanding diabetes) and retained libido.

There are two types of prosthesis available, of which semi-rigid devices were the first to be developed. They are relatively cheap and simple to implant into each corpora cavernosum, and are less prone to the complications described below. After insertion the penis remains permanently 'erect' but because they are malleable they may be concealed in the dressed patient. They are occasionally associated with patient and partner dissatisfaction, especially in the longer term. Complaints include a decrease in penile sensitivity, poor concealment, and some persistence of penile deviation in patients with Peyronie's disease.

Inflatable prosthetic devices are more expensive, technically more difficult to insert and more prone to complications. They comprise inflatable rods implanted into the penis which can be inflated via scrotal pumps when the patient desires an erection. The vast majority of patients are satisfied with these devices – reports suggest up to 96% of patients. In the minority of patients in whom the prosthesis fails, the usual cause is either major unresolved sepsis or ulceration of the prosthesis from the penis.

Specific complications will occur in up to 10% of patients. They include: incorrect length of prostheses resulting in painful or smaller erections (8%); accidental inflation on exercise (4%); mechanical failure (2–4%) and sepsis (2%).

Hyperprolactinemia

This condition is often seen in patients receiving treatment for psychiatric illness. Neuroleptic medication often results in raised prolactin levels, and where necessary and clinically indicated, dose reduction or substitution should be the first consideration. Where this is not possible several other options exist and are considered below. The other common condition causing hyperprolactinemia is a benign pituitary adenoma, which unless large usually responds well to bromocriptine.

Erection impaired by medication

Tricyclic antidepressants, monoamine oxidase inhibitors (MAOIs), and selective serotonin reuptake inhibitors (SSRIs) have all been implicated in affecting erection capability. The action is presumed secondary to blockade at the serotonin and possibly alpha-adrenergic receptors. There may be a central effect of decrease of libido, increased sedation and raised prolactin levels. The mainstay of treatment is to decrease the dose or change the agent.

Certain drugs are considered more likely to cause problems with erectile dysfunction, which is increased with MAOIs and the SSRI fluoxetine (Brock & Lue, 1993). The antidepressants bupropion, desipramine and fluvoxamine are least likely to cause sexual dysfunction. A rare complication of trazodone is priapism. Up to 25% of patients receiving antipsychotics report sexual dysfunction, with the rate as high as 60% for those on thioridazine. Drugs commonly associated with MED are thioridazine and fluphenazine. Lithium has been reported to cause MED and a decrease in libido.

Benzodiazepines have little effect on sexual function; however, beta blockers commonly used to treat anxiety do have a detrimental effect. Reports suggest that up to 15% of patients receiving propanolol may experience impaired sexual function. Beta blockers also cause a reduction in serum testosterone. For patients receiving beta blockers for hypertension, advice can be given to the prescribing physician to try to avoid beta blockers in general (although lower rates of side-effects are seen with the beta-1 selective agents such as atenolol), diuretics and methyldopa. Digoxin decreases serum testosterone, as well as increasing oestrogen. The latter effect could cause MED by central activity.

In patients who smoke or misuse alcohol, advice should be given regarding the effect of nicotine on erectile dysfunction as well as the effect of alcohol. Other drugs that may have an effect include cimetidine (due to its anti-androgenic effects leading to raised prolactin), clofibrate and corticosteroids.

Miscellaneous treatments

Patients who are able to attain erections but then lose them typically 5–10 minutes afterwards may find the use of penile rings of benefit. This can be helpful for patients with both venoocclusive disease and psychogenic erectile loss. By application of a tight ring around the base of the penis, the erection can be maintained sufficiently long enough for lovemaking. As with the rings in vacuum devices, the ring cannot be applied for more than 30 minutes. Ring loading systems can be bought from various companies as well as in sex aid shops. Care must be taken that the ring is applied as close to the shaft base as possible, otherwise pivoting will occur proximal to the ring. Lubricating jelly or shaving pubic hair may be useful, particularly in hairy patients. If there are problems with ejaculation, pressure can be released on the ventral side when appropriate by use of finger rings.

The role of pelvic floor training has been found to be a useful alternative to surgery for patients with mild venous leakage (Claes & Baert, 1993). Surgery was not found to be superior to the pelvic floor training programme, either subjectively or objectively after 12 months; 58% of patients receiving physiotherapy instruction improved so much that they did not wish to proceed with surgery. Instruction along the lines of Kegal instructions given to women post-natally can easily be provided to the patient in clinic or from an interested physiotherapist.

The value of acupuncture remains under consideration in patients with erectile dysfunction. It has been my finding that there often exists an opportunity, while needles are being inserted and in place, for patients to discuss their sexual anxieties. Relaxation and anxiety control training may augment this response if carried out simultaneously. It remains unclear whether it is this or the acupuncture process *per se*, or both, that helps the patient. Other alternative treatments may have some value to the patient, including homeopathic remedies.

Ejaculatory and orgasmic problems

Premature and retarded ejaculation

Clomipramine was first reported as beneficial in the treatment of premature ejaculation (PE) two decades ago (Eaton, 1973). Since then it has become evident that serotonin reuptake inhibitors, including clomipramine, paroxetine and fluoxetine, may all be beneficial in the treatment of this condition by having the side-effect of delayed ejaculation and orgasm. Topical anaesthetic sprays and gels have been suggested as useful in some patients. There has been recent interest in neurotomy of the dorsal nerve for primary cases of PE.

For retarded ejaculation, behavioural techniques of superstimulation should be attempted using the bridging manoeuvre described by Masters & Johnson (1970). If this is insufficient, increased stimulation using a high-speed vibrator on the undersurface of the penis may facilitate ejaculation. These can be purchased from sex aid shops, or body massagers can be purchased from many high street chemists. Desipramine, neostigmine and yohimbine may be of benefit. When these techniques fail it is often necessary to discuss options like digital prostate massage, which if unacceptable or unsuccessful can be supplemented by rectal vibratory excitation (with caution) or electro-ejaculation techniques in specialist centres. This often provides some chance of ejaculation occurring when fertility aspects are important. Differentiation from retrograde ejaculation with failure of emission is useful, as specific treatments will then be indicated.

Anorgasmia

Kegal exercises to strengthen the pubococcygeus muscle can improve sexual sensation and response, including orgasm. A variation on this (for women) is the use of vaginal cones developed for stress incontinence. There is increase in pelvic muscle tone as well as cognitive awareness of sensations from the lower vagina and vulva. Riley (1993) reports that vaginal and penile sensations might be improved by the use of such cones.

Impairment by medication

The SSRI group of drugs are reported to cause sexual dysfunction, most commonly being delayed ejaculation and/or anorgasmia. Serotonin may centrally inhibit orgasm and has a relaxing effect on peripheral smooth muscle, so inhibiting orgasmic contractions. Dopamine is thought to facilitate ejaculation. Centrally-acting antihypertensives (e.g. clonidine and methyl dopa) may impair orgasm. Management can be along several lines: discontinue the drug; reduce the dose; postpone the daily dose until after sexual activity (reported beneficial with clomipramine); await spontaneous remission (or improvement of the depression); substitute another drug; or add another drug (see below).

Various reports exist suggesting that sexual functioning can be restored by the use of cyproheptadine (4–16 mg a day), yohimbine or amantadine. Cyproheptadine is a serotonin antagonist and antihistamine. The use of this may precipitate symptom relapse of the underlying psychiatric disorder. Yohimbine increases central noradrenergic tone and should not result in symptom relapse. It is useful to advise patients to take yohimbine 2–4 hours ahead of sexual activity, when used as a treatment for sexual dysfunction caused by the SSRIs. There appears to be a narrow therapeutic window which must be monitored for beneficial effect when yohimbine is used in this way (Hollander & McCarley, 1992). Amantadine is a mild dopamine agonist.

Bethanechol, a cholinomimetic agent, has been found to be useful in relieving sexual dysfunction created by the anticholinergic effects of some antidepressants. It is reported as helpful in MED due to MAOIs, anorgasmia secondary to amoxapine, and imipramine-induced ejaculatory dysfunction. Neostigmine 7.5–15 mg, 30 minutes before sexual intercourse, has been reported to increase libido and reverse retarded ejaculation.

A recent paper (Power-Smith, 1994) has suggested that fluoxetine may have the advantageous benefit of improving erectile and ejaculatory status in depressed men. Despite there being some discrepancy here with previous reports, withdrawal of the fluoxetine resulted in return to the pre-treatment level of sexual functioning in both cases.

Libido and desire disorders

Augmentation techniques including medication

The management of disorders of desire is often heavily reliant on psychological therapies. However, augmentation by maximising sensory stimulation can be helpful. In addition to tactile stimulation (e.g. self-focus, sensate focus and vibrators), the use of sensual clothing, aroma-therapy, incense and perfume can be considered.

It has been reported that increased libido might be experienced in patients taking imipramine, trazodone, viloxazine and trimipramine as well as moclobemide. However, it is not clear that these will be useful in patients without depressive illness. The use of hormone augmentation, particularly in perimenopausal women, is gaining acceptance. Androgen depletion in women was first documented in 1959, when it was found that libido and the ability to respond to sexual stimulation was lost in patients with advanced breast cancer treated by surgical ablation of the ovaries, adrenals and/or hypophyses (so losing all endogenous androgen). The benefit of replacement testosterone and oestrogen for menopausal symptoms, as well as more specific symptoms of depression and libido loss, has been documented but remains contested (Reynolds, 1993). Kaplan & Owett (1993) found that women with demonstrable testosterone deficiency (e.g. following bilateral oophorectomy) showed a significant decrease in libido and that testosterone supplementation (usually as subcutaneous implants) could return libido to previous levels. Clitoral erotic sensitivity has also been shown to be dependent upon androgenic and/or oestrogen stimulation. Increase in the subjective sensitivity of the clitoris is considered an important prognostic occurrence and is associated with a greater chance of successful outcome in women with lack of sexual drive.

Sex drive has been linked with zinc deficiency (in some studies), and nutritionists may advise plenty of red meat, chicken and fish as well as supplements of the mineral itself.

Impairment by medication

Many of the antidepressant drugs as well as lithium have been noted to decrease libido. Trazodone has been reported to increase libido in both depressed men and women. Libido was increased to levels greater than during euthymic states. It is unlikely that this was due to hypomania as an antidepressant response was not reported. Viloxazine is also considered an antidepressant that might specifically improve sex drive (either by disinhibition or increasing libido *per se*).

Moclobemide, a noncholinergic reversible inhibitor of monoamine oxidase-A (RIMA), was found more often than doxepin to lead to an improvement of reduced libido in patients with major depression. The increased sexual desire seen in recovery from depression may often be hidden as a result of drug-induced sexual dysfunction. Other reports suggest that yohimbine can reverse fluoxetine-induced low libido, and substitution of bupropion (with its low incidence of sexual side-effects) is of general value in this group of patients.

Other sexual problems

Dyspareunia

The majority of cases of dyspareunia are due to identifiable organic causes (e.g. endometriosis, vulval dysplasia, post-episiotomy scar tissue and vaginal infections) and require appropriate gynaecological management. Older patients often present with superficial dyspareunia, usually as the result of vaginal atrophy. This is secondary to a reduction of circulating oestrogens in menopausal women. In a few cases dyspareunia may be due to drug treatment, particularly in women receiving labetalol, thiazides and spironolactone.

Discomfort from penile penetration affects one in seven women over 35 years of age, usually as a result of vaginal dryness. Failure to treat the condition can lead to loss of sexual interest. In pre-menopausal women an infectious cause (e.g. trichomonas or candida organisms) must be excluded. Non-oestrogen lubricants include Replens gel inserted into the vagina 2–3 times a week or Senselle applied topically as required, and are improvements upon KY gel. In particular, Senselle is similar to vaginal transudate. Neither products are reported as harmful to latex. In post-menopausal women, dyspareunia can be alleviated by use of oestrogen creams or pessaries. Dienoestrol cream or 'Estring' is effective in over 70% of women, but should not be used long-term without considering the need for progestogen supplementation (in women with a uterus). Patients using hormone replacement therapy rarely report such problems.

Vaginismus

The approach to this condition is usually a graded desensitisation programme. This usually follows examination by the doctor and an initial attempt to allow entry of one gloved finger. Patients and/or partners are then encouraged to enter the vagina using their finger(s). In patients unable to adopt this routine, use of vaginal dilators or 'trainers' is encouraged. It is possible for patients to purchase a set of trainers for personal use (under £50.00), and may be an improvement over the loan of glass dilators from the hospital clinic. However, by purchasing a set for home use, there may be reduced opportunity for exploration of the psychological issues that are often crucial in the treatment of such cases.

Urinary incontinence

Urinary incontinence that can lead to vaginal dermatitis and urinary frequency is amenable to treatment. Patients may report incontinence during intercourse or at the time of orgasm. If it is associated with orgasm, it is likely to be due to detrusor instability, and if not, it is more likely to have a mechanical aetiology (Stanton, 1994). Advice includes emptying the bladder before lovemaking, pelvic floor exercises, and considering the use of oxybutynin hydrochloride (2.5–5 mg) an hour before (predicted) intercourse. Mechanical problems such as urethral sphincter incompetence (genuine stress incontinence) can be managed with pelvic floor exercises or colposuspension. Incontinence around the menopause may respond to topical oestrogens.

Paraphilias

While behavioural therapy is considered by many as essential for long-lasting treatment of these conditions, concurrent use of antiandrogens like cyproterone acetate and medroxyprogesterone has proven value, particularly in reducing sex drive. There is some evidence that the SSRI group of drugs may be of benefit in the treatment of paraphilias, with increasing reports appearing in the literature (e.g. fluoxetine for exhibitionism and voyeurism). A more comprehensive review of this subject can be found elsewhere (Wylie, 1994).

Penis size dissatisfaction

Penis enlargement has been advocated to some patients who fear that they have a small penis and whose partner complains that they cannot feel their partner during penetration. Other men simply want the operation in an attempt to improve self-esteem. Although there is often no abnormality found on examination, sexual problems may remain until some treatment is offered. The problem may even remain after treatment! Vacuum developers are available in various sex shops which work on the same basis as VCDs. Royal Jelly is advocated by some as beneficial, although this has never been substantiated. As far as surgical intervention is concerned, elongation is achieved by division of the fundiform and suspensory ligaments from the symphasis pubis. In addition, enlargement of penile girth is achieved by transfer of body fat (around 100 cc) which is obtained from hips, inner thighs, abdomen and buttocks. Up to 40% may be reabsorbed within eight weeks, necessitating further surgery. Both operations require private consultations outside of the National Health Service.

Transsexualism

After an appropriate period of psychological assessment, hormonal therapy precedes any realignment surgery. The first effects of hormones will become apparent after a couple of months, but it may take several years before the changes are complete. The interested reader is referred to Asscheman & Gooren (1992) for a detailed article on hormone treatments.

References

Asscheman, H. & Gooren, L. J. G. (1992) Hormone treatment in transsexuals. *Journal of Psychology and Human Sexuality*, 5, 39–54.

Brock, G. B. & Lue, T. F. (1993) Drug induced male sexual dysfunction. *Drug Safety*, 8, 414–426.

Chancellor, M. B., Rivas, D. A., Panzar, D. E., *et al* (1994) Prospective comparison of topical minoxidil to vacuum constriction device and intracorporeal papaverine injection in treatment of erectile dysfunction due to spinal cord injury. *Urology*, 43, 365–369.

Claes, H. & Baert, L. (1993) Pelvic floor exercise versus surgery in the treatment of impotence. *British Journal of Urology*, 71, 52–57.

Eaton, H. (1973) Clomipramine in the treatment of premature ejaculation. *Journal of International Medical Research*, 1, 432–434.

Freedman, A. L., Neto, F. C., Mehringer, C. M., *et al* (1993) Long-term results of penile vein ligation for impotence from venous leakage. *Journal of Urology*, 149, 1301–1303.

Goldstein, I. (1986) Arterial revascularization procedures. *Seminars in Urology*, 4, 252–258.

Gregoire, A. (1993) Pharmacological treatments for impotence. In *Impotence: An Integrated Approach to Clinical Practice* (eds A. Gregoire & J. P. Pryor), pp. 165–184. Edinburgh: Churchill Livingstone.

Hollander, E. & McCarley, A. (1992) Yohimbine treatment of sexual side effects induced by serotonin reuptake blockers. *Journal of Clinical Psychiatry*, 53, 207–209.

Kaplan, H. S. & Owett, T. (1993) The female androgen deficiency syndrome. *Journal of Sexual and Marital Therapy*, 19, 3–24.

McClure, R. D. (1988) Endocrine evaluation and therapy. In *Contemporary Management of Impotence and Infertility* (eds E. A. Tanagho, T. F. Lue & R. D. McClure), pp. 84–94. Baltimore: Williams and Wilkins.

Masters, W. H. & Johnson, V. E. (1970) *Human Sexual Inadequacy*. Boston: Little, Brown and Co.

Power-Smith, P. (1994) Beneficial sexual side effects from fluoxetine. *British Journal of Psychiatry*, 164, 249–250.

Reynolds, J. E. F. (ed.) (1993) *The Extra Pharmacopoeia*. London: Pharmaceutical Press.

Riley, A. (1993) Pelvic exercise: men can benefit too. *Journal of Sexual Health*, 3, 123–125.

Stanton, S. (1994) Incontinence on intercourse. *British Journal of Sexual Medicine*, 21, 10.

Steif, C. G., Djamilian, M., Truss, M. C., *et al* (1994) Prognostic factors for the postoperative outcome of penile venous surgery for venogenic erectile dysfunction. *Journal of Urology*, 151, 880–883.

Turner, L. A., Althof, S. E., Levine, S. B., *et al* (1989) Self injection with papaverine and phentolamine in the treatment of psychogenic impotence. *Journal of Sex and Marital Therapy*, 15, 163–176.

——, ——, ——, *et al* (1991) External vacuum devices in the treatment of erectile dysfunction: A one year study of sexual and psychological impact. *Journal of Sex and Marital Therapy*, 17, 81–93.

Virag, R., Shouukry, K., Floresco, J., *et al* (1991) Intracavernous self-injection of vasoactive drugs in the treatment of impotence: 8 year experience with 615 cases. *Journal of Urology*, 145, 287-293.

Vrijhof, H. J. E. J. & Delaere, K. P. J. (1994) Vacuum constriction devices in erectile dysfunction: acceptance and effectiveness in patients with impotence of organic or mixed aetiology. *British Journal of Urology*, 74, 102–105.

Wylie, K. (1994) New approaches to paraphilias. *British Journal of Sexual Medicine*, 21, 18–21.

6 Child abuse

Gerry Doyle

*Definitions • Historical aspects • Descriptions of abuse •
Epidemiology • Risk factors • Consequences of abuse •
Intervention • Childhood sexual abuse • Consequences of
childhood sexual abuse • False memory syndrome • Summary*

Definitions

Child abuse is a highly emotive term which can conjure a variety of horrors to the imagination. The expression is used to cover a multitude of sins and is poorly defined by the general public. This is not surprising as there are considerable cultural and subcultural differences in what is accepted as normal child-rearing practice. As the child ages and gains some autonomy, different standards of behaviour are expected from the parents. In general people will judge parental behaviour by their own personal experience of childhood and parenthood.

The 1989 Children Act of England and Wales defines child abuse in terms of acts or omissions which cause or are likely to cause "harm to the child" physically, mentally or developmentally. The parents' intentions are not of key importance; a parent who shakes a crying baby is unlikely to intend brain damage.

The broad categories that are widely used to describe abuse are physical, emotional, sexual and neglect. Each has its own definition problem.

The concept of harm is easily applied to physical abuse; the tangible results include bruising, burns, pinch marks and bone fractures, some of which are characteristic. The psychological results must not be overlooked as they can take much longer to heal.

Finkelhor & Korbin (1988) described emotional abuse in terms of chronic rejection, with a chronic lack of attention to the child, threats of abandonment, inappropriate methods of childcare, and age-inappropriate demands placed upon the child.

Neglect involves depriving a child of the resources that are essential (and available) for its welfare and development. The damage caused by emotional maltreatment and neglect may be less visible than a bruise or burn mark, but the harmful effects can be much more handicapping.

Sexual abuse will be discussed later.

Historical aspects

From a historical point of view it is possible that children are better treated now than ever before, with the abolition of child labour, the provision of compulsory schooling and statutes protecting their rights. Maltreatment of children is not a recent phenomenon; the National Society for the Prevention of Cruelty to Children was founded in 1884. It may be that the standards we expect in childcare are rising and our threshold for concern is lowering. Corporal punishment was widespread in British schools until the 1970s. Such acts might now be considered as physical abuse, but not long ago this form of discipline was seen as an important part of a child's education and essential in the formation of the British ruling class. Now a broadly similar debate rages over parents smacking children.

In a similar way our views on emotional care are changing. In the 1950s parents were advised to limit their visits to children in hospital, where now we encourage them to stay as long as possible. Children's homes have also seen a change in attitude towards the amount of individual attention a child should receive.

Descriptions of abuse

All forms of child abuse involve a degree of emotional ill-treatment and point to a breakdown in the parent/child relationship. Inevitably the four categories overlap, but they do provide a useful framework.

Physical abuse can take many forms; as well as direct acts of violence, the child may be deliberately poisoned or suffocated. Non-fatal smothering may present as "near cot death" and it is worth noting that families with a child on the child protection register have a higher than expected incidence of cot death. Deliberate poisoning in toddlers can be difficult to detect, as accidental poisoning is common in this age group. Münchausen syndrome by proxy is an unusual form of abuse where the mother falsifies illness in a child and then seeks medical attention.

Primary healthcare workers and casualty staff may suspect physical abuse when they see a suspicious injury on a child. They then have the difficult question to answer: was the injury sustained by accidental or non-accidental means?

A new concept of physical abuse is 'foetal abuse'. In North America successful prosecutions have been brought against mothers who abuse drugs while pregnant and so harm their child.

Emotional abuse can also take many forms and can involve acts of omission or commission. Characteristically the parents are consistently rejecting and hostile to their child, both verbally and non-verbally. A key feature of neglect is a sustained pattern of behaviour by parents who fail to supply the essential love and nurture, and who may also ignore the child's physical needs.

A diagnosis of physical abuse is usually made by examining the child and interviewing the parents. Diagnosing emotional abuse and neglect rely more on observations of the child's emotional and behavioural adjustment.

Epidemiology

In 1991, 45 200 children were on child protection registers in England. This corresponds to a rate of 4.2 per 1000 children under 18 years. About a quarter of these children were in local authority care. The reasons for registration were as follows (Meadows, 1993):

Grave concern	47%
Physical abuse	20%
Sexual abuse	12%
Neglect	12%
Emotional abuse	6%

It is likely that many cases of abuse go unnoticed, as professionals fail to recognise the symptoms of abuse, or fail to connect the symptoms with abuse. Most attention is focused on young children, but is worth remembering that adolescents can also be victims. In fact, sexual and psychological abuse may be more common in children over 10 years of age than those under 10 years (Garbarino, 1989).

What are the risk factors?

A large number of studies have shown a strong relationship between abuse and low socio-economic status (e.g. Straus & Gelles, 1986). Large disadvantaged families with few social supports who are coping with a number of stresses appear to be most at risk.

Some characteristics of the child may increase its risk of being abused. Spending time in a special care baby unit may impair parent/child bonding. A child who cries continually or who has a "difficult temperament" may be difficult to love. Children with chronic illnesses and handicaps (physical or mental) may exhaust the coping skills of stressed parents.

The parent's own personality and emotional needs are important factors which, along with their expectations and interpretations of their child's behaviour, shape how they function as parents.

Consequences of abuse

When assessing the effects of abuse it is important to remember that the clinician sees a biased population of abused children. A psychiatrist will see suspected or proven cases where someone has been sufficiently concerned to make a referral. Unsuspected cases by definition go unnoticed, and well-adjusted victims are not referred, hence clinical experience and research will reflect this bias.

There are a number of variables to consider in each case of abuse. The nature, severity and duration of the maltreatment are important, as is the relationship that exists between victim and perpetrator. An assault by an uncle may have less emotional impact than a similar assault from a parent. A key factor determining psychological damage appears to be the age and developmental stage of the child.

Healthy development is thought to arise from specific attainments within critical age periods. Unsuccessful negotiation of a developmental stage can disrupt future developmental progress. For example, attachment theory suggests that children gain confidence to explore their environment and meet unfamiliar people by being securely attached to their parents – the primary attachment figures. Failed primary attachments can damage the child's ability to form new relationships, and so abnormal patterns of social interaction can follow (Crittenden & Ainsworth, 1989). Clinical experience reflects this model, as socially inappropriate behaviour is frequently displayed by abused children. However, this may be due to their parents being poor role models of normal social behaviour.

Before attributing behavioural or emotional difficulties to abusive experiences, it is worth bearing in mind that most victims come from socially disadvantaged families. It is not easy to tease out the effects of abuse from the effects of poor housing, overcrowding, poverty and the many other hardships such families face. It seems likely that these two forms of adversity have a cumulative effect on a child's well-being.

Taking all the above points into consideration, it does still appear that sustained maltreatment can adversely affect a child physically, emotionally and developmentally. Physical abuse can leave permanent deformity or brain damage, which may handicap a child directly or indirectly by stigmatisation. Emotional abuse can lead to failure to thrive. In severe cases, "psychosocial dwarfism" is said to follow, with growth below the 3rd centile, immature body proportions and microcephaly. Inadequate provision of nutrition may be an additional factor retarding growth.

Low self-esteem is a common finding among abused children. Depressed mood, anxiety symptoms and psychosomatic symptoms are also often present. Nightmares, enuresis and encopresis may occur as a distressed child regresses to developmentally less mature patterns of behaviour. Severely abused children may display the 'reactive attachment disorder' (ICD–10 F94-1; World Health Organization, 1992), a syndrome characterised by persistent abnormalities in the child's social relationships, and a fearfulness and hypervigilance which does not respond to comforting. Other patterns of abnormal behaviour include antisocial acts and incompetence with everyday social relationships. These may disrupt school performance, which can be further hampered by impaired cognitive development.

Child abuse has been linked to disorders of attention-span and language development, and it seems likely that other cognitive functions are similarly affected.

These handicaps are fortunately not an inevitable consequence of child abuse; some children appear to cope remarkably well with adversity. Protective factors were proposed by Rosenberg (1987) and include positive adult relationships, intelligence, emotional resilience and involvement in community activities. These and other unknowns may mitigate the harmful effects of abuse.

The long-term effects of child abuse are not clearly understood; it has long been suspected that the victims would go on to have impairments in social, emotional and cognitive functioning in adulthood, but proof is lacking. Research is hampered by the biases already mentioned, and most studies are further devalued by being retrospective.

Another key area for research is whether abused children grow up to abuse their own offspring. 'Intergenerational transmission' is a much debated concept. Although it is not uncommon for perpetrators of abuse to report being victims themselves, it remains unclear whether their disclosures should always be believed, and whether their own experience makes them any more or less likely to act in the same way.

Intervention

Any person who suspects abuse should contact local social services to discuss their concerns. The childcare teams investigate possible cases, arrange case conferences for multidisciplinary discussion, and liaise with the police.

Abuse can be very difficult to prove in court, but does not have to be proven for the child to be entered on the child protection register. Once a child is registered the parents must accept the allocation of a social worker, and the registration must be regularly reviewed.

Once abuse is discovered, social services are often faced with a difficult choice. Should the child remain with the family, or would finding a new home be better for the child? Staying entails a risk of further abuse, but fostering and adoption are potentially traumatic experiences which can worsen feelings of victimisation and alienation. Important factors include, will the parents:

(1) accept responsibility for their actions?
(2) work with the childcare team?
(3) critically appraise themselves?
(4) identify their problem areas?
(5) make the appropriate changes?

A previously abused child can flourish in a loving family, and dramatic improvements in all areas of the child's development can follow, giving hope for the future. The child may also benefit from individual therapy, and siblings who may themselves be victims should not be forgotten.

Childhood sexual abuse

Although it is likely that children have been used by adults for sexual gratification since time began, the general public's awareness of the situation is poor. Research would suggest it is not a rare occurrence, but it receives little public discussion. Compare the public's consideration of adult sexual abuse (rape/indecent assault) with their consideration of childhood sexual abuse, and one might conclude that denial is the preferred approach to this distressing topic.

Cultural issues

Different cultures have a variety of opinions regarding childhood sexual activity. In some countries a child bride is highly prized. In England and Wales the age of consent is 16 years, but a distinction is made between under 13-year-olds and under 16-year-olds. It is always unlawful to have sexual intercourse with a girl younger than 13, but with a girl aged between 13 and 16 a man under 24 years of age can put forward a defence.

Adolescents appear to be becoming sexually active at a younger age than previous generations, and it is estimated that 20% of girls in Britain have first intercourse before their 16th birthday. Many adolescents believe that the age of consent is unrealistically high and perceive pressure from their peers and magazines to have intercourse at an early age. This raises the question that if a 15-year-old couple choose to have sexual intercourse, should this be considered sexual abuse, and who is the victim?

What is childhood sexual abuse?

A number of definitions have been put forward, each with the core concept of sexual acts involving a child. Differences exist in the upper age limit of childhood and whether acts committed by adolescents and children should be included. Most definitions do not specify the nature of the sexual acts involved. Consequently a wide range of sexual experiences can be brought together under the heading of childhood sexual abuse.

Non-penetrative acts (exposure, fondling, masturbation) appear to be the most common types of sexual abuse. Penetrative acts seem over-represented in clinical populations. It may be that they are more psychologically damaging to the child, and so are more likely to lead to referral.

All studies suggest that females are more commonly the victim than males. Most perpetrators are men, with an estimated 5–15% of sexual abuse being committed by women. Women appear more likely to abuse boys than girls; their role as co-abusers is not clear.

An important distinction is often made between abuse that occurs between family members and that occurring outside the family. Intrafamilial abuse commonly involves father and daughter or stepfather and stepdaughter over a period of time. Because of the breach of trust involved in such cases, disclosure poses a major threat to the continued existence of that family. Extrafamilial abuse may involve a trusted family friend or a stranger. After disclosure the family can rally together to support the victim and so disclosure may be less of a threat to the family unit. This form of abuse often presents earlier.

How common is childhood sexual abuse?

This is an extremely difficult question to answer. Most studies have involved asking adults about their childhood, avoiding the question "how reliable are adult's memories of childhood events?" (Doyle, 1994). Problems with definition complicate the picture, and sampling biases within study populations compound the problem.

Smith & Bentovim (1994) estimated that "between 15–30% of women will have been subjected to an unwanted experience of sexual contact at sometime during their childhood", with double that figure experiencing an unwanted non-contact sexual experience in childhood.

Risk factors

The strong correlation that exists between physical/emotional abuse and low socio-economic status is not so obviously present with sexual abuse. Different risk factors appear to apply, most notably being a stepdaughter. It may be that the stepfather is attracted to the household by the daughter rather than the mother.

Children living in chaotic families who lack clear boundaries appear to be at risk, especially if the mother is sexually unavailable to the father and where alcohol loosens inhibitions. Poorly supervised children who crave the adult affection their parents fail to supply can become vulnerable to the attention of paedophiles.

Presentation

Sexual abuse can present in many guises, but possibly the most common is for the child to tell a friend, relative or trusted adult. Another common method of presentation is via a change in behaviour. Sexualised behaviour in a young child is highly suggestive of sexual abuse; other changes seen include regression to less mature behaviour, antisocial acts, deliberate self-harm, eating disorders, and running away from home. Emotional distress may be the first sign of abuse; the child may display low self-esteem, low mood, anxiety symptoms and psychosomatic symptoms.

Physical disorders can be related to abuse; sexually transmitted diseases, pregnancy and genital trauma are obviously pathognomonic, but the paediatrician must remember sexual abuse when treating children with urinary tract infections, enuresis and encopresis.

An 'accommodation syndrome' has been described where a child sexually abused from a young age displays no symptoms from their experience. These cases can come to light when the child is surprised to learn that its peers are not sexually active, and that the acts they have been involved in are not a normal part of childhood.

What are the consequences of childhood sexual abuse?

This is also a difficult question to answer with any authority. As clinicians we see a biased population of suspected or proven cases that someone chose to refer. When dealing with intrafamilial abuse, another complication is to separate out the consequences of being sexually abused from the consequences of being in that family. It seems reasonable to suggest that intrafamilial abuse will occur most commonly in dysfunctional families where boundaries, dynamics and relationships are unusual, if not frankly abnormal. Hence membership of such a family in itself may be damaging.

A further problem for the researcher is to separate the effects of being abused from the effects of the investigation process. Following disclosure a child can be subjected to considerable potentially harmful attention, with interviews, examinations and possible court appearances. The family may be broken up and the children taken from home and accommodated by the local authority.

How the mother reacts in intrafamilial cases appears especially important. She may be faced with a choice: to stay with an abusing partner and reject her child, or reject her partner and support her child. Thus the mother's own emotional needs enter the equation, and surely the saddest cases are when the abused child is further traumatised by maternal rejection. All this can be a large burden to fall upon a small pair of shoulders.

The expression childhood sexual abuse can be used to cover a variety of abusive experiences. Features of the abuse itself are likely to modify its damaging potential. The exact nature and duration of the act are important, along with the use of threats, violence and coercion. In addition, details of the victim and perpetrator combine to make each case unique. The victim's age and developmental stage, their premorbid personality and relationships with the abusers are key points, as are the abuser's age and gender.

Once again we must consider whether there are any protective factors which may mitigate the harmful effects of this childhood trauma. If sexual abuse is as common as research suggests, there must be a large group of individuals who appear to escape into adulthood largely unscathed. We can only speculate what it is about these people and their experiences that prevents damage.

Traumagenic dynamics

With so many variables and unknown factors to consider, one soon realises why so little is known in certainty. Finkelhor & Browne (1985) wrote "unfortunately the sum total of literature adds up to little more than a list of possible outcomes". They went on to put forward a useful model concerning the traumatic impact of child sexual abuse.

They postulated four trauma-causing factors or "traumagenic dynamics" which may alter the child's cognitive and emotional orientation to the world: powerlessness, betrayal, stigmatisation, and traumatic sexualisation. The dynamics can act to corrupt the normal development of autonomy, trust, self-esteem and sexuality.

This model emphasises the developmental factors that can make childhood traumas so different from adult traumas, and it reminds us how important it is to keep a developmental perspective when discussing childhood adversity.

Effects

The emotional, behavioural and physical disorders by which childhood sexual abuse can present are themselves the effects of abuse. A post-traumatic stress disorder type syndrome has also been described (Wolfe *et al*, 1989).

Guilt and low self-esteem are commonly prominent in victims. Guilt may stem from the child feeling responsible for the abuse. It is not uncommon for the perpetrator to blame the child, and unfortunately members of the public sometimes do the same. The child may feel responsible for the breakup of the family, and rejection by mother and siblings will only aggravate their distress.

The act of abuse can be demeaning in itself, and the secrecy which usually surrounds abuse can further convey a sense of shame. With disclosure a private tragedy can become public conversation, and self-esteem can be further damaged.

The possibility of the child carrying these deficiencies into adulthood and of them handicapping adult life has been explored by many researchers. A large number of studies have tried to confirm a correlation between childhood sexual abuse and adult mental illness and impairments in adult social, interpersonal and sexual functioning. Unfortunately, most of these are retrospective studies relying on unvalidated self-reports from adults attending psychiatrists.

For some children the damage does appear to be life-long, but at present, predicting in which individuals that will be is not possible.

Intervention

Investigations into suspected cases of childhood sexual abuse need to be handled tactfully and by professionals. Once again, any person suspecting abuse should inform social services who will arrange the appropriate response. The Butler-Sloss Report (1988) outlined some of the potential pitfalls of investigation and highlighted the importance of multidisciplinary work.

The child's safety is paramount and a child may need to be removed from their home during the investigation. It is important to recognise the child's distress and vulnerability, and to assess the impact any abuse has had. The child must be interviewed alone, since if intrafamilial abuse has occurred the child may feel inhibited speaking in front of family members. Anatomical dolls can be used to assist young children, and video-taped interviews may be accepted in court, so, in theory, saving the child the ordeal of a court appearance.

A full assessment of the family is necessary. This involves exploring how abuse could have occurred and whether the parents will support and protect their children in future. It is also important to ascertain if other children are at risk.

Treatment

The child involved may require individual attention and a variety of thera-peutic styles have been advocated. Age-appropriate sex education and relearning of social norms may also be necessary. A major concern of all therapists working with abused children is the cycle where victims go on to become perpetrators, either shortly after their own abuse or as adults.

Sexualised behaviour can be very difficult for families to cope with, and they may need advice on dealing with public masturbation and other inappropriate behaviours. Involving the school is often advisable.

In cases of intrafamilial abuse especially, the mother requires additional consideration. Her emotional needs for a partner may restrict her ability to support her child, and if she too was a victim in her childhood, her ability to cope may be severely handicapped. Guilt feelings in either parent can paralyse their leadership of the family.

Siblings should not be overlooked; they may themselves be victims and can be angry at the abused child, especially if disclosure leads to the family's breakup. They are likely to be upset by the upheaval their home has witnessed.

Legal considerations

Successful prosecutions are unfortunately infrequent in cases of child sexual abuse. Children generally do not make good court witnesses, and most cases occur in private under a veil of secrecy. Independent eye witnesses are therefore rarely available to support the prosecution. Paediatricians and psychiatrists can give evidence on their certainty that abuse has occurred, but proving who was the perpetrator is a different matter. It may also be difficult for jurors to believe that a person who appears ordinary could commit such an abhorrent act.

A guilty verdict gives the judge a range of possible disposals. Custodial sentences may involve prison, or a secure hospital if the perpetrator satisfies the criteria for mental impairment or psychopathic disorder. A probation order can be made conditional on receiving treatment.

Work with offenders can follow a number of approaches, but common themes include: taking responsibility for offending; identifying patterns of offending behaviour; learning preventative measures; victim empathy; and recognising how personal experiences of abuse may be shaping abusing behaviour.

False memory syndrome

Disclosures made some time after the event raise the difficult issue of false memory syndrome. Here the passage of time and its effect on memory further complicate any attempt to discover the truth.

Much has been written about enthusiastic therapists who are able to uncover "memories" of abuse the individual was never previously aware of (Merskey, 1995), and the question remains whether these are truly "repressed" memories or merely "implanted" memories. Opinion varies regarding whether false memory syndrome is a product of unscrupulous therapists taking advantage of suggestible clients, or whether it is a shield used by guilty adults to escape conviction.

An adult psychiatrist faced with a disclosure of childhood abuse is advised by Mullen *et al* (1994) to consider other adversities the individual may have faced as a child. Childhood sexual abuse generally does not occur in isolation, and may possibly serve as a marker to indicate a traumatic childhood; hence a therapeutic approach that focuses solely on abuse is likely to be too narrow.

Summary

The concept of childhood events affecting adult life is not a new one. Over 150 years ago, Wordsworth famously wrote "The Child is Father of the Man". Hence it is widely held that childhood adversity can impair adult functioning. Does it then follow that previously abused children will attend general adult psychiatrists? Clear proof is lacking, but such a supposition is supported by a large body of research. Jehu (1991) investigated the sexual functioning of women who reported sexual abuse in childhood; 94% of the studied population described sexual problems. Other studies have yielded similar findings, and 'traumagenic dynamics' provides a mechanism by which a traumatic childhood can lead to distress in adulthood.

References

Butler-Sloss, E. (1988) *Report on the Inquiry into Child Abuse in Cleveland.* London: HMSO.

Crittenden, P. M. & Ainsworth, M. D. S. (1989) Child maltreatment and attachment theory. In *Child Maltreatment, Theory and Research on the Causes and Consequences of Child Abuse and Neglect* (eds D. Cicchetti & V. Carlson), pp. 432–463. New York: Cambridge University Press.

Doyle, G. (1994) Child sexual abuse "looking in the wrong direction?" *British Journal of Psychiatry*, 165, 406.

Finkelhor, D. & Browne, A. (1985) The traumatic impact of child sexual abuse: a conceptualisation. *American Journal of Orthopsychiatry*, 55, 530–541.

—— & Korbin, J. (1988) Child abuse as an international issue. *Child Abuse and Neglect*, 12, 2–24.

Garbarino J. (1989) Troubled youth, troubled families – the dynamics of adolescent maltreatment. In *Child Maltreatment, Theory and Research on the Causes and Consequences of Child Abuse and Neglect* (eds D. Cicchetti & V. Carlson), pp. 685–706. New York: Cambridge University Press.

Jehu, D. (1991) Clinical work with adults who were sexually abused in childhood. In *Clinical Approches to Sex Offenders and their Victims* (eds C. R. Hollin & K. Howells), p. 243. Chichester: John Wiley.

Meadow, R. (1993) Epidemiology. In *ABC of Child Abuse* (2nd edn) (ed. R. Meadow), p. 4. London: BMJ Publishing Group.

Merskey, H. (1995) Multiple personality disorder and false memory syndrome. *British Journal of Psychiatry*, 166, 281–283.

Mullen, P. E., Martin, J. L., Anderson, J. C., *et al* (1994) The effect of child sexual abuse on social, interpersonal and sexual function in adult life. *British Journal of Psychiatry*, 165, 35–47.

Rosenberg, M. S. (1987) New directions for research on the psychological maltreatment of children. *American Psychologist*, 42, 166–171.

Smith, M. & Bentovim, A. (1994) Sexual abuse. In *Child and Adolescent Psychiatry: Modern Approaches* (3rd edn) (eds M. Rutter, E. Taylor & L. Hersov), p. 235. Oxford: Blackwell Scientific.

Straus, M. A. & Gelles, R. J. (1986) Change in family violence from 1975–85. *Journal of Marriage and Family*, 48, 465–479.

Wolfe, V., Gentile, C. & Wolfe, D. A. (1989) The impact of sexual abuse on children – a PTSD formulation. *Behaviour Therapy*, 20, 215–228.

World Health Organization (1992) *The ICD–10 Classification of Mental and Behavioural Disorders*. Geneva: WHO.

Further reading

Meadow, R. (ed.) (1993) *ABC of Child Abuse* (2nd edn). London: BMJ Publishing Group.

Skuse, D. & Bentovim, A. (1994) Physical and emotional maltreatment. In *Child and Adolescent Psychiatry: Modern Approaches* (3rd edn) (eds M. Rutter, E. Taylor & L. Herson), pp. 209–229. Oxford: Blackwell Scientific.

7 Psychiatric aspects of HIV infection and disease

Massimo Riccio

---

*Non-organic psychiatric manifestations in people infected with HIV •
HIV and brain disease • Treatment of HIV-related psychiatric
disorder • Treatment of HIV brain disease • Conclusions*

The human immunodeficiency virus (HIV) is known to be associated
with progressive immunodeficiency, leading, in some people, to the
development of characteristic physical symptoms, opportunistic infections
and/or tumours. HIV is also known to infect directly the central nervous
system (CNS), thus leading to neurological, cognitive and behavioural
abnormalities in those affected. With its widespread impact on people's
lives it is hardly surprising that HIV infection is associated with a wide
range of psychosocial, psychiatric and neuropsychiatric morbidity.
Psychiatrists and mental health professionals will therefore be called upon
to deal not only with the emergence of such morbidity, but also to help
prevent further spread of HIV, in particular by developing interventions
aimed at reducing the prevalence of risk behaviours, particularly in
populations traditionally under their care, such as injecting (IV) drug
users. This chapter will deal both with the non-organic and the organic
psychiatric aspects of HIV infection. It will not specifically deal with the
psychiatric aspects of HIV infection in children nor with the complex area
of HIV infection in people with personality disorders or learning difficulties,
sexual offenders and survivors of sexual abuse.

Non-organic psychiatric manifestations in people infected with HIV

Despite the clear stresses associated with contracting HIV infection and
developing disease, the great majority of people affected do not require
specialist mental health intervention. Most appear to cope remarkably
well, especially if notification of the infection is handled with the
appropriate sensitivity and support is offered in the form of pre- and post-
test counselling (Green & McCreaner, 1989). Of those who do develop
psychological disturbance, the majority suffer from minor morbidity in
the form of adjustment reactions and disorders, with symptoms such as
free-floating anxiety and transitory depression of mood most commonly

noted. A minority will present with more severe psychiatric syndromes, such as major affective disorders and less commonly psychotic illnesses. Other problems such as the development of eating disorders or of sexual dysfunction have also been described in HIV sero-positive people. The latter appear to be related to the psychosocial impact of the infection, but also to physical and iatrogenic causes, especially in more advanced disease (Catalan *et al*, 1995).

Adjustment disorders in HIV sero-positive individuals

The diagnosis of HIV infection can lead to manifestations of despair, high levels of anxiety and guilt ruminations, sometimes associated with manifestations of protest, leading to uncharacteristic behaviours. Those affected may develop hypochondriacal preoccupations. All the symptoms are, however, characteristically short-lived (Miller & Riccio, 1990)

The same minor affective disturbances characteristic of adjustment disorders in people with HIV disease are associated with the onset of episodes of illness. Here, not surprisingly, individual coping styles play an important mediating role. In keeping with research in other physical diseases, such as cancer, psychological morbidity in people with HIV infection is associated with using more avoidant coping styles, with denial and hopelessness/helplessness being the coping mechanisms more often associated with psychological morbidity.

A large research effort has gone into attempting to determine whether HIV infection *per se* predisposes to greater psychiatric morbidity. The majority of controlled studies show that people with HIV infection are not very different in levels of distress and psychological morbidity from comparable HIV sero-negative controls. Most of the studies confirm that the levels of distress and psychological morbidity are generally low in people infected with HIV. These findings appear to hold across different groups of people infected with HIV, such as gay or bisexual men, IV drug-users, heterosexuals and women. Interestingly, injecting drug-users appear to have higher levels of psychiatric morbidity than other groups of individuals with HIV infection, regardless of their HIV sero-status (Catalan *et al*, 1995).

It is arguable that the negative findings of these studies may be due to methodological problems. Most studies take place on populations of well educated, compliant, white males. The whole issue of whether people participating in long-term prospective studies are representative of the general population needs also to be taken into consideration.

In any case, it is safe at present to state that the majority of people with HIV infection do not appear to be at greater risk of psychological distress and morbidity. Some, however, are, and factors associated with psychological morbidity in HIV infection and disease include the stage of the notification of the infection, the onset of physical symptoms, the start of early antiretroviral treatment, a previous psychiatric history, lack of social support, accommodation, financial or employment difficulties, different coping styles, belonging to a particular transmission group (e.g. IV drug-users), and having experienced repeated losses due to HIV (Catalan *et al*, 1995).

Depression

Some HIV sero-positive people will develop a more significant affective disturbance. Moderate and sometimes severe depressive episodes are observed in this population. Lack of social support, adjustment to diagnosis and the development of physical symptoms are powerful mediators. Although depression can present itself in people across the disease stages, as HIV disease progresses so does the prevalence and severity of depressive episodes. Patients typically present with markedly depressed mood and preoccupation with ideas of guilt, hopelessness and suicidal intent. The severity and persistence of these symptoms are more useful in reaching a diagnosis of severe depressive episodes, while the more characteristic and 'biological' symptoms of depression, such as loss of weight, loss of appetite, poor sleep, anergia and slowness, need to be taken more cautiously as they might be correlates of the underlying physical disorder (Miller & Riccio, 1990).

Not uncommonly, people with HIV infection may, at some point, experience suicidal ideas or even engage in suicidal behaviour. For most, suicidal ideation may be a passing and fleeting phase in the adjustment to the infection and/or the disease. For others they may be more persistent and lead to the suspicion of a severe psychiatric disorder, such as a major depressive episode. Many researchers have attempted to answer the question of whether suicide and suicidal behaviour are more common among HIV sero-positive people. Such studies are fraught with methodological difficulties, but most suggest an increase in suicide risk when compared with age and gender-matched controls. Interestingly, the increase in suicide risk appears to be less in Europe (suggested increase about 10 times) than in the US (suggested increase between 16 and 36 times) (Pugh *et al*, 1993).

Psychotic disorders

While there is ample evidence that major psychiatric disorders such as manic and schizophrenic episodes can occur in people with HIV infection across all stages of the disease, their meaning in relation to the infection with HIV is more uncertain. Very few HIV sero-positive people will develop a psychotic illness, but it is suggested that the prevalence of psychotic illnesses in these populations may be marginally higher than the general population. Once again, people with a previous history of psychotic illnesses are most at risk, but interestingly those without a previous history may have a poorer prognosis in terms of survival (Catalan *et al*, 1995). The presence of a psychotic illness in a HIV sero-positive person gives rise to a number of diagnostic questions which will need to be addressed. The presentation could be entirely unassociated with any aspect of the concomitant HIV disease. Manic and schizophrenia-like psychosis should be diagnosed in the absence of symptoms suggestive of an acute or chronic brain syndrome, such as clouding of consciousness or cognitive impairment. Even so, however, it is important and essential to widen the differential diagnosis and consider the possibility of an underlying organic cause. In the short-term the outcome appears to be favourable, but there are suggestions that the onset of a psychotic illness marks the beginning of cognitive decline in some patients, in addition to poorer survival. The question of causality often arises in cases of psychotic illnesses in HIV sero-positive people; can and does HIV infection of the brain cause psychotic illnesses? If the answer was unequivocal we would by now see a huge rise in psychotic illnesses among the population infected with HIV. This is not the case. While some degree of causality cannot at present be totally excluded, one must remember that psychotic illness and HIV may accidentally coincide in the same individual. Life-time prevalence rates of psychotic illnesses in the general population also apply to people with HIV infection and disease, thus justifying the emergence of new cases of psychotic illnesses in the HIV-infected population.

HIV and brain disease

HIV has been demonstrated to enter the CNS early on in the infection. Neuropathological studies have found the presence of abnormalities in the majority of cases of advanced HIV disease, even in the absence of significant neurological syndrome. Neurological and neuropsychiatric symptoms develop in more than 50% of cases of advanced HIV disease. These include acute and chronic disorders, central and peripheral nervous system involvement, and can be either primarily attributable to HIV infection or a secondary consequence of the immune-deficiency. In most cases, the CNS manifestations of HIV disease are secondary to the immune-deficiency and caused by opportunistic infections or tumours. The direct impact of HIV on the brain may lead to some individuals' cognitive decline which, in the worst cases, may result in a clinical dementia (Burgess & Riccio, 1992).

The term 'AIDS dementia complex (ADC)' was coined in the first detailed report linking *in vivo* cognitive impairment in people with AIDS to *post mortem* encephalopathic changes not ascribable to other pathogens (Navia *et al*, 1986*a,b*). The authors suggested that ADC was a syndrome characterised by a triad of cognitive, motor and behavioural symptoms with typical neuropathological findings. While the term ADC is still widely used, especially in people with advanced HIV disease, its use in descriptive terms is more controversial. Only a third of the patients described by the authors actually complained of forgetfulness, while dementia is an established diagnosis which requires demonstrable impairment of short and long-term memory. Since the description of ADC, the AIDS literature has become inundated with a variety of descriptive and assumptive terms referring to the cognitive impairment seen in people with AIDS. Unfortunately many of these have been poorly defined and sometimes contradictory and often used interchangeably (Catalan, 1991). This terminological confusion has not helped research methodology. In the early 1990s, the World Health Organization(WHO) operationally defined 'HIV 1 associated dementia' based on the ICD–10 definition of dementia. The WHO suggests that this term should be used to describe the dementia seen in people with AIDS (WHO, 1990).

Early reports suggested that about 30% of people with AIDS would develop dementia. This relatively high prevalence was probably due to the fact that the reports came from specialist neurological centres where samples were unrepresentative or arose from very liberal definitions of the term dementia. More recent and better designed studies suggest that the prevalence of dementia in people with AIDS is much lower. The WHO Consultation Meeting (1990) concluded that for unselected subjects, the point prevalence ranged from 8–16%. Our own clinical and research experience suggests a prevalence of around 5% (Chiesi *et al*, 1996). It has been suggested that the differing rates may also be due to the fact that in the western world the prevalence may have fallen since the introduction of effective anti-retroviral treatment. Zidovudine has been shown to have an impact on reducing the prevalence of dementia in HIV-infected individuals (Portegies *et al*,1989).

Many people with advanced HIV disease will show some significant neuropsychological impairment, short of dementia. The cognitive functions most commonly appearing to deteriorate in people with advanced HIV disease are psychomotor control, speed of information processes and executive functions, such as planning, problem-solving, sequencing and concept formation (Tross *et al*,1988). Memory and language impairment are also common but tend not to be as severe as in other dementias such as Alzheimer's disease. In other words, the pattern of cognitive decline appears to be more similar to the so-called sub-cortical dementias (Burgess & Riccio, 1992).

The existence of cognitive impairment in people with asymptomatic disease is, however, more controversial. Grant *et al* (1987) reported in an influential paper that 44% of asymptomatic HIV-positive gay men were cognitively impaired. Not surprisingly their paper caused enormous anxiety among HIV-infected individuals as it suggested that cognitive impairment may be independent of immune deficiency. Since that paper many studies have been published attempting to answer the question of whether HIV infected asymptomatic individuals are more likely to be cognitively impaired than matched sero-negative controls. On the whole, the larger and better designed studies have failed to find any impairment with the symptomatic HIV infection, although some have (Grant *et al*, 1987; Maj *et al*, 1994*b*). The evidence for significant cognitive impairment in asymptomatic HIV-1 infection among adults is weak or non-existent (Burgess & Riccio, 1992). Where differences are seen, although statistically significant, the absolute differences are small and of little, if any, significance and are unlikely to have any impact on activities of daily living (Riccio & Burgess, 1994). Furthermore, when evaluating cognitive performance it has been suggested that the effect of HIV is often secondary and overshadowed by the effect of other factors that may interfere with performance, such as low levels of education, psychiatric illness, other neurological disease, and drug and alcohol usage (Wilkins *et al*, 1990). Most studies suggest that, while the impact of HIV on the brain during the asymptomatic infection is minimal, there appears to be a disproportionate effect on those who are very young, very old or socially disadvantaged (Maj *et al*, 1994*a,b*).

Neuropathology

HIV enters the brain within the first few months of infection and once in the brain it infects monocytes, microglia and macrophages. Up to 90% of people who die of AIDS show some neuropathological abnormality regardless of the presence of *in vivo* neurological disorders. In addition to neuropathological abnormalities secondary to opportunistic infections and tumours, HIV can cause a distinct encephalitis and leuco-encephalopathy (Everall & Lantos, 1991). Apart from macroscopic evidence of cerebral atrophy, white matter pallor, multi-nucleated giant cells of macrophagic origin with perivascular infiltrates and diffuse astrocytosis are the hallmark of HIV-induced brain disease. Although there is so far no evidence that HIV directly infects neurones, it is well established that HIV infection does cause substantial neuronal loss. Interestingly, none of the above-described neuropathological changes bears correlation with the severity of the clinical picture of cognitive or neurological abnormalities.

Neuroradiology

Both CT and MRI scans of the brain are useful in detecting abnormalities in people with HIV brain disease. The most common ones are cerebral atrophy with widening of the cortical sulci and enlarged ventricles. The MRI will show defused white matter pallor with high intensity signal which is, however, of unproved significance. The aspecificity of the above changes, however, is further highlighted once again by the lack of correlation with the severity of the clinical picture. It would appear that the most important use of MRI and CT scanning in people with HIV disease perhaps lies in the differential diagnosis of opportunistic infections and tumours of the CNS (Catalan *et al,* 1995).

PET and SPECT scanning also show promise in further defining the quantity and quality of abnormalities of brain function in people with HIV disease. Presently, however, they remain instruments of research rather than of direct clinical use.

Electrophysiology

Routine electroencephalography (EEG) has been shown to be abnormal especially in people with advanced HIV disease. The most common finding is pronounced generalised slowing of theta and delta rhythms. Overall, while EEG abnormalities in the advanced stage of the disease have frequently been reported, abnormalities during the asymptomatic infection are not well established and when found appear to be associated with neuropsychological impairment (Baldeweg & Lovett, 1991).

Treatment of HIV-related psychiatric disorder

In view of the range of psychiatric diagnoses, it is hardly surprising that psychological interventions are the most useful therapeutic tools for the majority of people with HIV infection. Most HIV sero-positive people referred to specialist mental health services will require appropriate psychotherapeutic help, either problem or symptom-specific. As such, HIV sero-positive and sero-negative people should be treated in exactly the same way. Care needs to be taken with the particular challenges of possible gradual or sudden changes in personal autonomy, work, social life or income. Therapists will need to be aware of the developments in the rapidly changing field of HIV infection and AIDS and be able to take a reassuring, educational as well as supportive role. Psychological interventions may need to be aimed at individuals, couples and families. Particular problems, which go beyond the scope of this chapter, are presented by those people in palliative or terminal care and those affected by multiple losses due to HIV.

For the minority of HIV sero-positive people with more serious psychiatric disturbance, psychopharmacological interventions may, however, be appropriate. Once again HIV-infected individuals should not be treated differently from sero-negative people presenting with similar problems. Therapeutic nihilism should be avoided. HIV-infected individuals have been successfully treated with the whole range of psychopharmacological and other physical methods of treatment such as electroconvulsive therapy (ECT). Of particular importance is the need to consider the possibility of interactions with other drugs the individual may be taking. Furthermore, clinical experience suggests that individuals with HIV infection are particularly prone to side-effects of all medication. Particular care should therefore be taken to select compounds with a lower side-effect profile, in order to minimise discomfort and maximise compliance. Adequate dosage should be prescribed, but possibly gradually reached in view of the need to minimise side-effects. Antidepressants are to be used where the clinical indications require them. The appropriate therapeutic dosage is to be reached, considering newer antidepressants such as SSRIs as first-line treatments, in view of their lower, especially anticholinergic, side-effect profile.

In psychotic illnesses neuroleptic drugs are to be used, once again with great care taken to avoid unnecessary side-effects. The need to limit the use of anxiolytics and hypnotics in order to avoid dependence remains unchallenged, but it is also important not to deny patients with a potentially fatal condition and high levels of distress the undisputed advantage that these drugs offer in the short term. Lithium augmentation and maintenance for cases of resistant depression or bipolar affective disorder, anti-convulsants such as carbamazepine or sodium valproate, as well as ECT have all been tried and tested successfully in people with HIV infection. Less orthodox treatments such as psychostimulants have also been advocated as helpful in some cases (Catalan *et al*, 1995).

Treatment of HIV brain disease

Zidovudine either as the sole agent or in combination with other anti-retrovirals remains the only well established treatment of HIV-associated dementia. The evidence for this comes mainly from clinical and circumstantial evidence. Double-blind placebo-controlled trials are few and mostly with short follow-up times. They do show, however, a clear advantage for those subjects taking zidovudine compared with controls in improving their cognitive performance. The question of whether zidovudine or other antiretrovirals may prevent development of cognitive impairment as the disease progresses, if given in the asymptomatic stage of the infection, remains unresolved. On balance, the evidence suggests that zidovudine has a beneficial effect on cognitive functioning in advanced HIV disease, although this appears to be quite short-lived and probably not lasting longer than six months (Catalan *et al*, 1995).

Conclusions

Psychiatrists and mental health professionals have a great role to play in the management of HIV-infected individuals. In order to be effective we must be aware of the range of presentations, refine our differential diagnostic skills, and attempt to distinguish the organic from the non-organic presentation. We must avoid being taken by therapeutic nihilism and prescribe, where appropriate, medication at therapeutic dosages, remaining aware of the potential for increased sensitivity to side-effects. Psychiatrists are well placed to ensure that HIV-infected individuals presenting with psychiatric or behavioural disturbances are appropriately nursed either on a medical or a psychiatric ward according to the prominence of the physical or psychiatric symptomatology. Advice on the correct use of the Mental Health Act, where appropriate, is also naturally our role. Most importantly, psychiatrists ought to ensure that HIV-infected individuals receive the highest standard of mental health care regardless of HIV sero-status.

References

Baldeweg, T. & Lovett, E. (1991) Psychophysiology and neurophysiology of HIV infection. *International Review of Psychiatry*, 3, 331–342.

Burgess, A. & Riccio, M. (1992) Cognitive impairment and dementia in HIV-1 infection. In *Neurological Aspects of Human Retroviruses* (ed. P. Rudge), pp. 155–174. London: Bailliere Tindall.

Catalan, J. (1991) Neuropsychiatric disorders and HIV-1 associated dementia: conceptual and terminological problems. *International Review of Psychiatry*, 3, 331–342.

——, Burgess, A. & Klimes, I. (1995) *Psychological Medicine of HIV Infection*. Oxford: Oxford University Press.

Chiesi, A., Vella, S., Dally, L. G., *et al* (1996) Epidemiology of AIDS dementia complex in Europe. AIDS in Europe Study Group. *Journal of Acquired Immonodeficiency Syndromes and Human Retrovirology*, 11, 39–44.

Everall, I. & Lantos, P. (1991) The neuropathology of HIV infection: a review of the first 10 years. *International Review of Psychiatry*, 3, 307–320.

Grant, I., Atkinson, J. H., Hesselenick, J. R., *et al* (1987) Evidence for early CNS involvement in AIDS and other HIV infections. *Annals of Internal Medicine*, 107, 828–836.

Green, J. & McCreaner, A. (1989) *Counselling in HIV Infection and AIDS*. Oxford: Blackwell.

Maj, M., Janssen, R., Starace, F., *et al* (1994a) WHO Neuropsychiatric AIDS Study – Cross Sectional Phase I. *Archives of General Psychiatry*, 51, 39–49.

——, Satz, P., Janssen, R., *et al* (1994b) WHO Neuropsychiatric AIDS Study – Cross Sectional Phase II. Neuropsychological and neurological findings. *Archives of General Psychiatry*, 51, 51–61.

Miller, D. & Riccio, M. (1990) Psychiatric syndromes associated with HIV infection and disease without evidence of cognitive impairment. *AIDS*, 4, 381–388.

Navia, B. A., Jordan, B. D. & Price, R. W. (1986a) The AIDS dementia complex: I. Clinical features. *Annals of Neurology*, 19, 517–524.

——, Cho, E.–S., Petito, C. K., *et al* (1986b) The AIDS dementia complex: II. Neuropathology. *Annals of Neurology*, 19, 525–535.

Portegies, P., de Gans, J., Lange, J., *et al* (1989) Declining incidence of ADC after introduction of AZT. *British Medical Journal*, 299, 819–821.

Pugh, K., O'Donnell, I. & Catalan, J. (1993) Suicide in HIV disease. *AIDS Care*, 4, 391–399.

Riccio, M. & Burgess, A. (1994) AIDS and dementia: ten years on (editorial). *British Journal of Hospital Medicine*, 51,144–147.

Tross, S., Price, R. W., Navia, B., *et al* (1988) Neuropsychological characterization of the AIDS dementia complex: a preliminary report. *AIDS*, 2, 1–88.

Wilkins, J. W., Robertson, K. R., van der Horst, C., *et al* (1990) The importance of confounding factors in the evaluation of neuropsychological changes in patients infected with human immunodeficiency virus. *Journal of Acquired Immune Deficiency Syndromes*, 3, 938–942.

World Health Organization (1990) *Report on the Second Consultation on the Neuropsychiatric Aspects of HIV–1 Infection* (11–13 January 1990). Geneva: WHO.

8 Problems of sexuality among people in mental health facilities

D. J. West

The need for a sex policy • Policy points to be considered • Powers to discipline patients • Control of offending • Problems of learning disability • Prisons and special hospitals • Conclusion

---

The sexuality of mentally disordered patients in hospital or residential care used not to be of such concern as it is today. When institutions were run on authoritarian lines, with the sexes strictly segregated, wards locked, movements restricted and surveillance pervasive, the idea of patients having rights to sexual expression scarcely arose. Indeed, sexual behaviour among them was viewed as inappropriate, or a symptom of their disorder, something to be suppressed by disciplinary action. Contacts between men and women were kept to a minimum; even the staff were segregated, male nurses looking after male wards.

When male homosexual behaviour was in all circumstances a serious criminal offence, sex contacts between male patients could never be officially countenanced, although it might be privately viewed as less disruptive than contacts involving risk of pregnancy. Young women from deprived backgrounds with limited intelligence or social skills, if they were inconveniently inclined to promiscuity, were at risk of indefinite detention in mental institutions as moral defectives, defined under the Mental Deficiency Act 1927 as defectives "with strongly vicious or criminal propensities and who require care, supervision and control for the protection of others". It was not until the Mental Health Act 1959 that the statutory criteria for compulsory hospitalisation explicitly excluded detention "by reason only of promiscuity or other immoral conduct". That same Act ensured that the majority of mental hospital patients became informal and, at least in theory, had the same rights and freedoms as normal citizens or ordinary medical patients (Jones, 1993).

As late as 1950, the traditional mental hospital was a rambling structure housing thousands of inmates, characterised by locked wards, jangling keys, bare dormitories, miles of empty corridors, a dreary institutional timetable and innumerable rules discouraging individual enterprise. A 'them and us' tradition kept a yawning social chasm between staff and patients. Patients generally lacked money for personal luxuries and were often to be seen scavenging in bins for cigarette butts. Laundry and cleaning were largely done by patient labour. Those too ill for regimented activity or domestic chores remained idle, sometimes left for hours in statuesque poses of catatonia. The worst aspects of these 'total institutions' became notorious through the writings of authors such as Goffman (1961) and Scull (1989), whose experience came from American state hospitals where conditions were even worse than in the UK. In hospitals for the mentally impaired, issues of sexual freedom were even less likely to appear on any agenda. Sex with or between impaired patients was regarded with horror. Most of the inmates had been brought up from childhood to think of any overt manifestation of sex, including self-masturbation, as punishable behaviour.

The need for a sex policy

Attitudes have changed radically. In an age of equal opportunities and respect for the individual's rights and freedom, the guiding principles in dealing with the mentally disordered are to restrict liberty only when truly necessary and to encourage normal activities as far as possible by providing opportunities for pursuing them. This liberal approach can present carers with dilemmas when a patient's behaviour appears unwise but they lack sufficient means or authority to control it. A patient compulsorily detained under the Mental Health Act 1983 can be prevented from leaving and obliged to take medication, but powers to regulate behaviour in other respects are limited (Creighton, 1995). Ignoring sexuality is no longer appropriate. Agreed policies are needed as never before.

Mental disorder may impair judgement and this, combined with unfamiliar circumstances, limited privacy and closeness to strangers, increases vulnerability to sexual molestation, harassment or exploitation. Some patients, by reason of their disorder, become sexually disinhibited or sexually aggressive, causing other patients embarrassment, annoyance or fright. This occurs notably in conditions of hypomania, but also in cases of brain damage, personality disorder, mental impairment and, of course, in paraphilias. Illness does not necessarily eliminate pre-existing predatory sexual habits and may sometimes exacerbate them.

Many situations arise that require a regulatory policy. Patients, and sometimes staff, may be found behaving in ways that contravene the criminal law on sexual behaviour. The institution may well be blamed for lack of care if a patient is sexually assaulted. Concerned relatives or spouses may also feel aggrieved and blame staff for a patient's voluntary but disapproved participation in sexual activity, or exposure to sexual advances by other patients, arguing that such things would not have happened had the patient remained well and at home. The voluntary organisation MIND, which campaigns on behalf of patients, has drawn attention to complaints by women of inadequate protection from sexual abuse or harassment on mixed hospital wards.

When mentally disordered patients become pregnant further problems arise. The woman may be insufficiently stable to cope with the situation, the man unable to fulfil the social or financial obligations of parenthood, and the baby may be at significant risk of genetic vunerability to schizophrenia or other serious disorders. The prospects of the parents themselves providing a sound home and upbringing for the child may be remote. Medico-legal issues and differing moral views concerning abortion are additional complications. An institution may be held lacking in duty of care for not preventing an obviously undesirable and costly outcome.

Institutional policy should set out ground rules for patients and staff, stating what action will be taken in the event of infractions. It should not be just a list of prohibitions and sanctions. Sexual outlets that are allowable should be specified. The policy should also be sufficiently flexible to allow for the differing requirements of individual patients and for positive advice and counselling as appropriate, particularly with regard to measures of contraception and protection from infection. The development of independent mental health trusts bound by contracts and the utilisation of voluntary agencies, also working to a contract, have increased the opportunity for legal action by or on behalf of patients, and caused some local authorities and hospitals to realise the advisability of establishing formal policies which can be cited when their way of dealing with situations is criticised. Not all NHS trusts have taken adequate action, but without clear policy guidance, ad hoc decisions in particular instances can be arbitrary, ill-considered, unfair, insensitive to ethnic issues and more readily open to challenge.

Breaking the law

In considering policy, managers of institutions must not be so liberal that they permit behaviour on their premises that contravenes criminal law. Any bodily contact with sexual intent involving a person of either sex who is not consenting to it constitutes an indecent assult and carries a maximum penalty of ten years' imprisonment. Males or females, adults or juveniles, patients or staff are all liable to be found guilty if they attempt even the mildest sexual touching or groping of a non-consenting individual. Should such behaviour be directed towards someone aged 15 or less it counts as indecent assault, even if the boy or girl is a willing participant, for persons under 16 are legally incompetent to give consent to sexual contact.

Sexual intercourse without the consent of the female concerned is rape, rendering the guilty male liable to a maximum penalty of life imprisonment. If the man is a hospital patient this does not itself affect his liability. If the female is under 16, but consenting, the male's behaviour is not rape, but it is still unlawful and an imprisonable offence, although the maximum penalty is only two years' imprisonment if the girl is aged 13 or older.

Adult female patients with mental disorders, even if consenting, are protected from sexual intercourse with hospital staff, since it is an offence for a male member of staff of a hospital or mental nursing home to have intercourse with a woman (not his wife) who is under treatment there, or to have intercourse on the premises with an out-patient (Section 128, Mental Health Act 1959). In addition, it is an imprisonable offence for a man to have sexual intercourse with a woman who is severely mentally impaired.

Sexual contact between consenting males is regarded by many people as offensive. If either participant is under 18, if the acts take place in situations accessible to the public or if a third party is present, the behaviour amounts to the imprisonable crime of gross indecency. If the behaviour includes anal intercourse (buggery), the possible penalties are greater. Anal intercourse with a woman is in all circumstances a criminal offence. The law is unconcerned with lesbian behaviour, unless it involves children, when it comes under the category of indecent assault.

Prostitution, that is promiscuous trading of sex for money or material favours by males or females, is not in itself a crime, but the owners or leaseholders of premises in which it occurs are liable to prosecution, as are persons who facilitate contacts (procuring) or who benefit in a material way from the prostitution of others (immoral earnings). It would seem that managers of institutions have some vicarious responsibility for their clients' behaviour.

Since, under the Indecent Displays (Control) Act 1981, it is an offence to display, or permit to be displayed, any indecent matter in a place to which the public have access, pornography left around on an open ward could be in breach of the law. It is also an offence to take, show, distribute or possess indecent material featuring children (Protection of Children Act 1978; Criminal Justice Act 1988, Section 160).

Policy points to be considered

The suggestions which follow are the result of personal observation and scrutiny of some extant policies, or policies in preparation, drawn from some of the trusts or authorities who have them.

Some house rules are necessary in any institution. They do not have to be the same for every unit. The gender and gender distribution of the clients, their mental condition, their length of stay, their legal status, the degree of security required, the type of treatments on offer and the physical characteristics of the accommodation all impinge upon the amount of freedom it is reasonable to aim for. Although it may be viewed as unfair, the nature of their illness or their particular vulnerability call for special restrictions for certain individuals. Staff need to be both familiar with and accepting of whatever policies are to be implemented. This entails specifying opportunities for discussion and training and, where feasible, consultation with patient groups and patient advocates. Information about sexual relationship counselling can be obtained from such agencies as RELATE.

Behaviours that are a nuisance or offensive to others have to be stopped even if they are not actually criminal. These might include inappropriate fondling and intimate contact in view of other patients, use of crude sexual language, verbal importuning and other forms of sexual harassment, wandering into others' rooms or dormitories, failure to respect others' privacy in the toilets, unseemly intimacy or masturbation in the presence of others, and public displays of or sharing of pornographic materials. Homosexual propositioning or innuendoes can be very provocative and, among males especially, may cause retaliatory violence. Guidance and education to reduce these unacceptable behaviours is an important part of therapy. It has to be kept in mind that the residents of a ward or hostel are likely to include a mixture of generations, subcultures and ethnicity, including some who may be peculiarly sensitive to impropriety. For example, a young Moslem woman accustomed to very modest dress and habitual segregation from the opposite sex may find living on a mixed ward particularly stressful.

Some units may find it necessary, while encouraging heterosexual friendships and socialising, to impose an absolute ban on sexual intercourse on the premises, ostensibly because there are no suitable private places or because the provision of facilities would be incompatible with the unit's surveillance and security rules. For example, the policy guidelines issued by one NHS trust point out that "There are situations where the expression of one's sexuality is both normal and desirable", it urges a caring and understanding approach and suggests that masturbation is an acceptable behaviour if carried out discreetly and in private, but declares that "sexual intercourse is not acceptable within the psychiatric unit". Such a blanket ban, when imposed in long-stay institutions housing patients who cannot be given home leave, may be thought unduly harsh. It risks provoking covert acts under uncivilised conditions. In an atmosphere of sexual frustration the more vulnerable are open to coercion. Total prohibition of sexual intercourse over long periods is incompatible with the aim of encouraging normal activities as far as the limitations of illness permit.

Patients' relationships while on leave from hospital may be thought to be their own affair, but even that generalisation, like almost any rule concerning the contentious business of sex, is open to dispute. At one hospital, the behaviour of a woman patient given regular home leaves, who used these opportunities to have regular sexual relations with a new acquaintance, caused sharp differences of opinion among nursing staff, some feeling she had a right to pursue her customary lifestyle, others wanting to curtail her liberty. The dispute might have been avoided had there been a policy in operation specifying that action to curtail a consensual relationship outside the hospital should be taken only if the clinical team agrees that it is demonstrably damaging to the patient's mental health.

A balance has to be struck between the rights of patients to self-determination in their sexual lives and the need to protect those individuals whose disorder renders them vulnerable. Relationships that are clearly not based on informed consent or are the result of undue pressure must be stopped. Patients who are volitional and choose to engage in sexual contacts with other patients may have to be discouraged if it is evident that the behaviour is having a detrimental effect on the well-being or social circumstances of either party. Behaviour may be consensual in a literal sense, but only because the individual's views of the situation and its consequences are clouded by illness. A patient may fail to appreciate the serious implications or even the sexual nature of approaches made to them, or their judgement may be so impaired they see nothing inappropriate in exchanging sexual favours for cigarettes or other small bribes. In such cases it is incumbent upon staff to recognise the situation and shield the patient from predators.

The decision to discourage or forbid a relationship should be taken after multidisciplinary discussion among the clinical staff. A useful yardstick is whether the relationship, or the activity in question, is such as might reasonably have occurred had the patient been well and living in the community. Advice and persuasion or the threat of discharge are the only means of securing the compliance of informal patients, but these can be very powerful in the context of a multidisciplinary therapeutic environment, especially if support from relatives is forthcoming. Policy guidelines should specify who is responsible for making decisions to permit or restrict the behaviour of individuals. Where the character of a unit makes it feasible, patients whose behaviour is acceptable, or at least tolerable and not illegal, should be supported by staff to the extent of providing opportunities for privacy, for example by allowing the couple access at reasonable times to one of their bedrooms. The use of rooms for group sex is another matter, but restrictions intended to force conformity with the moral views of particular members of staff are unjustified. For instance, discrimination between otherwise acceptable relationships because they are homosexual, or prohibitions based on age differentials between adults or on marital status, should not be part of official policy.

Where sexual contacts are permitted it is essential that sexual counselling should also be available, particularly in relation to contraception and sexually transmitted diseases. It should also be made explicit who is responsible for providing condoms, hormonal contraceptives and mechanical barrier methods for females. Agreed policies may help, but some disputes are inevitable where discretionary decisions cannot be avoided, as the following example shows.

A young schizophrenic woman in-patient met up with a male patient she had known previously in another hospital. She telephoned him frequently and encouraged him to visit her on the ward. He entered unobserved by staff and the couple began a sexual encounter in her room. They were discovered and interrupted by staff, much to the woman's annoyance. Her parents complained that she had been insufficiently restricted in view of her vulnerable state and that the police should have been called to the incident. Her consultant pointed out that since the activity was consensual the police would not be concerned and that the patient needed to be allowed some freedom to act as an adult, albeit with guidance and supervision, which was why the staff had seen fit to intervene. The relatives remained unconvinced and pursued a formal complaint against the hospital.

Modern wards normally accommodate both sexes. The recent Department of Health directive that patients should have a choice may alter this. The problems of maintaining bodily privacy apply less in psychiatric hospitals than in medical and surgical wards, although MIND has been hearing increasingly of women concerned about being in mixed mental hospital wards.

In formulating rules about observation and protection of vulnerable patients the layout of a ward needs to be considered. Sleeping areas are generally kept apart, but the proportions of men and women may change unpredictably and adjacent rooms may house persons of opposite sex.

Ideally, single rooms should be lockable from the inside but accessible by means of master keys held by staff, yet this simple arrangement is often lacking. Large dormitories are undesirable and all dormitories should have beds well spaced and curtained off if not separated by cubicle partitioning. Until recently some special hospital male patients with criminal propensities were locked in crowded dormitories overnight. Such arrangements are unacceptable. Whether bedrooms and dormitories remain open to patients throughout the day or are available only at set times has to depend on the level of patient disturbance, the availability of staff and the facilities for observation. The traditional 'race track' layout of many wards, with rooms leading off a winding corridor that parallels the perimeter of the building, makes observation especially difficult. Where day and night facilities are on separate floors, rules about visits to bedrooms may need to be stricter, but there is always a tension between the provision of near-normal freedoms and civilised privacy and the need to guard against abuse and risk of self-harm. The common practice of having all bathroom and lavatory facilities open to both sexes is coming into question as many female patients express dissatisfaction. Unisex arrangements acceptable elsewhere may not be appropriate where the patient mix can include some with histories of sexual assault.

Powers to discipline patients

Policies need to be realistic in terms of what powers of regulation are available. Patients admitted informally comprise the majority in most hospitals. Rules introduced in the interests of safety and preservation of reasonable standards of propriety cannot be imposed by force on informal patients. Patients who have agreed to behaviour modification regimes, with token rewards and disincentives (such as a period of 'time out' on their own following inappropriate conduct), can be trained in this way in sexual as in other matters. If patients refuse to accept necessary regulation, or if they persist in causing disruption and annoyance, they have to be discharged. Even if their behaviour is the result of illness they cannot be physically restrained or prevented from leaving, except under common law to forestall immediate harm to self or others. However, if discharge would endanger a patient's own health and safety or the safety of others, he or she can be detained, forcibly if necessary, using powers conferred by the Mental Health Act 1983. Section 5 allows a registered mental nurse to detain for up to 6 hours pending a doctor's arrival, and a doctor to detain for up to 72 hours pending an order for compulsory detention for assessment or treatment under Sections 2 or 3. This requires recommendations from an approved social worker and two doctors.

Patients detained compulsorily under the provisions of the Mental Health Act 1983, whether by civil procedures, via the criminal courts or by transfer from prison, can be controlled by staff acting in a reasonable manner in pursuit of the requirement to detain and treat, using force if necessary. The Department of Health periodically issues a *Code of Practice* as a guide to the management and treatment of detained patients, but it is silent on the topic of the control of sexual conduct.

What it is reasonable to do to control detained patients is open to dispute. There could be little objection to restricting the movement of a patient, under the influence of delusions or mania, who was making dangerously provocative sexual advances to all and sundry. On the other hand, complaints can be caused if attempts are made to prevent relationships that would not be restricted were the individual not a patient. In the exercise of their discretion, staff enjoy some protection from frivolous complaints. Staff cannot be proceeded against for alleged assaults on detained patients without leave from the High Court (Mental Health Act 1959; Section 139). In a leading case on the issue, Poutney *v.* Griffiths ([1975] 2 All ER, 881), an appeal was upheld from a Broadmoor nurse who was accused of unwarranted force in removing a patient from his visitors. In practice, where a complaint that staff behaviour was excessive or unnecessary appears to have any merit, leave to sue is likely to be granted and nurses dealing with informal patients enjoy no special protection for legal action for assault (Hoggett, 1990, p. 366).

When action to control inappropriate behaviour, sexual or otherwise, of a detained patient becomes necessary, it is often cloaked in the language of treatment, although to the recipient it will certainly be interpreted as punishment. If the action taken is perceived as excessive or unwarranted it may incite the patient to violence and rebound on the staff involved. A sad example of this kind, leading to official criticism of staff, was that of Sean Walton, a young patient in Ashworth Special Hospital. His case is detailed in the report of an official inquiry into complaints against the Hospital (Blom-Cooper, 1992).

> The incident began when a nurse investigated noises coming from the toilets. Finding Sean there with another male patient, he concluded that Sean had been making improper sexual advances. "To cool his ardour", as a partially obliterated comment in the nursing notes put it, Sean was given a mop and bucket and made to clean the toilet floor, supervised by a nursing assistant. Although he did not admit it, this assistant was said to have aggravated Sean by kicking over the bucket so that the mopping-up task had to be repeated. However that may be, there was a confrontation and Sean was shut into a seclusion room where, although he calmed down, he was kept overnight and into the next day. This may have been because, as another note recorded, he showed "no remorse for his actions". By lunchtime he was dead, having been found suddenly collapsed in the seclusion room, presumably from the toxic effects of his recently increased dosage of psychotropic medication, possibly aggravated by the stress of forced confinement.

The Ashworth Inquiry had little difficulty in concluding that the treatment Sean received was punishment rather than therapy. The distinction is not always so easy to draw, especially on wards where seclusion (being placed alone in a locked room), or 'time out' (being segregated from other patients), are frequently used techniques. The Mental Health Act Code of Practice (Department of Health, 1993) is clear that physical restraint and placement in seclusion should be used as last resorts in emergencies and for as short duration as possible, and never as punishment. The use of seclusion rooms has been discontinued in many hospitals in favour of intensive nursing, close observation and the deployment of safe methods of restraint, learned and practised in regular training courses.

Well-trained mental hospital staff should normally be able to bring under control incidents where detained patients have become assaultative, without needing to call in the police. The arrival of an intimidating posse of uniformed police, particularly if they appear in riot gear, risks a catastrophic escalation of patient aggression. Sexual incidents are rarely so uncontrollably violent, but whenever a significant sexual incident takes place and someone is injured or seriously offended, police should be notified of what has happened and invited to investigate.

Control of offending

Sexual contact of any kind between any member of staff and a patient should be explicitly prohibited and defined as a serious disciplinary offence. This necessarily goes beyond what is forbidden by criminal law, which penalises intercourse with a patient only if the perpetrator is male and the patient female and is silent on the issue of consensual acts other than intercourse. Nursing staff have to remain in close proximity to patients and sometimes need to help them with personal hygiene. Male staff should not be required, on their own, to supervise female dormitories overnight or be involved in procedures requiring intimate physical contact with female patients. Proper arrangements help reduce the scope for both real and unfounded complaints. Since complaints of sexual misconduct against a nurse will generally involve temporary suspension or transfer while the matter is investigated, a spate of accusations can be very disruptive as well as extremely stressful for the staff concerned.

Complaints from patients of sexual impropriety by fellow patients or by staff are quite common. Often allegations are unjustified, arising from morbid fantasies, suspicions or misinterpretations that are part of an illness. Nevertheless, it is unsafe to ignore or fail to record complaints. A degree of sexual paranoia does not preclude a real incident having occurred.

All institutions need a written policy with procedures clearly laid down for recording and swiftly investigating complaints by patients, whether made verbally or in writing. A distressed victim has a right to have the incident properly established since this can determine eligibility for criminal injuries compensation. The seriousness of the situation may not be immediately obvious. Even in the absence of any significant physical damage, sex assaults can produce lasting psychological trauma and compensation orders take this into account.

The following is a typical example of an incident that could have been taken more seriously and investigated more thoroughly, had its full implications been appreciated at the time.

> The complaining female patient was sleeping in a two-bedded room with another woman. During the night a disturbed male patient was brought in by police. Two nurses were on the ward, but while one was taking details from the social worker and the other was ushering out the police the new patient, left momentarily in the company of his relatives, unexpectedly broke away, entered the unlocked bedroom and groped the complainant in an indecent manner. A nurse came swiftly to the scene and he was led away. A doctor was called, but the victim was not complaining of any physical hurt and appeared to have regained her composure. It emerged subsequently, however, that the incident had reactivated trauma from a previous assault, as a result of which the patient, after she had been discharged, felt she had a case for demanding compensation from the hospital on the grounds of failure to protect her from a damaging and avoidable experience.

There should be a procedure set out for action to be taken by staff when a sexual offence is known or suspected to have occurred, regardless of whether a complaint has been made. Suspicions of sexual victimisation may be aroused by odd remarks from a patient, sudden antipathy towards someone on the ward, unusual sexual behaviour or ano-genital soreness. The appropriate manager needs to be informed and decisions taken about further observation in cases of doubt or, where there appears to have been a definite assault, immediate investigation, recording and reporting to police.

Where one patient is alleged to have sexually assaulted another, the demeanour of both and any comments they make should be carefully recorded and one of them should be moved out of the ward. Staff who were in the vicinity or witnessed the incident should record promptly any information they have. Where an incident may have left physical traces, the area should be cordoned off for subsequent forensic examination, the victim's clothing and bedding set aside and the victim asked not to wash or drink. Spermatozoa can be detected in swabs from the vagina for up to six days afterwards, from the anus for up to three days and from the mouth for up to twelve hours.

The decision to report to the police a suspected offence by a mental patient presents managers with difficult issues. The supposed victim may not wish it. Minor indecencies towards nurses can be, perhaps wrongly, tolerated as all part of the generally disturbed behaviour of the mentally disordered, and the nurse concerned may have no wish to press charges. Relatives of a patient who has behaved badly, already aggrieved and feeling that inadequate care or observation was the cause, may be further annoyed at police involvement or threatened prosecution. Relatives of victimised patients are likely to complain of inadequate protection from molestation. Rights to compensation for criminal injury, which includes psychological trauma, may be lost if there has been no police investigation. The reporting of trivial matters, however, even though technically offences, would endanger relationships with the police and produce no material result.

In practice, police do not always treat complaints of misconduct by patients with mental disorders in the same way as they might handle similar complaints by others. Allegations of sexual assault, in the absence of witnesses or physical damage, are peculiarly difficult to substantiate at the best of times. When the complainant is a confused mental patient it becomes still more difficult. If the only witnesses are other mentally disturbed patients, their statements will be treated with reserve. Police are aware also that patients may not have been fully responsible for their offending actions. If they are already in hospital, especially if compulsorily detained under a section of the Mental Health Act, prosecution can seem pointless. If the victim does not want to press charges the police may consider any action unnecessary. Even if the police bring a charge there is no guarantee that the Crown Prosecution Service will consider a prosecution in the public interest.

Notwithstanding the difficulties, wherever there has been a serious assault there is no question but that police should be informed. Any serious incident that reveals a patient's hitherto unsuspected dangerous propensities should be on record for future reference.

Problems of learning disability

The difficult issues surrounding the sexuality of the mentally ill apply with even greater force to the care of persons with learning disabilities, many of whom used to spend the best part of their lives in hospital. Now they are more often looked after in sheltered accommodation under the supervision of local authority carers or the employees of voluntary agencies. Unlike patients with episodic mental illness, their limitations are present throughout their developing years, through puberty and beyond, impeding age-appropriate sexual learning, but not necessarily lessening sexual impulses or the desire for sexual relationships.

Although some are physically malformed, many seriously handicapped individuals may be physically well developed, sexually attractive and sexually responsive. This, combined with lack of social skills and social experience and a learned habit of obedience to instructions, renders them vulnerable to predators. The risks to which children and young persons with disabilities are exposed in residential homes and hospitals has been repeatedly documented. Sobsey & Doe (1991), in an analysis of reported sexual assaults on persons with disabilities, note that they are liable to repeated and persistent abuse, often perpetrated by service providers, but rarely reported to authorities. Problems in communication and fear of not being believed or being punished discourage reporting, especially when the predator is an ostensibly caring relative or a staff member. Even hospital porters and physiotherapists have been implicated in sexual abuse (Westcott, 1993). In comparison with the small minority still occupying the dwindling supply of hospital beds, the activities of the majority who live in group homes or other community placements are subject to limited surveillance. They are therefore exposed to greater risk of molestation from fellow residents and from casual contacts in the community as well as from persons charged with their care.

Given a normal community environment, the mildly impaired mature physically at puberty and manifest much the same behaviour, desires and sexual expectations as their normal age peers. Much of the deviant behaviour seen in repressive institutions, such as obsessive masturbation and homosexual activity, is promoted by the artificial conditions. It is now acknowledged that given training, social support and adequate housing and finance, a much larger proportion of the moderately handicapped than was previously believed can live substantially independent lives in the community. The modern aim is to train as many as possible to do so. The concept of 'normalisation' implies giving the handicapped the respect due to any adult, the right to choose their way of life and encouragement for maximum integration into normal living, normal groups and normal activities. This necessarily includes preparation for coping with relations with the opposite sex. It is noteworthy, however, that a standard text on the subject, while acknowledging that normalisation includes the development of heterosexual relationships and the right to marry, has little to say about how this is to be achieved (Brown & Smith, 1992).

Policy guidelines should emphasise a sympathetic, non-judgemental and helping attitude on the part of staff. In practice this might include positive support for the maintenance or termination of current sexual relationships, a private, lockable bedroom with the right to an overnight visitor. There should also be support for persons wanting to cohabit, marry or become parents, without conditions being insisted upon which would be thought unreasonable if applied to normal citizens.

Traditionally, healthcare professionals have shared in the public perception of the mentally impaired as necessarily unsuited to marriage and child-rearing and hence to be discouraged from forming heterosexual relationships. As Ann Craft (1987), pioneer in the promotion of sexual rights for the mentally handicapped, pointed out, old myths linger on. There is a persistent notion that the mentally handicapped remain childlike and asexual, and if they are exposed to sex information or experience they become uncontrollably sexualised. Such fears underlie parents' opposition to sex education for their disabled offspring (Squire, 1989) and the resistance of some professional staff to allowing, much less encouraging, sexual contact between their clients. Staff also have a fear of permissiveness in case it should lead to public scandal and loss of reputation. The adverse genetic consequences of pregnancy among persons with learning disability have been exaggerated in the past. Some of the severely disabled who are least suited to child-bearing are infertile. Parenting can be problematic, since persons with disability who are capable of a sexualised relationship or a companionable marriage are not necessarily able to perform child-rearing tasks successfully.

Long-term psychological support and confidential, one-to-one counselling is an essential prerequisite for a policy that facilitates access to sexual intercourse. It should be coupled with the provision of contraceptives and insistence on effective instruction in how to use them. The contraceptives should be of a kind that do not require much advance preparation. Counselling is important, especially concerning voluntary sterilisation (which should be available to both sexes) or abortion in the event of an unintended pregnancy. Counselling rather than moralistic condemnation is also needed about the use of erotic literature and videos, mechanical sex aids, sex contact services in magazines or via the telephone, sexual massage or call girls (and boys). Advice on masturbation is a particularly sensitive matter, especially if clients need teaching how to achieve orgasm. Any attempt to help has to be a team decision.

In general, persons with learning disabilities have the same legal rights to decide about all these matters as do normal citizens, including the right to conduct themselves within the law in ways their relatives disapprove. The law concerning those who are truly incompetent to decide for themselves or to consent to medical interventions remains somewhat uncertain (Carson, 1987; Gunn & Rosser, 1987). Nowadays hospitals house only the most severely damaged and difficult to manage clients. Many of these, although *de facto* detained in closed wards, have the theoretical status of informal patients, compulsory detention under the Mental Health Act requiring that the subnormality of intelligence be "associated with abnormally aggressive or seriously irresponsible conduct".

Restrictions on the liberty of impaired patients can be legitimised as necessary elements of the duty of care or in their 'best interests'. The best interests criterion can be used, for example, if a patient is sexually active, but clearly unable to cope with a pregnancy or to undertake the care of a baby. Sterilisation may be the best option, being more effective than attempts to police behaviour. It can readily be carried out if consent is forthcoming, but if the patient is too disabled to give informed consent, the operation can still be performed if it is clearly in the patient's best interests. This was decided by the House of Lords in the case of F (Re F [1988] All ER, 193), a woman with severe mental disability, a general mental capacity of a four-year-old and a verbal capacity of a two-year-old. She was an informal in-patient and had formed a relationship with a fellow male resident. It was thought that she would be unable to cope with a possible pregnancy, which would be likely to have a deleterious effect upon her mental condition. The Lords ruled that, notwithstanding her inability to give informed consent, the operation could go ahead on medical evidence that it was in her 'best interests'. The consultant should in such cases confer with relatives and with other professionals concerned with the care of the patient. Application to the High Court for a prior declaration of approval is not a strict legal necessity, but may be a wise course (Mental Health Act Commission, 1989, p. 34).

Prisons and special hospitals

Although the staff are no longer all one sex, prison inmates are strictly segregated and the control of sex conduct in effect amounts to the repression of male homosexuality. The extent and nature of sexual behaviour within British prisons is a delicate subject which has never been fully researched, whereas in America much more is known and written on the subject (Propper, 1981). The British prison service holds that there is nowhere private in their institutions and that therefore sex contacts between males are against the law and subject to disciplinary punishments. It is argued by many who are concerned about the spread of sexually transmitted diseases, especially AIDS and hepatitis, that this total prohibition and refusal to acknowledge what happens inside male prisons constitutes an unwarranted risk to health (Strang, 1993). The prison service, however, will not condone illegal acts and, although this could change, it presently refuses to allow condoms to be made available, just as it refuses to allow access to clean needles for those injecting drugs. It must be acknowledged, however, that so long as conjugal visits by wives or girlfriends are not part of the prison system, the provision of facilities for homosexual relationships would appear a little anomalous.

Sexual assaults in male prisons often go unreported, but the Prison Reform Trust hears of some of them. Apart from inmate disapproval of 'grassing' to prison officers, the victim of sexual aggression may suffer secondary victimisation from the response of the prison authorities. He can be transferred to another prison, perhaps far from home, and be placed in a vulnerable prisoner unit among known sex offenders. At the time of writing a prisoner alleging violent sexual assault by a cell-mate is suing for the harm caused by the incident and the aftermath of disclosure.

The concern aroused by homosexuality in male prisons contrasts with the relative tolerance of relationships in female prisons. Only rarely do such matters come to public notice. An unusual example was the exposure of a prison officer who was having a lesbian relationship with the child-killer Myra Hindley and was planning to help her to escape.

The control of sexual aggression within male prisons is important. The literature on American prisons describe inmate cultures where sexual assault, or the threat of it, is used to maintain a brutal pecking order among prisoners. Men insufficiently tough to fend for themselves are forced to submit to the sexual demands of a protector to avoid being preyed upon by all and sundry. It is unlikely that English institutions are entirely free from such abuses. In young offender institutions, bullying in particular may sometimes take a sexual form. Young males perceived by others as weak or effeminate or suspected of homosexual inclinations are especially vulnerable. Some much-publicised suicides by youthful prisoners have been linked to sexual victimisation. For example, Lee Waite, who killed himself while on remand in Feltham Young Offender Institution, was found by the pathologist who examined his body to have suffered a brutal sexual assault causing bruising and internal tears to the anal canal, inflicted some hours before his death, possibly with a snooker cue (Howard League, 1993).

In adult male prisons violence, not necessarily sexual, is often threatened against men with a history of sex offences against children. When there are riots and prisoners take over, known sex offenders, who are usually in protective segregation, are at risk of being killed. In the 1990 riot at Strangeways, for example, sex offenders were threatened and some badly injured in violent mob attacks. One tried to hang himself before the mob could get to him (Woolf, 1991, p. 71–2). At the time of writing two prisoners have been charged with murdering one of the imprisoned killers of the rent boy Jason Swift.

The special hospitals house patients deemed dangerous and in need of high security, most of whom arrive via the criminal courts after being convicted of a serious offence, often homicide. The control of sexuality within these hospitals has much in common with the prisons. For example, the majority of inmates are male, some of them with histories of gross sexual violence; wards are segregated and contact with patients of the opposite sex is limited and for some patients prohibited; security is a high priority, both for the protection of the public against escapers and for the protection of patients from each other; many of the nurses belong to the Prison Officers' Association with all that implies as regards attitudes towards control and discipline and standards of sexual conformity.

As in prisons, sexual contact between patients in the special hospitals is not supposed to happen. Before its demise, the Special Hospitals Service Authority was reviewing policy and proposing a more liberal stance, at least towards conjugal visits. Some traditionally-minded staff hold strong contrary views and stories of illicit sexual acts by hospitalised rapists have reached the tabloid press (*Guardian*, 3 August 1994). It will be difficult to devise a policy generally applicable throughout the special hospitals. The patients on different wards vary in age, in severity of disturbance and in intellectual development, and some are detained specifically on account of assaultative sexual crime. Proposals to provide condoms meet with resistance. Requirements of privacy conflict with the imperatives of high security. Among the sexually segregated patients homosexual associations are inevitable, but some staff would find it particularly difficult to tolerate overt homosexuality.

In special hospitals some contact between the sexes in communal areas and at entertainments is allowed, and as a consequence there are occasions when long-stay patients form a close relationship and eventually ask to marry. Some have been permitted to do so, even though consummation while either of them remains in hospital has not been sanctioned. If a marriage appears grossly unsuitable it is open to the Responsible Medical Officer, or any other concerned citizen, to object by submitting a caveat to the superintendent registrar who has the power to refuse to issue a licence.

Given the efforts being made by the special hospitals to develop local environments of a more relaxed therapeutic character within the confines of perimeter security, there are signs of slow development of more liberal attitudes. The Government has endorsed the principles recommended by the Reed Committee, that mentally disordered offenders should be cared for "under conditions of no greater security than is justified by the degree of danger they present to themselves or to others...In such a way as to maximise rehabilitation and their chances of sustaining an independent life" (Department of Health & Home Office, 1992). Reasonable access to visiting sexual partners could well be argued to be an important part of rehabilitation in long-stay institutions claiming to be therapeutic. Unfortunately, the balance between the conflicting demands of security and therapy in the special hospitals inevitably swings back in favour of the former when some untoward event, such as the discovery of pornographic materials on wards at Ashworth and Broadmoor, gains media coverage, as happened in February 1997.

Conclusion

Standards of sexual morality in society are still in a state of flux and a multiplicity of norms coexist. The scope of sex education in state schools remains a source of political concern and public controversy. The behaviour of the mentally disordered or disabled in the community still arouses suspicion and anxiety, with their relatives fearing scandal and parents in the neighbourhood fearing for the safety of their children. It is only to be expected under these circumstances that some carers in the community and some staff in hostels and hospitals should prefer to play safe even if this means control overkill and denial of patients' rights to a sex life.

Recent public inquiries and notorious trials have shown that untoward sexual behaviours in institutions sometimes continues unchecked for years. Knowing the consequences of exposure and the tendency for the media to sensationalise events and whip up public outrage, authorities may be reluctant to face the situation and take the decisive action called for.

A partial remedy for all these ills is to have open discussion of potential problems and clear written policies, both for routine guidance of client behaviours and for swift and effective response to complaints or suspicions of sexual offences by or against clients of mental health services.

References

Blom-Cooper, L. (1992) *Report of the Inquiry into Complaints about Ashworth Hospital*. Command 2028. London: HMSO.

Brown, H. & Smith, H. (1992) *Normalisation: A Reader for the Nineties*. London: Routledge.

Carson, D. (1987) *The Law and Sexuality of People with Mental Handicap*. Southampton: University of Southampton.

Craft, A. (ed.) (1987) *Mental Handicap and Sexuality*. Tunbridge Wells: Costello.

Creighton, J. H. M. (1995) Is it time for a formal disciplinary code for psychiatric in-patients in England and Wales? *Medicine, Science and the Law*, 35, 65–68.

Department of Health & Home Office (1992) *Review of Services for Mentally Disordered Offenders and Others Requiring Similar Services*. London: HMSO.

—— & Welsh Office (1993) *Code of Practice, Mental Health Act 1983*. London: HMSO.

Goffman, E. (1961) *Asylums: Essays on the Social Situation of Mental Patients and Other Inmates*. New York: Doubleday.

Gunn, M. & Rosser, J. (1987) *Sex and the Law: A Brief Guide for Staff Working in the Mental Handicap Field*. London: Family Planning Association Education Unit.

Hoggett, B. (1990) (3rd edn) *Mental Health Law*. London: Sweet and Maxwell.

Howard League (1993) *Suicides in Feltham*. London: Howard League for Penal Reform.

Jones, K. (1993) *Asylums and After*. London: Athlone Press.

Mental Health Act Commission (1989) *Third Biennial Report 1987–1989*. London: HMSO.

Propper, A. M. (1981) *Prison Homosexuality*. Lexington, MA: Lexington Books.

Scacco, A. M. (1975) *Rape in Prison*. Springfield: C.C. Thomas.

Scull, A. T. (1989) *Social Order/Mental Disorder. Anglo American Psychiatry in Perspective*. London: Routledge.

Sobsey, D. & Doe, T. (1991) Patterns of sexual abuse and assault. *Sexuality and Disability*, 9, 243–259.

Squire, J. (1989) Sex education for pupils with severe learning difficulties: a survey of parent and staff attitudes. *Mental Handicap*, 17, 66–69.

Strang, J. (1993) Sexual and injecting behaviours in prisons. *Criminal Behaviour and Mental Health*, 3, 393–402.

West Berkshire Health Authority (1989) *All England Law Reports*, 545–571.

Westcott, H. L. (1993) *Abuse of Children and Adults with Disabilities*. London: NSPCC.

Woolf, Lord Justice (1991) *Prison Disturbances April 1990. Report of an Inquiry. Parts I and II*. Command 1456. London: HMSO.

9 The paraphilias: an evolutionary and developmental perspective

Raymond E. Goodman

Sadomasochism • *Fetishism* • *Other paraphilias* • *Conclusions*

The word paraphilia means a love of (philia) the beyond or irregular (para), and is usually used in place of terms such as perversion or deviance which today have pejorative implications that are not always relevant. The term itself is used to describe people with intense sexual urges that are directed towards nonhuman objects, or the suffering or humiliation of oneself or one's partner, or more unacceptably, towards others who are incapable of giving informed consent, such as children, animals or unwilling adults. People who are paraphiliacs often exhibit three or four different aspects, and clinical psychiatric conditions (personality disorders or depression) may sometimes be present.

The human brain reached its present size and proportions in modern man about 50 to 100 000 years ago. This has made possible the protean manifestations of human sexual behaviour. It is not the mere size of the human brain *per se*, however, that is important, but its organisation, especially the development of the neocortex, and the associated lower areas which have of necessity expanded to service this. The brain consists of regions which formed at different epochs in vertebrate evolution, each of which reflects an integrated phylogeny (Rapoport, 1990).

In most species sexuality and reproduction are of necessity tied together and overlap, but in modern humans it is the relatively recent separation of sexuality from reproduction that represents a crucial evolutionary phase. Despite huge sociological changes we are genetically still at the stage of hunter-gatherers, exemplified by the !Kung, the Bushmen of the Kalahari who are still extant. Significantly the girls here have their first period at the age of fifteen and a half, when they marry, but ovulation does not occur until they are nineteen and a half when they have fully matured. Pregnancy usually occurs at this time. Breast-feeding is undertaken for some four years before the infant is weaned, and this acts as a contraceptive. After four or five pregnancies, with an average of two or three children surviving to adulthood, the mother, now in her mid-30s, often dies. There is, therefore, no menopause. Perhaps because of better nutrition, and possibly exposure to electric light (which affects the hypothalamus), girls in the developed countries in the 1990s have their first period around 13 years of age, and ovulation

142

starts soon afterwards. This adolescent stage demands a cultural, not a natural, sterility, with birth control and abortion acting as failsafes. Modern western women usually limit their families to two or three children whom they bear and rear while in their 20s or early 30s. This leaves 20 or so years before the menopause and a further 20–30 years before senility or death. These sociological changes have given women a period of almost 50 years when sexuality and reproduction are separate, so that the former has taken on new meanings and fulfils other roles (Short, 1976). Similarly, men are at their most potent around the mid teens and early 20s, so that in our extended lifetime it is not so surprising that many men have erectile difficulties later on. Therefore in modern times it could be said that sex for both men and women has become largely a recreational activity divorced from procreation. This is perhaps why such a wide variety of sexual behaviour is exhibited today.

It is the hypothalamus that is largely concerned with the hormonal control of reproduction, but fantasy depends on the cortex. As the latter is not identical in any two individuals (even identical twins show differences), an almost infinite variety of mental responses is therefore possible and this gives a unique plasticity to the range of sexual behaviours (Prochiantz, 1989).

Sadomasochism (S & M)

Evolutionary considerations

Aggression is very much tied up with reproductive behaviours in many animals. Usually the male, who is bigger and stronger, has his aggression diverted by ritualistic appeasing behaviours exhibited by the female around the time of mating. The violence that often ensues at this period between the sexes serves to raise the level of excitement and facilitates the mating process, and may cause ovulation in the female. Indeed, in some species the male will not attempt to mate unless the female shows the appropriate resistance. During mating itself, the male mink, sable or big cat bites the female's neck, which stimulates his erection and causes her to adopt a suitable presenting position, so that penetration can occur (Ford & Beech, 1972).

Psychoanalytical theories

Krafft-Ebing (1886), in the last century, first described S & M as a syndrome, the salient points of which he took from a novel written by Leopold von Sacher-Masoch, a German professor of history. The novel *Venus in Furs* describes S & M behaviours in a graphic and informative manner.

Freud (1905) believed S & M to be a perversion, created through abnormalities of childhood in the affected individual. Most modern research shows this not to be true, as many S & M practitioners report no childhood traumas. Baumeister (1988) believes that these behaviours offer an escape from the self, for by undergoing such humiliations the here and now offers a relief from the cares of the everyday. He makes the point that before the 16 and 17th centuries, history does not record such behaviours, and he feels this reflects the ego and concept of individual self which developed at this time. The profusion of flagellation clubs that flourished in 17th century England onwards may offer support to this theory.

S & M behaviours

In humans, as described in the behaviour of animals above, erotic play can also consist of a struggle, which may include biting, slapping and tickling, all of which serve to heighten excitement. The addition of language adds another dimension to the possibilities of interaction and fantasy between couples, so that what is just mating behaviour in animals has been turned into something of a different order in humans. The surge in endorphins which is partly responsible for orgasm in humans is a reflection of the physical basis of this process.

S & M is usually taken to refer to sexual arousal that is associated with rituals of pain, bondage and humiliation. From what has been said above, these behaviours are linked with the mating processes in other species as well as humans. S & M rituals, however, reflect the dissociation between sex and reproduction in human behaviour and it is the ritual itself that gains increasingly in importance. The pain between couples who are involved in S & M may be caused by whipping, usually around the buttocks, biting, pinching and slapping, whereas bondage usually consists of the victim being rendered immobile and helpless. The humiliation is acted out in a mistress/slave fantasy, where one partner is dominant and the other submissive. In a study by Spengler (1977), most couples were found to alternate these roles. Furthermore, he noted that a mere 15% of the men questioned could achieve orgasm by S & M behaviours alone. Perhaps it is this population only to whom the concept of paraphilia should really apply. Spengler also showed that half the reported S & M practitioners had fetishistic interests, especially associated with leather, boots and jeans. It had been assumed that the only women to take part in these behaviours were prostitutes at the behest of their male clients, but more recent studies (e.g. Breslow *et al*, 1985; Baumeister, 1988) found that women who are not prostitutes do indeed actively participate. There are differences, however, in the patterns of male and female S & M practitioners, which may reflect both biological and sociocultural factors. Men may cross-dress, but women rarely do. In fact, women often become more stereotypically feminine by stylishly dressing in exaggerated fetishistic clothes, which are usually fashioned in leather or rubber. Women S & M practitioners, although consenting to some slave identities, rarely choose the purely masochistic roles of babies in nappies, infants or animals, whereas men often assume these subservient identities. A not uncommon female masochistic behaviour is for the woman to be displayed naked in front of strange men, so that she is in effect considered merely in terms of her body and genitalia. The dominant woman may involve other men in sexual acts in front of her partner. However, this activity is never allowed to be part of a dominant man's behaviour when with his female partner, for the woman, even in a masochistic situation, remains centre-stage. Men are often required to perform oral sex to order on the mistress, whereas for the female masochist forced coitus is the usual punishment.

The association between erotic piercing and S & M among gay men and some lesbians is reported in the literature. These erotic piercings usually involve the insertion of gold or silver rings or studs through nipples, perineum or penis.

The themes of dominance and submission consist of role-playing, the rules and rituals of which are usually discussed first, and sometimes written down. The essential component is trust between partners. It is the illusion of pain, involving fantasy and imagination that is at the core of S & M, not real pain or harm. The couple will have a signal to be used should anything go wrong, the use of which results in instant release and cessation of activities. The behaviour is considered as recreational, and has been likened to joining a sports club or having a hobby, rather than a product of developmental pathology. One should mention perhaps that S & M devotees dislike dentists and migraine as much as anybody else.

Variations on the S & M theme

Sadistic murder

Although it is not actually known whether this form of behaviour is in any way related to the diversions practised by S & M devotees, there are qualitative differences between the two which suggest that they are actually totally different entities. Sexual sadists who commit violence and murder seem to be driven by fantasies of domination, they feel an overwhelming urge to control the victim completely, whereas the S & M group have predominantly fantasies of bondage and pseudo-rape. Furthermore, the former report very disturbed family backgrounds, with physical and sexual abuse, and a pathological sense of isolation, none of which is found in the S & M population. It is not that sexual sadists do not empathise with their victims, they do, but it is the wrong sort of empathy, which leads to sexual arousal rather than pity (Grubin, 1994).

Autoerotic asphyxia

This variety of masochistic behaviour has come into the news recently. It comes to notice when a body, usually male, is discovered in bizarre circumstances. The deceased is often found bound and gagged, evidence of cross-dressing may be present, and some method of asphyxia is in evidence, often in the form of scarves or ropes that have been elaborately knotted around the victim's neck. Pornographic magazines, which sometimes depict similar scenarios, are often present. Sometimes the deceased has video-taped the proceedings. There is inevitably evidence that ejaculation has occurred. There is also evidence that these behaviours have been practised over a period of time and that death is accidental. In young men this is commonly from asphyxia, whereas in older practitioners a myocardial infarction or a cerebrovascular accident may be responsible. Sometimes associated drug and alcohol use is in evidence. Gay practitioners are more likely to meet like-minded partners, and fatalities usually occur when the activity is practised alone. Most of the men who like this form of sexual arousal practise in secret, and are often found to be lonely, single and under stress. Their families are unaware of their activities, and if they are the first to find the body they may remove the various accoutrements out of an understandable feeling of shock and embarrassment. The association with partial asphyxia and enhanced orgasm is well known in the literature and in some cultures, for example among the Eskimo, it is used as part of normal love-play (Goodman, 1985).

Fetishism

Evolutionary considerations

The sexual behaviour of lower mammals is heavily dependent on smell. This acts through the production of pheromones (called copulins in humans), which are small volatile chemicals that are associated with the genital areas. In dogs, for example, the female at oestrus secretes substances in her urine that stimulate luteinising hormone and testosterone production in the male. Krafft-Ebing (1886) noted that in humans the nasal tissues resemble the erectile structure found in the penis, clitoris and nipples, and indeed smell often plays a part in arousal in many couples. The olfactory system in man works via the vomeronasal organ (also called Jacobson's Organ), which is situated in the nasopharyngeal septum. The terminalis nerves, in intimate association with the olfactory nerves, link the volmeronasal organ with various specific nuclei of the hypothalamus. These nuclei produce gonadotrophic-releasing hormones, which establish a link between pheromones and hormones. Although much of the role of olfaction in sexual attraction in humans has been taken over by the visual system, it still plays some part. The proportion of the different pheromones produced in the urine and sweat glands is linked to the major histocompatibility system in many animals and man. This gives a variability that may govern such factors as partner choice and the prevention of incest by the male who tends to avoid his own genetic subtypes. Understanding these factors make it easier to see why smell could become dissociated from the other sexual processes in fetishists, and therefore their preference, for example, for worn as against clean female underwear (Novotny, 1987).

In addition to olfaction, animals use many visual and sound cues to signal availability for mating, and we have inherited aspects of these behaviours. As our human interactions are now so complex it is therefore not surprising perhaps that these can become disorganised in some people.

Once our ancestors discovered the use of tools the stage was set for depictions of the environment which led eventually to symbolic art and writing. Sexual acts and genitalia were often depicted, perhaps with a magical significance. Fetishism therefore possibly developed from these depictions which were seen as an association between sexual arousal and the various objects. The sights, sounds and smells that the subject experienced in his environment became linked presumably by some type of conditioned reflex. The flowering of the neocortex in humans allowed a great number of associative linkages between cognitive ideas, which was further enhanced by the development of language so that a picture of the world was able to be internally projected. Such representations of past and present events, especially when of a sexual nature with strong affect, sometimes became linked. Repeated recall of these in fantasy, say during masturbation, would reinforce the established circuits.

Fetishistic behaviours have been observed in some lower primates. A gibbon, a baboon and a chimpanzee have been so described. This last was an animal of 17 years of age that had been born into captivity. It would gaze at a particular rubber boot and become sexually aroused, and then masturbate (Epstein, 1987). Animals do not bring the associative and cognitive fantasies that occur in humans to their behaviours, but that they exist at all in other species highlights the biological basis to much of our own sexuality.

Psychoanalytic ideas

There are numerous formulations, but it is usually assumed that the male fetish has developed because the youth developed a severe castration complex in his childhood. This supposedly arose when he saw that his mother did not have a penis and assumed that she had been castrated by the powerful father. The fetish object then acts to give him reassurance that his own penis is safe. He is usually described as obsessional and fixated at the anal–sadistic phase of development (Greenacre, 1979). Attempts have been made by modern feminists to explain female fetishism in analytic terms, and most have offered reworkings of this model, in which they challenge the idea of the castration complex as central to the development of fetishism (Gammon & Makinen, 1994).

Behavioural constructs

Behavioural constructs assume that in many circumstances there is a conditioning experience. This may be a quite accidental association that links intense sexual arousal and orgasm with an object, which later develops into the fetish. Rachman (1966) was able experimentally to condition a fetish in a group of young male psychology students by showing slides of a woman's boots followed by slides of nude females which each had chosen as being sexually stimulating. Eventually they became aroused by viewing the slides of the boots alone.

Medical models

Some epileptics with temporal lobe lesions do exhibit fetishistic behaviours, which may suggest that these regions of the brain are involved in this behaviour (Epstein, 1961). Furthermore, paraphiliac behaviours have been reported in otherwise normal individuals who misuse psychoactive drugs such as amphetamines or cocaine. These substances act through dopaminergic neurones in the limbic system, which play some part in the control of sexuality (Buffum, 1988).

Current fetishistic behaviours

Fetishism is defined as sexual arousal by one part of the human body or by inanimate objects rather than by the whole person. More men than women are affected. If the fetish involves clothing of the opposite sex, it may resemble transvestism, but transvestites have to specifically cross-dress to obtain arousal. Fetishists, however, unlike transvestites, use a wide range of objects for arousal. To some extent all sexual behaviours have elements of fetishism about them. Some men prefer blondes, others brunettes; reputedly there are breast, bottom or leg men, depending on which part of female anatomy excites them most. Today women also profess to be excited by specific parts of male anatomy, such as the shoulders, thighs, crotch and bottom. In many couples the wife may dress up in provocative underwear to increase the sexual tempo, and such behaviour is common in S & M rituals as described above. Gebhard (1969) graded fetishistic behaviours along a spectrum that ranged from a slight preference to a stronger one, proceeding to a point where the fetish is a necessity for sexual activity, and finally to the stage where the fetish substitutes for the partner entirely. He felt that only the final two stages should be regarded as clinical fetishism.

Fetishists use a wide variety of objects which commonly include items of female clothing, such as underwear (especially if it has been worn and is unwashed), gloves, shoes and stockings. They have fantasies about parts of the female body, such as ankles, breasts, buttocks and hair – pubic or head. Rubber, fur and silk are common items of veneration and are sought after. The use of leather as a second skin has its devotees. However, the fetish can be quite bizarre, and cases have been described where a motor car (Bergler, 1946) and tractors (O'Halloran & Dietz, 1993) served this role. In the former case the exhaust pipe had to emit fumes, and an element of intoxication was involved, whereas in the latter the fetishist became romantically involved with the tractor, gave it a name and wrote poetry to it. Equally strange, perhaps, is the case described by King (1990) of a young man who developed a fetish to other people sneezing.

Pygmalionism refers to a type of fetishism in which the object has the form of a person but the content of a thing. It is named after the Greek sculptor who reputedly fell in love with his own creation, the statue of a beautiful woman, and examples of this condition do occur in the writings of antiquity. The term fetishism does not strictly apply to those individuals who use sex aids (i.e. vibrators or dolls), as these have been specifically made for sexual purposes.

Today the fashion industry makes much use of fetishism in its designs. Magazines such as *Skin Two* cater for a whole range of people, both gay and straight, with fetishistic and S & M interests. A survey showed nearly 40% of readers were female, but this may include men who adopt female gender identity personae. Relatively new phenomena have appeared in recent times, such as 'Vogueing'. Here the devotee dresses up as a facsimile of an admired personality, either of the same sex (homovestism), or of the opposite sex (the well-known transvestism). Common examples are Elvis Presley and Madonna lookalikes. Voguers compete with each other for realness. Fans who obtain objects, such as articles of clothing or signed photographs from their idols, or who in the US search the dustbins of stars for trinkets (so-called trashcanners) and later use these in their sexual fantasies, resemble classical fetishists in their behaviour (Gammon & Makinen, 1994).

Cases often come to light if there has been an accidental death, as described above, or if the fetishist is caught stealing items of women's clothes, or cutting hair off women whom he may meet at random or by design. Others may present to marital or sex therapists because of their inability to have a reasonable sex life, the fetish either getting in the way of arousal for coitus or preventing it altogether. The decision to treat the problem will depend on how much personal distress is being caused by the fetish to the patient or his partner, or whether it is causing legal problems. Usually the behaviour can be incorporated into the couple's love-life, but sometimes various psychological procedures are necessary to diminish its significance (de Silva, 1993).

Other paraphilias

Bestiality (also called zoophilia)

This term applies to individuals who use animals for sexual purposes. Depictions of such acts occur in carvings from the Bronze Age, in the 2nd millennium BC. Many different animals are used for these purposes. Often the behaviour is done out of curiosity but it is usually used as an alternative to human contact, especially if the latter is not available. Liliequist (1991) reviewed these behaviours among young men in 17th and 18th century Sweden. He described pull factors as the familiarity with animals, and the fact that the youth was often alone with them for long periods, and the push factors as high male sex drive and the absence of women. Kinsey *et al* (1948), furthermore, found that 17% of boys who lived in rural areas had sexual contact with animals, but they also found that it occurred even among those who lived in urban areas, albeit to a lesser extent. Kinsey *et al* (1953) noted that these behaviours do occur in females, although more infrequently; he cited a figure of 4% for the rural population of girls in his study. The animals involved include sheep, horses and dogs. The sexual activities include having intercourse, performing oral sex or masturbation on the animal, or training it to lick or rub the individuals' genitals. In other countries exhibitions of coitus between women and dogs or donkeys do take place for a predominantly male audience, while stag films also often depict these activities. Small animals (e.g. gerbils, snakes, etc.) have been inserted into the rectum of some individuals for sexual purposes (Tollison & Adams, 1979).

Necrophilia

This refers to people who obtain sexual gratification from the use of a dead body. The perpetrator may actually have coitus with it, and often some mutilation of the corpse takes place. Sometimes films are made of these behaviours which involve the actual killing of the victims. These are the so-called 'snuff movies'. Bodies may be removed from morgues or cemeteries for this purpose. Prostitutes may be called to act out such fantasies, which may involve their lying in a coffin and being made up to resemble a corpse, before they have some sexual act with the participant.

Urine and faeces

The use of these in the attainment of sexual arousal and orgasm is well known, and these behaviours are termed urophilia and coprophilia respectively. Sometimes urinating or defaecating on the victim is part of an S & M ritual. Some men find the sight of a woman urinating or defaecating extremely arousing. Objects of every variety have been inserted into the urethra of both sexes for the purpose of arousal and masturbation since time immemorial, and these behaviours are termed urethralism. Klismaphilia is the name given to the use of rectal enemas for sexual purposes; the resultant stretching of the rectal wall is perceived by some as erotic. Enemas in the form of dishwashing liquids or detergents irritate the colon and are sometimes used in S & M practices, and recreational drugs may be given in this way to ensure a rapid onset of action. Anal dilatation may be caused by nitrites, commonly used by gay men, which facilitate anal intercourse or other practices such as fist fornication (the insertion of the fist and forearm of a partner into the rectum), or the insertion of various other objects. Needless to say these behaviours can lead to risks of perforation, infection and the particular object becoming impacted (Agnew, 1985).

Apotemnophilia

This refers to individuals who become sexually aroused by people who are in some way crippled or have an amputation, or who themselves wish to obtain an amputation for these purposes. Various surveys have shown that, as with the other paraphilias, most apotemno-philiacs are men, although women do exist. The preferred amputee for such men was usually found to be a woman with an above-knee amputation of one leg, who used a crutch and had a stump. The individual usually became aware of his interest before puberty, and only rarely reported a triggering situation. Again, perhaps strangely, few apotemnophiliacs married partners with amputations. Requests for amputation from self-directed apotemnophiliacs for sexual reasons are obviously refused by the medical profession, so that some individuals have attempted self-mutilations. The condition has links to S & M and transsexualism, and is thought to represent an *idée fixe* rather than a paranoid delusion (Money *et al*, 1977; Dixon, 1983).

Conclusions

The complex processes of the cortex have been built up over evolutionary time-scales and probably have some genetic represent-ations (Epstein, 1987). Now that it has been found that homosexuality, both male and female, tends to run in families through the maternal line and involves minor genes (Bailey & Pillard, 1991; Bailey & Benishay, 1993), one can speculate whether this could also apply to the paraphilias. Indeed, cases have been described of fetishism occurring in identical twins (Gorman, 1964). It should be realised, however, that sexual behaviours depend ultimately on a host of interactions between, among others, genes, foetal hormones, early environments, learning, psychological factors and chance. These interactions are probably non-linear, and involve the mathematical concept of chaos. This process ensures an overall stability in spite of much internal variation. The range of human sexual behaviours positively reflects this process (Gleick, 1988). The relationship between the genotype and the phenotype is likewise non-linear; the developmental genes, for instance, are involved in interactions which in turn may affect them themselves and induce or inhibit other genes in a feedback system. Based on these factors, the concept of parameter space offers a picture of how different phenotypes may be constructed from the same genotype (Alberch, 1991; Goodman, 1997). This could explain the occurrence of sexual variant behaviour as a phenotypic rather than a purely genotypic phenomenon.

As computer technology advances, new interactions are possible which in turn modify sexual behaviour. Cybersex refers to sexual activities and games that are contained on various computer disk systems, which make it possible for people to interact in simulated sexual situations. This process has reached some degree of sophistication, and a wide variety of sexual outlets, including fetishism and S & M, are available. (This process of sex at a distance has been termed, with some humour, Teledildonics, which in the age of AIDS is the ultimate form of safe sex.) In the near future this will come into the realm of virtual reality.

> Imagine getting decked out in your cybersensual suit for a hot night....
> you can run your hands through virtual hair, touch virtual silk,
> unzip virtual clothing and caress virtual flesh. (Robinson &
> Tamosaitis, 1993)

New difficulties will arise in classifying people who, for example, live one sexual lifestyle in our reality and another in virtual reality, where only the imagination limits the sexual possibilities. The concept of self, sexuality and morality will have new meanings at the shared mind/machine interface. Can one's visual persona, for example, be held responsible for virtual abuse when cruising the computer networks (Rheingold, 1991)? These will be the concerns of the not too distant future.

References

Agnew, J. (1985) Some anatomical and physiological aspects of anal practices. *Journal of Homosexuality*, 12, 75–96.

Alberch, P. (1991) From genes to phenotype: dynamical systems and evolvability. *Genetica*, 84, 5–11.

Bailey, J. M. & Pillard, R. C. (1991) A genetic study of male sexual orientation. *Archives of General Psychiatry*, 48, 1089–1096.

—— & Benishay, D. S. (1993) Familial aggregation of female sexual orientation. *American Journal of Psychiatry*, 150, 272–277.

Baumeister, R. F. (1988) Gender difference in masochistic scripts. *Journal of Sex Research*, 25, 478–499.

Bergler, E. (1946) Analysis of an unusual case of fetishism. *Bulletin of the Menninger Clinic*, 2, 67–75.

Breslow, N., Evans, L. & Langley, J. (1985) On the prevalence and roles of females in the sadomasochistic subculture: report of an empirical study. *Archives of Sexual Behavior*, 14, 303–317.

Buffum, J. (1988) Substance abuse and high-risk sexual behavior: drugs and sex – the dark side. *Journal of Psychoactive Drugs*, 20, 165–166.

de Silva, P. (1993) Fetishism and sexual dysfunction: clinical presentation and management. *Sexual and Marital Therapy*, 8, 147–155.

Dixon, D. (1983) An erotic attraction to amputees. *Sexuality and Disability*, 6, 3–19.

Epstein, A. W. (1961) Relationship of fetishism and transvestism to brain and particularly to temporal lobe dysfunction. *Journal of Nervous and Mental Disorders*, 133, 247–253.

—— (1987) The phylogenetics of fetishism. In *Variant Sexuality: Research and Theory* (ed. G. D. Wilson), pp. 142–149. London: Croom Helm.

Ford, C. S. & Beech, F. A. (1972) *Patterns of Sexual Behavior*. Harper Torch.

Freud, S. (1905) *On Sexuality, Three Essays on the Theory of Sexuality and Other Works* (4th edn, 1977). London: Penguin.

Gammon, L. & Makinen, M. (1994) *Female Fetishism: a New Look*. London: Lawrence & Wishart.

Gebhard, P. H. (1969) Fetishism and sado-masochism. In *Dynamics of Deviant Sexuality* (ed. J. H. Masermann), p. 71. New York: Grune & Stratton.

Gleick, J. (1988) *Chaos*. London: Cardinal Sphere Books.

Goodman, R. E. (1985) Autoerotic death. *British Journal of Sexual Medicine*, 12, 17–19.

—— (1997) Understanding human sexuality, specifically homosexuality and the paraphilias, in terms of chaos theory and fetal development. *Medical Hypotheses*, 48, 237–243.

Gorman, G. F. (1964) Fetishism occurring in identical twins. *British Journal of Psychiatry*, 110, 255–256.

Greenacre, P. (1979) Fetishism. In *Sexual Deviation* (ed. I. Rosen) (2nd edn), pp. 79–108. Oxford: Oxford University Press.

Grubin, D. (1994) Fantasy, sadism and murder. *Bulletin of the British Association for Sexual and Marital Therapy*, 10, 5–6.

King, M. B. (1990) Sneezing as a fetishistic stimulus. *Sexual and Marital Therapy*, 5, 69–72.

Kinsey, A. C., Pomeroy, W. B. & Martin, C. E. (1948) *Sexual Behaviour in the Human Male*. Philadelphia: W.B. Saunders.

——, ——, ——, *et al* (1953) *Sexual Behavior in the Human Female*. Philadelphia: W.B. Saunders.

Krafft-Ebing, R. von (1886) *The Psychopathia Sexualis*. London: Panther.

Liliequist, J. (1991) Peasants against nature; crossing the boundaries between man and animals in seventeenth and eighteenth century Sweden. *Journal of the History of Sexuality*, 1, 393–423.

Money, J., Jobaris, R. & Furth, G. (1977) Apotemnophilia: Two cases of self-demand amputation as a paraphilia. *Journal of Sex Research*, 13, 115–125.

Novotny, M. (1987) The importance of chemical messengers in mammalian reproduction. In *Masculinity/Femininity, Basic Perspectives* (eds J. M. Reinisch, L. A. Rosenblum & S. A. Sanders), pp. 107–128. Oxford: Oxford University Press.

O'Halloran, R. L. & Dietz, P. E. (1993) Autoerotic fatalities with power hydraulics. *Journal of Forensic Science*, 38, 359–364.

Prochiantz, A. (1989) *How The Brain Evolved*. New York: McGraw-Hill.

Rachman, S. (1966) Sexual fetishism: an experimental analogue. *Psychological Record*, 16, 293–296.

Rapoport, S. I. (1990) Integrated phylogeny of the primate brain, with special reference to humans and their diseases. *Brain Research Reviews*, 15, 267–294.

Rheingold, H. (1991) *Virtual Reality*. London: Mandarin.

Robinson, P. & Tamosaitis, N. (1993) *The Joy of Cybersex*. New York: Brady Publishing.

Short, R. V. (1976) The evolution of human reproduction. *Proceedings of the Royal Society of London, Biology*, 195, 3–24.

Spengler, A. (1977) Manifest sadomasochism of males: results of an empirical study. *Archives of Sexual Behavior*, 6, 441–456.

Tollison, C. D. & Adams, H. E. (1979) *Sexual Disorders, Treatment, Theory, Research*. New York: Gardner Press.

Further reading

American Psychiatric Association (1987) Sexual disorders. In *Diagnostic and Statistical Manual of Mental Disorders* (3rd edn, revised) (DSM–III–R), pp. 279–296. Washington, DC: APA.

Goodman, R. E. (1987) Genetic and hormonal factors in human sexuality: Evolutionary and developmental perspectives. In *Variant Sexuality: Research and Theory* (ed. G. Wilson), pp. 21–48. Chicago: Chicago University Press.

Gosselin, C. C. & Wilson, G. D. (1980) *Sexual Variations*. London: Faber & Faber.

Marks, I. M. (1972) Phylogenesis and learning in the acquisition of fetishism. *Danish Medical Bulletin*, 19, 307–310.

Money, J. (1984) Paraphilias: phenomenology and classification. *American Journal of Psychotherapy*, 38, 164–179.

Weinberg, T. S. (1987) Sadomasochism in the United States: a review of recent sociological literature. *Journal of Sex Research*, 23, 50–69.

Wise, T. N. (1985) Fetishism – etiology and treatment: a review from multiple perspectives. *Comprehensive Psychiatry*, 26, 249–257.

10 Transgenderism and the psychiatrist

Jed Bland

The transgender spectrum • *The prescription of hormones* • *Surgery* •
Conclusions

For the purposes of this article, 'transgenderism' is a blanket term to describe people who challenge existing gender attitudes (transvestites and transsexuals). Before turning quickly to the next chapter, consider a moment. What is the difference between those who consciously challenge gender roles – feminists and 'new men', for example – and those who feel driven unthinkingly to do so?

The first confusion to dispose of is between sex and gender. The biological sex of a person is determined by whether he, or she, is chromosomally XX or XY. There are variations with this, and factors arising during prenatal development (Money & Ehrhardt, 1972), but the purpose of this article is not to deal with 'pseudo-hermaphroditism'. In practice, the newborn baby is sexually labelled by the midwife or doctor from an examination of the genital organs.

There is controversy about whether certain sexually dimorphic behaviours are present from birth. Some writers even seem to suggest that a baby 'knows' whether it is a boy or a girl. However, also from the moment of birth, certain behaviours and mental attitudes are encouraged or discouraged according to the child's sexual label. The personality of all children varies immensely. Being viewed by others as more or less masculine or feminine, they will come to see themselves in the same way. They will set out to become acceptably masculine or feminine, although it is easier for a girl to be a 'tomboy' than for a boy to be a 'sissy'.

The literature is extremely confusing in its use of the words 'sex' and 'gender', which is why the author has taken care to explain his own definition. In particular, some authors use the term 'gender identity' to describe something that a child is born with. Others use it to describe that part of the complex personality schema called the 'self' which contains subschemata of masculinity or femininity. Money & Ehrhardt (1972) have clarified the issue by referring to 'Gender Identity/Role' (GI/R). This is the process by which each child negotiates a compromise between itself, as masculine or feminine, and the role that its individual environment expects it to adopt: 'who' he is and 'who' he 'ought' to be.

However, if we view gender identity as an expression of personality, something that is extremely variable, we could, perhaps, think of natal gender identity as a locus, emphasising that it is not one of two directions, but a probability distribution (Bland, 1994*a*).

Thus gender is that part of our personalities, and of the attributions we make about others, which is associated with concepts of *being* male or female. For most people their gender identity develops and becomes modified as they grow, and their core personality becomes built on by experience. In the author's view, sex is functional, but gender is cognitive, even though it is a fundamental part of each individual's mind-set.

Transvestism, transsexualism and various cross-gender behaviours are not, then, simple issues. Rooted in personal and cultural construction, a complex of different psychological processes may be involved for different people at different times.

A psychiatrist may become involved with cross-gender behaviour for various reasons, three of which follow.

The person is in trouble with the law

A client may have been referred because of arrest by the police or an appearance in court. There is no law against cross-dressing in this country, but someone may take exception and make a complaint that ends in legal proceedings. If the person dresses soberly, and behaves quietly, most people, including the police, are fairly tolerant.

However, it is possible for a transvestite to run into trouble. Brierley (1979) reported a case where a transvestite had been assaulted by some youths. Despite the physical injury, the court held the transvestite responsible. In a recent case, a transvestite who was still 'in the closet' and dressed respectably, but not very passably, was teased by two girls. What happened is not clear, but he was charged with indecent assault. The charge was dismissed, but he was still bound over. It seems that in every court in the land, the fact of cross-dressing will cloud the real issues.

Most court cases involve more bizarre behaviour like walking through a shopping precinct with a short miniskirt and an erection. There have been several cases of men exposing themselves to women, while wearing female underwear. It seems likely that, for such people, there is a strong erotic component, and the motivation is not strictly transvestism but, perhaps, exhibitionism.

The person expresses feelings of guilt about cross-dressing

For the psychiatrist to imagine a big hairy man wearing a dress may be somewhat daunting. He may have to overcome negative feelings, particularly as these may be the feelings that the client is projecting. It may become apparent that someone in this position will seek help more because of family pressures than from any personal commitment. He is likely to ask to be "made to stop" cross-dressing; what will become apparent is that what he really wants is to be made to want to stop. The repression of the cross-dressing urge may result in other problems, like a greater tendency to depression in an already depressive personality.

The person expresses a need for gender reassignment

More people than ever, both men and women, are seeking this course of action, if the statistics are to be believed. Male clients, especially, may have considerable hidden agendas which create problems for the psychiatrist. Although the client may see the therapeutic path as a clear way out of confusion, it may not be the right solution. On the other hand, simply labelling people as unsuitable for therapy will not help them and may make their troubles worse. In the end, what matters is their future success as people, whatever their gender role, but, having settled on the idea of the 'sex change' as their goal, they are not often receptive to alternative suggestions. Indeed, they may see the general psychiatrist, or even the gender consultant, as a frustrating impediment to their progress.

The transgender spectrum

The *International Classification of Disorders* (ICD) and the *Diagnostic and Statistical Manual* (DSM) both have categories for various gender-disordered people. Bancroft (1989) lists fetishist transvestites; transsexuals; dual role transvestites; and homosexual transvestites.

However, the range of transgenderism is increasingly being referred to as a spectrum, something that this author considers an over-simplification. If gender is an individual experience, so is transgenderism. While setting definitions may be helpful in understanding the issues, they are likely to be counterproductive in the clinic. Many transsexuals have found cross-dressing extremely erotic at some time in their lives. There are some who have an unshakeable feeling of femininity, yet have never cross-dressed. Some are homosexual, many are heterosexual. Some homosexual cross-dressers feel that they are primarily homosexual, while others feel that they are primarily transvestites.

Instead of following the above definitions, therefore, we will consider the four main issues that may affect all transgenderists in different degrees: eroticism and sexual fantasy; sexual preference; expression of personality; and gender identity problems.

Eroticism and sexual fantasy

Everyone has sexual fantasies. Much media attention has been given to encouraging their expression within relationships. However, there are many people who are not in a relationship, for various perfectly valid reasons. Many others experience difficulties in relating, or have had dysfunctional relationships in the past. We all harbour deep-seated guilt from centuries of sexual negativism, especially regarding masturbation.

The origin of this may be traced to pre-biblical times. Until the discovery of the cellular structure of living things, it was thought that the male sperm was the carrier of life, and the female simply a convenient receptacle for nurturing it. With his first crude microscope, Van Leeuwenhoek even claimed to see a small person, or 'animalcule', within the sperm cell. In parallel with this was the idea that bodily secretions, especially the female monthly cycle and male ejaculation, drained the person's vital forces. The science of physics formulated the idea of conservation of energy, and attempts were made to transport the idea into human biology. In addition, the energy expended in orgasm, it was said, would overload the nervous system, especially in youth, and lead to feeble-mindedness. Money (1985) described findings by a certain Dr Graham who claimed support for this from his observations of mental patients in a home that he ran, many of whom were probably consumptive, or suffering from dementia or tertiary syphilis. The idea nowadays is that masturbation is natural, healthy and innocent.

But what about people who have difficulties in relationships? As children grow into puberty, they develop sexual scripts based on idealised relationships and specific stimulating experiences in childhood. If the child is sexually naïve, the script can contain little of a conventional sexual relationship. If it has suffered trauma, a script may contain elements that enable him, or her, to gain power over the event. The script may be played over and over, and orgasm may become an escape from confronting past emotional pain. As time goes by, it may be extended and elaborated.

Perhaps the wish that something might happen becomes the belief that it can happen. The sex industry, to an extent, reinforces this. Pseudo-medical potions to virilise or feminise people are sold unchecked. Advertisements by commercial organisations for such preparations as topical applications, said to contain oestrogen and to produce 'breast' growth at exorbitant cost, seem, in the author's view, to be little different from the sale of opium by the East India Company to the Chinese, or 'firewater' to the North American Indians.

We know far too little about the development of individual sexuality. Plainly it is a wide-open field for research, but in publishing the results of studies, even if one receives funding, one is up against people who shudder and say "We don't want to know about anything like that". As Reiss (1990) says: "Do we really want our scientists to be neutral and silent on issues that tragically impinge on our lives? ... It is time we rid ourselves of shame and timidity and started to speak out more honestly and openly about sexuality".

If the person has been referred as a result of a court appearance, the guilt and shame of the court process with the ostracism, even hostility, of family and neighbours, is likely to cause him to see the psychiatrist as one more punitive authority figure. He is likely to feel that, if he can say what the psychiatrist wants to hear, the situation will be over as quickly as possible, so that he can retire deeper into the 'closet', withdrawing into an even more secret and private world. The problem is that long-suppressed feelings demand acknowledgement. Eventually, he may be in even worse trouble.

Counselling may help to acknowledge the hidden issues, and address socialisation problems. This may help him to redirect or contain fantasies, but he is likely to need to continue acting them out. The loneliness that is intrinsic with the closet situation is difficult to redress. There are groups, such as the Forum Society, that meet and play out scenarios which are clearly fantasies and set boundaries that ensure safety. However, social attitudes and the likelihood of exposure in the press force them underground, among less trustworthy groups.

Sexual preference

Introducing a talk to a group of student community health nurses, the author asked them what was in their minds when they chose their clothes for the day. They looked nonplussed and said "I pick what suits me" and "I like to feel good". The suggestion that their intention was to 'catch' a man produced a murderous atmosphere. The question relied on the fact that no liberated woman would openly admit such a thought, at least not in those words. The trap was sprung: "Why do you, then, assume that a transvestite dresses only with the intention of attracting a man?" The idea has already been proposed that gender is to do with personality and self-expression and, for most transvestites, this is what it is all about.

Three kinds of homosexuality have to be considered. There are those whose locus of gender identity is followed logically towards a homosexual identity. Others emphasise a clearly masculine identity, but find relationships with men more comfortable. Among the former are some 'drag artists', who parody the female stereotype in an exaggerated way. These have generally been the most publicly visible, and form the public perception of transvestism, possibly a more comfortable one. Thus there is a dichotomy in gay culture that parallels the gender dichotomy in heterosexual culture. This is best illustrated by certain cultures in South America, where there are masculine 'hombres' and feminine 'homosexuals'.

There are still others who may not see themselves as gay, but are simply 'turned on' by men or male anatomy. For them, it is their erotic target, just as some people are heterosexual but are 'turned on' by rubber mackintoshes.

Most people's sexual target is the logical result of their sexual identity, which corresponds to their gender identity. That it does not always do so explains some of the confusion that many people feel. However, Kinsey *et al* (1948) suggested that people are each somewhere on a line between exclusively heterosexual and exclusively homosexual. Many people have had a homosexual experience at some time in their lives, although they are otherwise heterosexual.

Some transvestites, in exploring the female gender role, may follow it through into the sex role. They may fantasise a lesbian encounter with a woman, or a reversed heterosexual encounter with a man. In the former case, they may well antagonise their wives. A woman would feel, quite reasonably, that if she wanted to be lesbian, she would have found a real woman. In the latter case, a transvestite who had always thought of himself as heterosexual, but following the natural course of the 'female' role, may afterwards experience considerable emotional distress.

Expression of personality

Of the four kinds of transgenderists, the dual role transvestite is at once the most complex and the least understood outside the transgender community and professionals who specialise in them. They are a widely varying group. Some are simply men who like to wear dresses. Some are flamboyant, some demure – the 'twin set and pearls' people. Some are marginal transsexuals, or are transsexuals who have adopted a compromise.

Transvestites typically begin dressing around the age of eight or in puberty. Some begin later in life, sometimes after a trauma, such as loss of a partner. Usually the small boy cross-dresses in secret, not with any guilt, perhaps, but knowing he should not talk about it. If he manages to acquire a small collection of clothes, he will become an expert in finding hiding places for them.

Teenage years are, for most cross-dressers, an extremely erotic experience. Many continue as fetishists, extending their sexual scripts into formalised rituals, like the French maid or dominance/submission scenarios. Many others, however, find that, as the erotic component diminishes, they simply enjoy dressing for its own sake and find it tremendously relaxing; that is, except for the guilt that deepens with the knowledge that it is wrong to have certain feelings as a man, and even more wrong to express them as a woman.

So-called 'closet' transvestites cross-dress in complete secrecy, often without the knowledge of even their closest family. Their numbers are unknown, but a week's community service advertisements would typically bring 200 calls from that television area alone.

Many transvestites follow a very similar path, although it is followed without any knowledge of others, and there are clearly common issues. The enjoyment of experimenting with one's image and the enjoyment of personal adornment is, of course, a fundamental right of all human beings. Attempts have been made to market skirts for men and more decorative underwear. However, transvestites point out that, while this is a factor, at least part of the motivation comes from the fact that it is women's clothes that they are wearing. Bland (1994*b*) has offered some hypotheses, based on the male identity and its ability to form relationships, and also as a Freudian incorporative defence mechanism.

Usually they begin to accept that it is a need within them. Generally, a transvestite appears before the psychiatrist at the urging of his wife and family, having confessed or been discovered. Clearly the psychiatrist is in a quandary. If he, or she, urges the client to 'keep on dressing' but enjoy it a bit more, his family will be horrified. Aversion therapy is sometimes tried, but the general opinion is that it not very effective. Indeed, reasons have been put forward why it is counterproductive (Haslam, 1994).

A solution is to counsel both partners in an attempt to negotiate a compromise. There are several networking groups that offer support to transvestites, partners, or both. There are also some that may do damage. Helpful support can be given to transvestites and their families by the Beaumont Trust, which operates a telephone helpline. The trust was formed by a group of professional consultants, counsellors and others engaged in helping work. The feelings of isolation can be approached by joining the Beaumont Society, or one of the other groups with a postal membership. Lines of communication can be set up without the person revealing himself. Wives and families can also share feelings and experiences, either through the Beaumont Trustline, or the Women of the Beaumont Society.

With the opportunity to express their feelings more freely, the compulsion to do so is reduced, and reduces to a need. In giving himself permission to cross-dress, the transvestite gains the freedom to be himself, with the responsibility to avoid distress to others.

At the beginning, however, many transvestites are unbelievably sexist, even in their 'female' role and, too often, their wives eventually require psychiatric help. Fortunately there are an increasing number of couples who have made a success of their unconventional relationship, and have been willing to share their experience publicly. It requires a reappraisal of fundamental attitudes instilled from childhood, for both partners, yet, for both, it can be a liberating experience.

Some idea of this can be gained from the accounts of women who have cross-dressed, although a discussion about why there are few women transvestites is beyond the scope of this article. They speak of being free to express themselves in a more direct manner, of having greater personal space, of being free to assert themselves.

The transvestites who appear on talk-shows like *Kilroy* or *The Time and the Place*, seem perfectly at ease with their situation. However, it is clear from many of their accounts they have each gone through some period of distress and confusion at some point in their lives. In effect, they have done the psychiatrist's job for themselves. This may seem a startling thing to consider. Surely they are disordered, and need treatment? But they are living their lives very successfully – why change them?

Why is it so special to be male or female, when it is simply a result of nature's coin-toss? Perhaps the bizarre stereotypes portrayed by the media are a reaction to the social realisation that "Men and women, boys and girls, are more alike than they are different" (Gross, 1987, quoting Maccoby).

Perhaps transvestites challenge the established order more effectively than any feminist can and, perhaps, this is why the tabloid press reacts with ridicule – it is something so disturbing that it has to be cut down to size. Yet there is hope. A local paper recently reported a civic function without finding it necessary to report that one of the councillors was transsexual. BBC Television News recently showed an item about an alternative fashion designer without dwelling on the fact that he was a transvestite.

Gender identity

Clearly, at least part of what has so far been described can be classified as a gender identity disorder, in that some of those described can only express their full personality by constructing two different identities, living alternately in different roles. Diagnostic manuals classify it as such, rather than as a multiple personality disorder, where the move between roles is often involuntary.

It has been suggested that cross-dressing erodes the male identity. However, there is a world of difference between, on the one hand, a child having a, perhaps, too rigid role imposed on it and, on the other, gaining an internalised sense of value in being male. There is an untested hypothesis that most young transvestites follow a specifically male path in their everyday life. They enter male-stereotyped careers, such as building and lorry-driving, or enter the forces or the judicial system, and many are highly successful. Often they have accepted their fate at an early stage. Bullough & Bullough (1993) suggest that they protect their male identity by building a separate female one. If the person feels inhibited in assigning areas of self-expression to the alternative female identity, he may be more likely to become dissatisfied with his male life.

The usual clinical term is 'gender dysphoria', which is defined as a feeling of acute dissatisfaction with the gender of assignment. However, the rider is added that the person also seeks clinical assistance with hormonal or surgical treatment. This implies that he, or she, needs to change gender role permanently, that is, he or she is transsexual. The process, popularly called the 'sex change', is gender reassignment or, more recently, gender confirmation.

Many health workers refuse to take transsexuals seriously, and certain health managers have labelled the process 'elective surgery'. It is clearly more than a whim, if someone goes through hours of painful electrolysis to remove beard growth, takes powerful medication, then asks for major surgery. Not only that, but transsexuals risk losing families, friends and careers. They risk the prurient curiosity of Fleet Street and social rejection, becoming fourth class citizens outside the law as far as equal rights legislation is concerned.

In the majority of cases transsexuals are rational people, often highly intelligent. There are some who have achieved great fame, and have become extremely successful in their lives and their careers. One of the most famous is Caroline Cossey. Her success seems attributed to her gender change rather than her personality, but one does not become a top international model simply by being a pretty face. Stephanie Anne Lloyd, figurehead of a chain of sex shops, was once a highly successful salesman and is now a highly successful saleswoman. A transsexual acquaintance of mine has just landed a £250 000 order to write computer software.

It is probably the only condition where clients arrive at the psychiatrist's office with a ready-made self-diagnosis and a self-prescribed therapeutic path. It is often very difficult to persuade them to question it, but the simple fact is that there is no diagnostic measure. This is why reputable consultants are so keen on networking between individual clients and themselves, as happens with the Gender Trust and the biennial GENDYS conferences. By observing changing attitudes, and a community of people who have achieved success, or not, in various ways, they have a reference with which to compare their clients.

Transsexuals may present themselves to the psychiatrist at any age from 7–70. Many small children experiment with gender in dressing-up games. Some, from a very young age, persist in feminine-type play patterns. Green (1987), in a study of such children, found that most grew up to be homosexual, without any apparent gender disorder. Some others, by the age of 9 or 10, show great distress, with apparently insoluble emotional problems, until the truth comes out. St George's Hospital in London is carrying out a great deal of work on paediatric gender identity problems.

Often, however, transsexuals decide their future path during the teenage years. Since their secondary sexual characteristics have not fully formed, they are likely to have an easier passage than more mature clients. It is usual to place them on a hormonal regime that will hold their sexual development in stasis until they reach the age of majority. It is felt that they are then capable of an adult decision. If they decide to continue their original gender role, cessation of medication should allow their sexual development to resume.

People who had exhibited such symptoms from an early age were for a time called primary transsexuals, while others, who had progressed in their original gender role successfully until adulthood, were termed secondary transsexuals. This terminology has now fallen into disuse, since the main problem is that the psychiatrist has to rely on clients' accounts of their past lives. Blanchard & Steiner (1990) suggest that psychoanalysis is not usually successful, and, perhaps, clients see the therapist as simply an impediment in reaching their goal. However, the client is often highly defensive about his past, and may have unwittingly rewritten it.

This is particularly true of mature clients, who are also likely to have considerable problems in adopting the new role. They invariably have male speech patterns and mannerisms to unlearn, while they learn feminine ones. Usually they have developed an unmistakably masculine frame and facial bone structure. Middle-aged and older clients may be more successful, since many post-menopausal women develop more masculine facial features.

Unlike the transvestite, who can construct two separate vital identities, such people have often struggled to maintain a masculine identity and failed. Transvestites who appear in the media, and at social meetings, at ease with themselves, tend to project an aura of being happy to be 'men in dresses'. The person seeking to review his gender role may reject the idea and move more towards being a transsexual. To suggest to the client that he is a transvestite will invariably be counterproductive, for the term is just as pejorative as the term fetishist is to a transvestite. He is likely to leave and look for another psychiatrist. "An over-clinical or technical approach to classification and management by professionals can rob an individual of his or her true authorship of present acts and future possibilities" (Tully, 1995).

The psychiatrist's aim is to be sure that the person is realistic about his, or her, future life, emphasising "the quality of life for patients as the major measure of the effectiveness of health care" (Reid, 1995). In the process he is likely to antagonise the client, or the partner and family. He may also attract the unwelcome attentions of the press and the censure of professional peers. One might ask why psychiatric consultants would put themselves out on a limb in this way. The answer is that they know the depth of human suffering that gender confusion brings about, which cripples lives and, too often, leads to suicide.

Yet many clients bring mental baggage with them. As Tully (1995) puts it, there are many individuals "who have failed to find any commanding meaning for unhappy and unconsummated feelings. There, particularly, can be found a longing for a heroic and clear-cut career of transexual salvation".

Occasionally neuroses or psychoses are complicated by cross-gender wishes. The author has come across two people, one of whom had been diagnosed with borderline Münchausen syndrome, and the other a chronic exhibitionist. For the first, the 'other' was one of his alternative personas; for the other he had, it seemed, a need to shock, a need to gain attention.

Another had been diagnosed as a borderline paranoid schizophrenic, and the reluctance of consultants to entertain the idea of gender change made him resentful to the point of questioning, in public, the consultant's abilities. The psychiatrist has the unenviable task of deciding whether a given neurosis is the cause, or the result of, the cross-gender feelings, or simply incidental.

For instance, the years of frustration and confusion can bring about depression. Can the consultant be sure that the change will alleviate this, as the person is freed to become him or herself? Transsexuals can be as depressive as anyone else. A post-operative transsexual, writing in one of the community newsletters, freely admits that she suffers from clinical depression, yet she is much happier as a female clinical depressive than she was as a male clinical depressive.

This is the purpose of the 'real life test' in which the client is told, in effect, "Go out and try it". One of the criteria was that he/she should be able to gain employment, although in these times, it is difficult for anyone. The other is that the person should build up a good supportive social network, including, ideally, the family. Partners and parents are often in a dreadful situation, and attempts are being made to set up family counselling and support groups. There should, in any case, be a positive forward-moving approach. Often the client is dazzled by the glamorous vision of their new life, and sometimes they cheat in the real life test. The best criterion for the consultant is a subjective feeling that the client is being honest, and clients who express doubts and fears may well be more likely to achieve success.

The qualifications for a gender consultant and guidelines for therapy are provided by the Harry Benjamin Standards of Care (Walker *et al*, 1981), although they have a distinctly American flavour. They speak of a 'clinical behavioural scientist', which would seem to equate, in Britain, to a clinical psychologist. In this country, however, gender consultants are usually psychiatrists, not least because they can prescribe drugs. In addition, however, a gender consultant is required to have good counselling qualifications, with considerable experience of working in a gender identity clinic.

Clients often present with a range of body-image disorders. The years of dissatisfaction with a body that does not accord with the feelings about themselves as people causes them to reconstruct their internal mental body maps. Many men come to imagine themselves as having small feminine hands, broad hips and so on. Others come to imagine their genital area as female. The constant reminder of the presence of their male organ has, from time to time, led to self-mutilation. Female-to-male transsexuals often have a history of wearing tight bandages around their chests to hide and inhibit the growth of their breasts. In addition, most males also have a totally unrealistic view of their ability to 'pass' in public.

Among such people are those who reject their sexual body. Men, having received orchidectomy, or women, having received hysterectomy and bilateral mastectomy, often become content to express an androgynous personality. This is qualitatively different from transsexualism, as that is usually defined as where the person feels him or herself as being of the opposite gender, and wants a body to accord with it. Yet each case is individual. Clinical boundaries can be illusory, and some clients can find one or another compromise.

This article has concentrated on male-to-female transsexuals. The literature about female-to-male transsexuals is not as complete, for they were relatively rare until a few years ago, although their numbers have recently risen very rapidly. They are not generally considered as complex, and seem to be more sure of themselves. There is an illuminating, although fictional, account in Rose Tremain's *Sacred Country* (1992). Generally, they find it so much easier to 'pass' in the new role that they simply fade into the community and have little to say about themselves, or to each other. There is now, however, a Female-to-Male Network with about 200 members.

The prescription of hormones

The prescription of hormones is an area of great controversy. Some consultants will not prescribe them until the real life test starts. Others prescribe them earlier, although not usually before three months after the first interview. They reason that there is diagnostic potential, based on their effect in reducing the male libido, and usually low doses are prescribed at first. The idea is that, with the erotic element reduced, the urge to cross-dress will be reduced. This is a somewhat stereotyped view of transsexualism, since many clients may cross-dress rarely or never, but still have an unshakeable view of their femininity. However, reduction of the libidinal frustration can help the client to review his inner feelings, if he is willing to do so. It is clear that what happens is self-diagnosis.

The author's feeling is that, depending on the dose, they may be less dangerous than many other drugs in everyday use, which often can be bought over the counter. It may be that the controversy arises, in part, from negativity about the idea of a man sterilising himself, even temporarily. The effect of low doses, prescribed for a short while, is said to disappear in time.

Even in large doses, the effect on the client's secondary sexual characteristics is not as great as popular myth would have us believe. The usual size of the breast tissue that forms is around 24 cm hemicircumference (Asscheman & Gooren, 1992), somewhat less than an A size bra. Many clients later have silicone implants. Weight gain tends to be around the waist rather than the hips. Beard and body hair growth is slower, but the former has to be removed by many hours of electrolysis.

The primary effect in men is sterility and a considerable reduction in seminal emission. There may be mood changes, varying widely from one client to another, possibly related to the bases of personality which Eysenck suggests are a function of individual neurological difference. In so far as mood affects individual psychology, there may also be changes in cognition. Bancroft emphasises the distinction between sexual appetite and sexual interest, which are mediated by different parts of the central nervous system. While appetite is reduced, interest is not likely to change.

The central theme in transsexual sexuality is to be made love to as a woman, not as a gay man. Some male-to-female transsexuals were always openly sexually attracted to men. Others may give themselves permission to express previously repressed attraction. Some, previously heterosexual, may feel "If I am now a woman, then I ought to be sexually attracted to men". Some make the switch, perhaps because they think it will please their psychiatrist. However, the stability of the change is debatable. Others are content to remain attracted to women.

Possible side-effects of medication should be clearly explained, so that clients give informed consent. Regular blood tests should be carried out by the client's GP, monitoring liver function and blood lipids. When taken orally, a large proportion of the hormone is metabolised by the liver and does not enter the blood stream (Asscheman & Gooren, 1992). The liver has considerable extra work to do. There is usually weight-gain, including the possibility of fluid retention. The main danger is an increased chance of deep vein thrombosis of the legs, and medication must stop three months before any planned surgical operation involving a general anaesthetic.

Many of the issues discussed above apply in reverse to female-to-male clients. They may become more aggressive, or allow themselves to be so. They develop male secondary sexual characteristics, such as whiskers, and changes occur in their voices. However, an important point is that the effect of medication is not reversible. Once secondary male characteristics form, they are permanent.

Surgery

Like anyone else involved in gender therapy, the surgeon has to be able to overcome negative feelings arising from his own gender identity. It should not be attempted by someone who has not had considerable experience of carrying out, or assisting with, an operation which is a delicate blend of urology and plastic surgery. Even so, patient satisfaction is variable. There is a choice of two operations. The standard Philips operation needs a sufficiency of penile and scrotal skin, and prolapse has occurred from time to time, requiring the patient to return for the alternative colovaginoplasty. Nowadays, it is usual to use the latter procedure immediately if there is any doubt: if, for instance, the patient has been circumcised (Royle, 1994).

In male patients sexual appetite is reduced, but if interest is raised enough erection and climax can occur; this means that the nerves involved in male climax before the operation can be incorporated in the constructed clitoris. For female-to-male transsexuals, the procedure is bilateral mastectomy and hysterectomy. Great efforts have been made to devise a aesthetically acceptable penis, but without total success, and most patients decide to manage without.

Post-operative care

Under NHS procedures, the case is considered closed as soon as the operation is complete, and if more help is required, the client has to reapply as a new patient. Many post-operative transsexuals simply wish to disappear quietly into the community. This is against the Harry Benjamin guidelines. American practice being privately funded, they suggest that the client pay in advance, to ensure that they return for post-operative follow-up. In addition, a lifelong prescription of hormones, at a lower dose, will be needed to protect against osteoporosis.

Conclusions

Whatever a person does is reflected through the mirror of their individual gender schemas, a mirror that has often been given to them complete with distortions. Dictionaries traditionally suggest that transvestites cross-dress "for sexual pleasure" while textbooks usually define a transsexual as "someone who, throughout life, has seen themself as being of the opposite sex". The cliché is "a woman in a man's body" (or vice versa). The reader will have gathered that, in the study of gender, nothing is that simple.

It is a challenging but rewarding field to work in. For the therapist to seek out, and modify, the distortions in his or her own mirror can be a liberating experience. The traditional medical paradigm of treatment and cure may not be appropriate. Clients often feel liberated by simply having someone with whom they can discuss ideas and feelings that they have never broached before. As one client said, "it was the first time in his life anyone had listened to him" (Purnell, 1994).

This chapter has attempted to cover a very large area of human experience in a few thousand words. The author's hope is that, having engaged the reader's interest, the references will prove to be useful further reading. Too rigid social definitions of masculine and feminine may themselves be unhealthy and Gross (1987) proposes an ideal where men

and women can find the best in themselves, regardless of whether we
now consider it masculine or feminine.

References

Asscheman, H. & Gooren, L. J. G. (1992) *Hormone Treatment in Transexuals.*
Second International Gender Dysphoria Conference 1992, Manchester University.
London: The Beaumont Trust; Amsterdam: The Free University Hospital.

Bancroft, J. (1989) *Human Sexuality and its Problems.* Edinburgh: Churchill
Livingstone.

Blanchard, R. & Steiner, B. W. (1990) *Clinical Management of Gender Identity Disorders
in Children and Adults.* Washington, DC: American Psychiatric Press.

Bland, J. (1994*a*) Born that way ... or made? In *GENDYS 1994. Report of the Third
International Gender Dysphoria Conference.* Belper, Derbyshire: GENDYS
Conferences.

—— (1994*b*) *Transvestism: Four Monographs.* Belper: The Derby TV/TS Group.

Brierley, H. (1979) *Transvestism.* Oxford: Pergamon Press.

Bullough, V. L. & Bullough, B. (1993) *Cross Dressing, Sex and Gender.* Philadelphia:
University of Pennsylvania.

Green, R. (1987) *The Sissy Boy Syndrome and the Development of Homosexuality.*
New Haven, CT: Yale University Press.

Gross, R. D. (1987) *Psychology: The Science of Mind and Behaviour.* London: Hodder
& Stoughton.

Haslam, M. T. (ed.) (1994) *Transvestism: A Guide* (2nd edn). London: Beaumont
Trust.

Kinsey, A. C., Pomeroy, W. B. & Martin, C. E. (1948) *Sexual Behaviour in the Human
Male.* Philadelphia: W. B. Saunders.

Money, J. (1985) *The Destroying Angel: Sex, Fitness and Food in the Legacy of
Degeneracy Theory, Graham's Crackers, Kellogg's Corn Flakes and American
Health History.* Buffalo, NY: Prometheus Books.

—— & Ehrhardt, A. (1972) *Man, Woman, Boy and Girl: The Differentiation and
Dimorphism of Gender Identity from Conception to Maturity.* Baltimore: Johns
Hopkins Press.

Purnell, A. (1994) Gender counselling and its problems. In *GENDYS 1994, Report
of the Third International Gender Dysphoria Conference.* Belper, Derbyshire:
GENDYS Conferences.

Reid, R. (1995) *Transsexualism, The Current Medical Viewpoint.* London: Press for
Change, BM Network.

Reiss, I. L. (1990) *An End to Shame: Shaping our Next Sexual Revolution.* Buffalo:
Prometheus Books.

Royle, M. (1994) Gender confirmation surgery: male to female. In *GENDYS 1994,
Report of the Third International Gender Dysphoria Conference.* Belper, Derbyshire:
GENDYS Conferences.

Tremain, R. (1992) *Sacred Country.* London: Hodder & Stoughton.

Tully, B. (1995) Transsexualism and transhomosexuality as gender-identity 'career'
developments. In *The New Psychologist* (eds L. Brown & M. Benjamin), pp. 39–
44. Milton Keynes: Open University Psychology Society.

Walker, P. A., Berger, J. C., Green, R., *et al* (1981) *Harry Benjamin Standards of Care: the hormonal and surgical sex reassignment of gender dysphoric persons* (2nd revision). Sonoma, California: The Harry Benjamin International Gender Dysphoria Association.

11 Counselling and sex therapy for couples with psychosexual problems

Jane Roy

Theoretical approaches ● *Sex therapy* ● *Sex therapy or relationship counselling?*

This chapter looks at how couple counselling or sex therapy can help when a psychosexual problem is having an impact on a couple's relationship. If individuals asking for help with sexual problems are in relationships it can be more effective to offer help to the couple rather than the individuals. The two approaches are described and the relative merits of each are discussed using case examples.

Couples who ask for relationship counselling usually describe a particular presenting problem which has caused them to seek help. Sometimes this is very general such as "We are arguing a lot" or "We seem to have drifted apart". This type of statement implies the couple are accepting a shared responsibility for the problem. However, when the problem described is more specific, such as a sexual problem, the couple often label the problem as belonging to only one of them. The choice of partner to blame is usually based on their perception of what is normal in a relationship. The partner of a transvestite would probably say that it is his problem and he may agree with her. If one partner has lost interest in sex they will both often agree that it is that person's problem. Couples living together expect to be having a sexual relationship so the one who is asking for sex is considered 'normal' by both.

Counsellors are taught to explore the presenting problem in the context of the relationship as a whole, and to avoid labelling the problem as belonging to one partner or the other. It is often the case that the person accepting the problem as their own is actually quite resentful and will become angry with the counsellor for agreeing it is his or her problem. Exploring the wider context of the problem enhances the likelihood that it can be resolved.

Case 1
John and Mary Smith are in complete agreement that the problem is Mary's. Over the last two years she has lost all interest in sex. However, when the counsellor explores the couple's relationship in more detail she discovers that Mary is angry because she feels

her husband is more interested in his work than her. She is also left to cope with the children alone because John gets home from work so late. The counsellor helps Mary and John explore what would make Mary feel more valued by John and how John could play a bigger role in caring for the children. The counsellor finds that by helping them to explore these issues constructively, Mary's anger begins to reduce. John finds Mary is becoming warmer and more affectionate again as he shows his willingness to modify his working patterns. After several weeks of counselling the tension in their relationship is greatly reduced and Mary's sexual feelings begin to return.

If Mary's underlying resentments had not been addressed and resolved in the counselling it is unlikely that she would have recovered her sexual desire. If Mary and John's counsellor had accepted that the problem was purely Mary's loss of desire, Mary may well have become angry with the counsellor and been uncooperative. In fact, if Mary and John had a good sex life in the past the sexual issue might be resolved without the counsellor spending much time looking at the couple's sexual relationship.

Counsellors will also explore the couple's childhoods and experiences of previous relationships, as the root causes of the problem may pre-date the relationship. When the problem clearly pre-dates the relationship it can be tempting to see it as belonging to one client and to see the other partner as an 'innocent' victim or bystander. Help may then be offered to the 'sick' partner and the focus shifts from the couple's relationship to the individual. However, the relationship counsellor is interested in what attracted the couple together and why they both entered the relationship. It may be that the apparently innocent one is playing a role in keeping the problem going. If this is the case, focusing help on the sick person may not resolve the couple's problem. There is also some danger that it will create such tension in the relationship, as the healthy partner attempts to maintain the status quo, that the sick person will feel the only way to become healthy is to end the relationship.

Case 2

Roger and Janet Jones have come for counselling because Roger is not interested in sex. The counsellor discovers that Roger's lack of sexual desire stems from sexual abuse he suffered in his childhood from his aunt. Roger says that his sex drive has always been low and is nothing to do with Janet. When the counsellor explores why Janet was attracted to Roger, Janet says Roger was different from her previous boyfriends who had given her the impression they only wanted her for sex; Roger was kind and thoughtful and did not rush her into having sex with him. In other words, Roger's difficulty with sex was one of the reasons which brought them together.

The counsellor then explores what has changed to make them discontented with their sex life now. Janet says she thought Roger would become more interested in sex once they were married and this did not happen. Roger says he finds all sexual contact an effort and he was pleased that Janet appeared to be undemanding. He cannot understand why she seems to want more sex now they are married. The counsellor feels that Roger made an effort sexually to attract Janet but now he has married her he does not have the same incentive to continue to do something he has always found stressful. So as Janet's expectations were increasing, Roger's level of sexual activity actually reduced.

Counsellors do not always see couples together at every session. It is sometimes appropriate to see them separately or to give one client more sessions than the other. Roger and Janet's counsellor, for example, may feel that Roger needs some individual sessions to talk through his abuse. Roger may also feel more comfortable doing this without Janet present. However, the counsellor is likely to recommend that Janet attends one session in four so that they can look together at the impact on their relationship of the issues raised as Roger deals with his abuse. They would move back to regular joint sessions when Roger, Janet and the counsellor feel the couple are ready to focus on their relationship again.

Theoretical approaches

Object relations theory

This was first developed by Melanie Klein and looks at how babies deal with conflicting good and bad feelings towards their primary carer. The theory suggests that if the young child does not learn to cope successfully with these conflicting feelings, then in later life the individual is likely to suppress either one set of feelings or the other. Thus in a close relationship the individual will have a tendency to see their partner as all good or all bad. The unconscious feelings are then sometimes displaced on to other people. A couple may have a strong bond where they each see the other as good, and they both suppress their bad feelings and project them on to the rest of the world. A couple behaving like this may have an apparently close and intimate relationship but describe themselves as like brother and sister rather than lovers. This is because they have unconsciously associated sex with bad feelings and so it gets repressed along with other bad feelings. Alternatively the bad feelings are expressed and the good feelings are repressed or projected on to the outside world. The third alternative for the couple is that one partner is the good partner and the other the bad partner. It is important for the counsellor to recognise these processes if they are present. The counsellor is part of the outside world and may find the couple projecting their repressed good or bad feelings on to the counsellor.

Attachment theory

This was developed by John Bowlby and suggests that children need to form a secure attachment to their primary carer. If this process is damaged, for example by the death of the carer, the individual may grow up unable to form close attachments to someone else. If the process is disrupted because the carer is unable to care adequately, then the individual may never be confident that they can form a secure bond. Someone who forms an anxious attachment in adult life may make heavy sexual demands on their partner because it is their way of seeking reassurance. This can easily lead to loss of desire in their partner.

Psychodynamic theory

An aspect of psychodynamic theory which can be relevant to couples' counselling is Oedipal theory. As a child grows it begins to identify with the same sex parent, but also sees that parent as a competitor for the other parent's attention. If the parents have a good relationship then the child is able to work through the issues of identification and competition. However, if the parents' relationship is poor, the opposite sex parent may use the child as a substitute for their partner. For example, a woman whose husband is rather distant may turn to her son for closeness and emotional support. This can make it difficult for the son to grow up and form an adult sexual relationship. If he forms a relationship, his partner may be quite jealous of the closeness between him and his mother and feel excluded. In the counselling room the counsellor may then find the clients are competing for his or her attention.

Systems theory

This looks at where the couple or the family fit in their social context and what kinds of rules they have learnt about the right way to behave. The woman who has lost interest in sex may have picked up negative messages about sex from her family such as "nice girls don't enjoy it".

She may marry a man whose family also gave him this message. The counsellor is likely to find that attempts to help improve the couple's sex life are met with resistance from both partners because they are both uncomfortable at the idea of the wife enjoying sex.

For some couples insight and understanding alone can be enough to enable them to solve the problem between them. However, greater understanding of the problem does not always by itself make it go away. In this situation the counsellor needs to help the couple negotiate a solution that works for them.

Case 2 continued

Roger and Janet Jones find that exploration of Roger's abuse has brought them closer together and they understand themselves and each other a lot better. Janet is now more patient with Roger about sex. However, the frequency of their sexual contacts has not increased and Janet still feels she wants more from Roger. Roger is also beginning to feel he may be missing out on something. The counsellor helps them to explore their sexual relationship so that they can begin to decide how to increase the frequency of sexual contact in a way which would be pleasurable to them both. This negotiation leads to them trying out some of the ideas they have discussed. Roger begins to realise that when Janet starts caressing him when they are watching TV he distances himself, because this is what his aunt used to do. However, they discover that Roger can cope with Janet making advances to him in other situations. Roger discovers that he needs to start by talking to Janet about his feelings before he touches her so that she does not put pressure on him by assuming he is willing to have intercourse.

In the examples given so far the assumption has been that it is possible for the counsellor to help the couple find a way of resolving the difficulties between them. Unfortunately this is not always the case. Sometimes helping the couple explore their problem shows that the gulf between them is too wide for a satisfactory solution to be possible. In this situation the only option might be to help the couple separate as amicably as possible.

Case 3

Robin and Susan Roberts have come for counselling because Susan has discovered Robin dressing in her clothes and putting on her make-up. Now his secret is out, Robin wants Susan to accept his need to cross-dress. While their children are young he is willing to confine his cross-dressing to the house and only do it when the children are out. Susan is unable to accept this solution and feels he should stop cross-dressing altogether.

> The counsellor finds that there are no compromises that are acceptable to both Susan and Robin. The counselling then moves on to discuss separation and what to tell the children.

If a couple have a good relationship in areas other than sex, or in other words they feel that any rows or tensions between them are a result of the sexual problem rather than a contributor to its cause, sex therapy may be appropriate rather than general relationship counselling. Sex therapy is most effective with the specific problems of impotence, premature ejaculation, vaginismus, anorgasmia and dyspareunia, where there is no underlying physical cause. If the sexual problem has an organic cause, sex therapy can also be useful to enable a couple to explore alternative ways of giving each other sexual satisfaction and enjoying a physical relationship. Sex therapy can be appropriate for disorders of desire in both men and women so long as the loss of desire does not reflect an underlying dislike of the partner.

Couples asking for sex therapy are carefully assessed for their suitability. This usually involves a joint interview followed by an individual interview for each partner. The joint interview enables the therapist to see how the couple interact, so that he or she can assess whether the relationship seems to be sound, apart from the sexual difficulty. The purpose of the individual sessions is to allow each person to talk freely about their past sexual experiences and their sexual experiences in the relationship. It also enables the therapist to explore wider issues which may have an impact on the person's self-perception and hence their views about their sexuality.

Behavioural theory

This is the principal theory underlying the therapeutic approach in sex therapy. The theory can be used to explain why the dysfunctioning individual has a problem. The man with premature ejaculation may have learnt to come quickly when he masturbated in his teens. This may have been his way of minimising the risk of being found masturbating by his parents. Unfortunately, having learnt to come quickly he may find it hard to unlearn this behaviour when he gets a partner, particularly if his early sexual experiences with partners involved a risk of discovery. A man with retarded ejaculation may have used a very vigorous masturbation technique and he may find that the friction between his penis and the walls of the vagina is not sufficient to enable him to reach a climax.

The learning can be more general. A woman who grows up in a family where the television is switched off every time something sexy or erotic is on, and whose mother gives her the impression sex is something women have to put up with rather than enjoy, may learn to be inhibited about sex.

She will then take this learnt inhibition into her adult sexual relationships. Sometimes the learning does not appear to be directly connected to sex. A boy may be taught that it is unmanly to show emotion or be physically demonstrative. He may have been given messages that sex is a normal healthy activity for a man. Unfortunately, when he is in a relationship as an adult this may mean he focuses all his needs for affection and attention into sex. His partner might complain that he is sexually demanding and rarely shows her affection at other times. This can easily lead to her feeling resentful and losing her sexual desire.

Although some sex therapists adopt a purely behavioural approach to the therapy and to explaining the client's problem, many do not. Therapists also use the theories described earlier to help understand the couple's problem and what is maintaining it. It is important for the therapist to understand the 'normally' functioning partner's role in maintaining the sexual problem. It is very common for couples to show resistance to the therapeutic tasks at some point in the therapy, and the more general theories of marital interaction can be useful in helping the therapist understand what the resistance is about.

Sex therapy

The therapy itself is task-centred, based on providing the couple with a new positive learning experience. This is achieved by giving the couple tasks to do at home, starting with a non-sexual touching exercise designed to be non-threatening. The tasks get slowly more sexual as the weeks progress, until intercourse is resumed. The couple are normally banned from attempting intercourse until the therapist gives permission. Typically they are asked to spend one hour three times a week on the set task. They then tell the therapist at the next appointment how they got on, and on the basis of the discussion of this feedback the therapist sets a new task.

The early sexual tasks are called 'sensate focus' and their aim is to help the couple learn how to get pleasure from touching their partner's body without performance anxiety. The partners take it in turns to touch; while one is touching the other lies passive, but thinks about what they are enjoying and why. The couple are encouraged to share information about what has pleased them. The individuals may also be given tasks to do on their own, aimed at helping them feel relaxed and comfortable with their own bodies. This is particularly important for people who have never masturbated or who have developed masturbation techniques which are a hindrance to their pleasure with their partner. As the therapy progresses the therapist will take into account not only the couple's feedback but the specific dysfunction being treated and relevant information from the individuals' backgrounds.

The man suffering from premature ejaculation will be taught how to recognise the point of inevitability so that he can stop stimulation, or signal to his partner to stop stimulation, until the feeling of urgency has eased; then the stimulation can be resumed. The man who has difficulty maintaining erections is encouraged to stimulate himself until he has a firm erection and then stop until the erection fades and then restimulate himself. This enables him to gain confidence that if an erection goes he can get it back again. When he can do this confidently on his own his partner will then do the stimulating. Sexual intercourse will only be resumed when he is confident that lost erections can be regained. The woman with vaginismus is encouraged to put a finger or small vaginal trainer into her vagina to gain confidence that penetration is possible. She will only be asked to insert the penis when she is comfortable with three fingers or a large trainer in her vagina. When she is comfortable with her own fingers her partner will be asked to insert his fingers.

If one partner has been abused, care will be taken to ensure that the couple develop a sex life which does not involve doing anything the abused person might find too difficult. If the abuse involved oral sex the couple may agree that this would be something they would not do. The abuse survivor may prefer to avoid certain intercourse positions, keep the lights on and to be in a position where he or she can see their partner's face. Different solutions will be appropriate for different couples.

When the dysfunction is specific and not a disorder of desire it is possible to take an individual through a sex therapy programme without his or her partner. However, there can be a limit to what can be achieved when only the dysfunctional individual is seen. A woman with vaginismus can become confident that her vagina is large enough for the penis to fit by inserting fingers or trainers; however, if she has a phobia about the penis, using fingers or trainers may not be enough to enable her to cope with intercourse. It also ignores the couple's relationship dynamics. The man in a relationship with a woman with vaginismus may be able to be very patient and understanding because it enables him to avoid confronting his own fears about intercourse or the vagina. If this is the case, 'curing' the woman's vaginismus may mean her partner starts losing his erections or develops premature ejaculation. If he is part of the therapy this is much less likely to happen. Similarly, the man with impotence can learn to gain confidence that he can keep erections during masturbation. However, part of the problem might be the performance pressure from his partner who sees his inability to sustain an erection as proof he does not find her desirable. This pressure will increase, not reduce, once his partner is aware he can masturbate successfully. If the couple attend sessions together, the woman's fears and anxieties can be tackled in the therapy so that the pressure is minimised.

Sex therapy or relationship counselling?

Deciding whether sex therapy or more general relationship counselling is the most appropriate approach is not always easy. Generally speaking, if the couple have a basically good relationship and a specific sexual problem, then sex therapy is the best approach. When the problem is less specific, such as a disorder of desire, careful assessment is essential to ensure the couple receive the most appropriate help. Two case histories where the problem is superficially the same – the woman's loss of interest in sex – illustrate this.

Case 4

Peter and Angela Brown requested a sex therapy appointment because Angela had found sex getting progressively more difficult for her. Their sex life had now reached a point where Angela could not bear to be touched by Peter. Peter was very hurt by this and would alternate between trying to be sympathetic and understanding, and when this did not make a difference, getting angry and threatening to leave. They were adamant they had no other problems. Angela said she had recently seen a TV programme about survivors of sexual abuse where one woman had described how the abuse had affected her adult sex-life. Angela had never told anyone about her own abuse; she had wanted to forget it. After the programme she had told Peter who had been shocked but understanding at first. However, when there was still no improvement in their sex life, his anger had returned.

While taking the couple's histories, the therapist discovered that Angela's problem with sex had become worse as her daughter grew older; her daughter was now the same age as she was when the abuse happened. Angela confessed that she did worry about Peter's relationship with his daughter even though she knew this was irrational. She had not dared say this in front of him because she knew how hurt he would be. There were no major issues in Peter's background, but it was clear that although he desperately wanted to help Angela he had no idea how to do it. The therapist felt the couple had a strong relationship, but that Angela needed to talk through her abuse and explore the issues it raised for her. The therapist decided counselling was more appropriate for this couple at this stage.

Counselling helped Peter to understand what the abuse must have been like for Angela and enabled him to be more patient. Angela found exploring her fears about her daughter very helpful. Peter did feel hurt and angry, as Angela had feared, but the counsellor helped them both deal with these feelings constructively. Angela found she was able to be more relaxed and open with Peter and talk to him about sex. However, she could not stop herself freezing when he approached her. At this point the counsellor referred Peter and Angela back to the sex therapist.

The therapist realised that Angela needed to take an active part in deciding what the tasks should be each week, as she was very fearful of any sexual situation where she felt she had no choices. Peter could see that completing the tasks some weeks was very difficult for Angela. He was often anxious that they were not making enough progress, but he was mostly able to be patient with Angela and take his anxieties to the therapist. She was able to help them both see the progress they were making. Angela's abuse had involved her being forced to perform oral sex. She felt that she really would not be able to tolerate fellatio with Peter. Peter was very disappointed about this, since he saw fellatio as a sign that Angela loved him enough "to give everything" sexually. However, over the course of the therapy he could see that Angela was much more relaxed and could enjoy being caressed and masturbated. She was also able to caress him and became comfortable stroking his penis. This was something she had never done in the past. Peter eventually came to accept that their sex life was so much better that it was not worth risking damaging it by asking for oral sex. At the end of therapy Angela felt she had become much more comfortable with her sexuality and did not feel so threatened by Peter's. She felt things would continue to improve if Peter was able to continue being patient with her.

Case 5

Robert and Susan Green came for sex therapy because Susan had lost interest in sex. At their first assessment interview Robert was angry and defensive, insisting Susan could not love him because she did not want sex. Susan was in tears because she felt so pressurised. She sometimes woke up in the night to find Robert trying to have intercourse with her. In spite of the tension between them they were both agreed that there were no other major issues in their relationship. History-taking confirmed this. Susan had had no previous partners and sex had been "OK but not brilliant" initially. Susan had had a rather inhibited upbringing and was sexually passive. She did not initiate sex, but in the past had always been willing to say yes when Robert made an approach. She felt things had changed when she went back to full-time work. She had been very tired and sex seemed an effort, so she started to say no to Robert. The more she said no the more he began to pressurise her and the more she said no.

Robert agreed in his history that sex had started to deteriorate when Susan had gone out to work full-time. He felt that Susan had begun to lose interest in him and was anxious that she might be having an affair. His history showed that his parents' marriage had split up when he was 8: the age his son was when Susan started full-time work. He said that he knew pressurising Susan was counterproductive but he "couldn't stop himself". The therapist decided there really were no other major issues troubling this couple. The problem was probably a combination of Susan's sexual passivity and Robert's need for reassurance that she would not leave like his mother had. Susan's job meant that she had some financial independence and the opportunity to meet other men.

The therapist therefore decided to offer them sex therapy. The first few weeks of therapy were very difficult for Robert. He did not like the ban on intercourse and found only being allowed to touch sensually rather than sexually very frustrating. Susan found the boundaries a relief. At first she found touching Robert difficult as she was not used to doing it. She began to enjoy being touched as long as Robert "didn't take liberties". After a few weeks Susan found she could begin to enjoy touching Robert; he noticed this and really appreciated it. He was also beginning to realise that although they were not having intercourse they were having three hours a week of intimate physical contact, which was a lot more than they had had for a long time.

As Robert eased off the pressure, Susan found herself more able to open out and enjoy the tasks. By the end of therapy they had settled for a pattern of sex once or twice a week. Robert had accepted that sex would not always end in intercourse, and it was not the end of the world if Susan said no sometimes. Susan was able to be much more active sexually which Robert found very reassuring. She did not feel that she had to make instant decisions about whether she wanted intercourse when Robert touched her. She still found it difficult to take the initiative but she was able to acknowledge she had sexual feelings. She could also hint that she might be interested, for example by being affectionate when they were watching TV together in the evenings.

These two case histories show how what appears to be the same problem can have very different underlying causes. In the case of Peter and Angela it could be argued that the problem is Angela's and she is the one who needs help. However, seeing both partners enables Peter to understand Angela's problems better and to support her more effectively; he also has an opportunity to express his own feelings of anger or resentment and for these to be dealt with constructively. Robert and Susan's problem is more clearly in their interaction and it is difficult to see how they could have been helped effectively if one or other of them had been labelled the patient and seen for individual therapy.

Couple counselling and sex therapy enables the partners to share the responsibility for the solution of their problem, whatever its origins are. This can be a more effective method of resolving a sexual difficulty for someone who is currently in a relationship than treating that person as the patient and offering individual help. If confronting their difficulties together brings the couple to the realisation that it will not be possible to find a mutually acceptable solution, then counselling can help them to part as amicably as possible and minimise the harm to any children in the relationship.

12 An investigation of partnership problems in sex therapy

Patricia Gillan

Therapy for partnership problems ● *Sabotage of sex therapy* ●
Psychosexual disorders in relation to partnership problems

Various forms of sex therapy are available, but the more successful
therapy courses are based on behavioural or desensitisation methods.
In the late 1970s, sexual dysfunction clinics were set up in the UK for
couples. Historically the approach to sex problems had been for one
partner to be treated: the female partner would attend the gynaecologist
or family planning clinic if pain was involved; the male partner with an
erectile problem would most likely seek the services of a genital-urinary
specialist.

The new 'couple approach' was based on research by Wolpe (1958)
and Masters & Johnson (1966, 1970). The latter approach was too
complicated and time-consuming for the UK so a modified Masters &
Johnson approach was devised by clinics in Oxford (Bancroft, 1976), and
the Maudsley Hospital, London (Crowe *et al*, 1981). Couples were treated
on an out-patient basis and this movement spread from the NHS to marriage
guidance (now called Relate). The structure of the standardised sex
therapy course is well researched, although some clinics adopt more
modified techniques than others.

Therapy for partnership problems

Assessment

Some clinics send case history forms for couples to complete and this can
be the first test for a couple wishing to be screened for sex therapy; if only
one partner returns the forms this is a bad sign. During assessment each
partner talks in private with the therapist. Assessment can usually be a
good indicator of whether each partner is committed to therapy; is one
partner having an affair that they will not suspend for the sake of therapy?
If this is the case, some clinics will refuse to treat the couple until the
affair has been suspended or ended.

Are both partners consistently reporting facts? The Woody Allen film
Manhattan shows the male, on one side of the screen, bemoaning the fact

that "they almost never have sex" while simultaneously on the other side of the screen the female partner says that "he is always at it, wanting sex more than three times a week". Who should the therapist believe over the frequency of sexual intercourse? Another discrepant factor is "who usually initiates love-making?"

Sensate focusing or massage

The first stage in the modified Masters & Johnson therapy is an excellent indicator of what is happening in the relationship, especially regarding communication. It is helpful for the therapist to have some idea of how the couple behave when touching and how anti-massage they are in the clinic setting. The couple can be asked to hold hands or gently stroke one another's arms. If they fail to do this in the clinic, this is the first therapy 'danger signal' and care needs to be taken to get them to massage one another very gradually at home, starting with relaxing on the bed, sitting opposite one another with feet touching and maybe drinking a cup of tea. Homework could continue with a hand or foot massage in the bedroom. Some couples might complain about the cold conditions of British bedrooms. If this is the case a hot bath may be recommended before the massage; the bath may even be shared.

During this early stage of sex therapy some marital therapy tasks are included, such as 'give-to-get' tasks in which each partner requests a non-sexual task for the other to do on a daily basis. These tasks can be set one week and discussed the week after at the next therapy session. One useful task during therapy is to ask each partner to say three things that please them about their partner. This is good positive reinforcement for the start of therapy. Feedback the next week will highlight any communication problems.

At this stage it is good to suggest a back massage for one partner, then a changeover, so the giver becomes the receiver. The couple take it in turns to massage each other's fronts, not touching breasts or genital areas. The couple are asked to enjoy touch and appreciate giving as well as receiving: listening to what their partner wants, not what they think their partner ought to want, and experimenting with firm or light pressure. Often touch becomes pleasurable for the first time because nothing further is allowed; during these stages sexual intercourse is forbidden.

Resistance to massage could be due to fear or bad conditioning in the early years of the relationship. If this is causing a problem and the couple are making no progress after several massage sessions, then other homework focusing on 'orgasmic reconditioning' needs to be introduced before going on either to self-pleasuring or sensate focusing together.

Orgasmic reconditioning

During orgasmic reconditioning the man or woman starts masturbating with any fantasy that produces pleasure, but as orgasm becomes imminent the patient is instructed to switch to the image of the partner so that positive pleasure is associated with the partner during orgasm. The partner's image can be introduced progressively earlier during the task until the partner becomes a 'conditioned stimulus' and just thinking of him or her produces sexual arousal. For a fuller account of this method see Gillan (1987).

Self-focusing or masturbation

Masters & Johnson (1966) followed the massage exercises with mutual masturbation which they called genital sensate focusing. In the UK various therapists found that patients needed an in-between stage of 'self-exploration' before progressing to mutual masturbation with a partner.

Lobitz & LoPiccolo (1972) extensively researched masturbation methods for clients, especially women, with little sexual confidence, and devised a programme of "finding, looking at and touching genitalia, including fantasising if necessary". Initially individuals touch their genitals in private and then invite their partner to be present when they feel confident. Then the patient shows their partner where and how they like to be stimulated.

It is sad that even in these days some women and many men do not know about the existence of the clitoris. Maybe Freud (see Ernest Jones, 1955) instilled a feeling of guilt in women when he suggested that focusing on the clitoris was masculine and immature.

General sensate focusing or mutual masturbation

The couple progress to sensuous massage and learn to communicate what they want. Sometimes one partner is asked to guide the other partner's hand to the erogenous zone. There are pitfalls which the therapist can warn about, such as uncaring or rough touching of the genitals. Again the emphasis is upon caring, pleasure, relaxation, communication and feedback, with instructions to avoid striving for orgasms. This stage can last several sessions as partnership problems are highlighted and worked through.

Oral sex

Some therapists would suggest that the couple should now proceed to intercourse, but Gillan & Gillan (1976) recommend bridging genital sensate focusing with oral sex. This stage brings out guilt and fears. Some couples find oral sex embarrassing and need reassuring that it can be pleasurable and fun. Jam or honey can be spread on the genitals to make them more palatable.

Sexual intercourse

By this stage hopefully partnership problems will have been investigated and sorted out. If there are continuing problems over the genitals and the couple need reassurance and sex education, it is advisable to give them a physical examination before this last stage.

The first recommended position is the female superior position (FSP) or the 'woman on top'. If there are problems associated with power and control, this position could cause trouble, i.e. "I do not feel comfortable with her on top of me", "I think if I am on top of him this is too masculine". Direct objections are easy to cope with, as the therapist can point out that the position relieves the man of the need to check whether his penis is erect enough and of finding the entry: the woman takes care of this. The woman can be reassured about this position when the therapist explains that she can move more freely and her orgasms will be better.

In cases of vaginismus the therapist can point out that the woman is in control of penetration and she is not trapped by the man lying on top of her. More subtle problems are when the woman complains of pain; this could be caused by too brief genital sensate focusing, or by the woman kneeling too upright. The therapist should recommend the woman to lean forward more, to avoid deep penetration.

Other positions can be tried like the 'feel free position' in which the woman lies on her back with her legs over her partner, who is lying sideways. This is good for women with orgasmic problems who need some direct manual clitoral stimulation during penetration.

The 'animal position' can be pleasurable for many couples, with the woman kneeling and the man mounting from behind. The 'missionary position' could be described as 'the graduation position'.

Sabotage of sex therapy

At all stages of sex therapy one or both partners might sabotage the therapy. Typical methods of sabotage are by smelling of alcohol, nicotine or garlic, smearing the face with a thick greasy face cream, or wearing perfume that the partner hates. One of the most common sabotage problems is refusing to wear items that turn on the partner, for example black knickers and suspenders or a karate jacket. Refusing to make love in the nude is another type of sabotage. If this is a problem the therapist can suggest 'give-to-get' contracts: "If he will wash before lovemaking, I'll wear the frilly purple satin knickers he bought me". If the same lady continues to sport pink knickers and her partner is washing enthusiastically, then this is unfair and the contract is failing, and the therapist should point this out to the couple.

Some men genuinely find it difficult to be romantic during foreplay and whisper 'sweet nothings' in the woman's ear, or tell her what she wants to be told. Some women find it hard to be crude and talk dirty. This type of resistance is not usually sabotage, it is more like embarrassment, and role-playing can desensitise either partner to things that embarrass them. Role-playing can also help a couple to become more aware of their behaviour and how they appear. The therapist can play the role of one partner and exaggerate the characteristics that are spoiling the therapy, for example passive aggression, lack of assertion or constant criticism. Often getting partners to exchange roles is a good method of coping with sabotage.

Psychosexual disorders in relation to partnership problems

Vaginismus

Vaginismus is a spasm of the muscles surrounding the vaginal introitus, the effect of which is to prevent entry into the vagina. The spasm is not confined to the vaginal inlet but may affect the whole body. During initial examination the therapist may well find that inserting a finger is impossible.

Women with primary vaginismus have usually had a repressive upbringing. Secondary vaginismus cases may be the result of unpleasant experiences or physical trauma. In both types of case the women tend to choose partners with a certain type of personality: passive, gentle, unassertive. The women know they are safe with such a man, as he will not trap or overpower them and they can be controlled. Often the partner of a woman with vaginismus suffers from premature ejaculation; he tries to push his penis in and gets stimulated at the same time and becomes over-aroused and ejaculates before insertion. This can result in erectile problems for the man. This is an easy disorder to treat, although some clinics might question the 100% success rate that Masters & Johnson (1970) report. Plastic dilators can be given to the woman to insert when she is relaxing at home, and her partner can help to insert these size-graded dilators until she is ready for his penis. A physical examination can help in the presence of the male partner, and the therapist can show him where to place his finger.

Role-playing can be a good method to bring home some of the personality interactions between the couple. The man can learn how to be more personally effective by saying 'no' more often and trying to encourage his partner to try out the dilators: "You know the therapist said that you are responsible for change in yourself, but I do want to help you".

Anorgasmia

There are different types of anorgasmia. A woman suffering from primary anorgasmia has never experienced an orgasm under any condition. American therapists refer to this condition as 'pre-orgasmia' and this seems a more sympathetic label. Women who suffer from this often have had a strict upbringing, both from the family and religious point of view, and this often makes them feel guilty about sex. They probably never have masturbated. With partners they are often very inhibited and shy, some of them might not even get sexually aroused at all and their vaginas could remain dry during intercourse, and they could be quite tense. Other women complain that they get very excited and aroused and reach what Masters & Johnson call the 'plateau phase' but they are unable to "tip over into orgasm"; some of them admit they do not like losing control or making a fool of themselves.

The male partner can often become unsympathetic and demanding saying: "Well, have you come yet? Are you frigid or something? You do not seem to get turned on whatever I do". Some male partners have complained that they can get erectile problems as they cannot go on and on thrusting. Some men, however, report that it can lead to premature ejaculation as often the female message comes over as "Hurry up and come, dear, I do not want to be lying here for too long, experiencing little pleasure".

This condition is easy to reverse using therapy programmes devised by Lobbitz & LoPiccolo (1972) or Barbach (1975). Some homework on fantasies is helpful, and studies have been reported on the use of a vibrator (see Gillan, 1987). Some group therapy for women is usually available and this is effective for women, as they can become sexually confident and orgasmic before proceeding to sex with a partner. Once the course of therapy is underway the prognosis is excellent.

Secondary anorgasmia is when a woman ceases to be orgasmic, although she has experienced orgasms before. Often the woman finds that this is situational anorgasmia (i.e. she can masturbate to orgasm when alone, but with a partner difficulties arise and maybe she 'turns off' at the wrong moment). Some women can have orgasms with other men but not with their partners. Often in such cases there is a poor marital relationship which needs to be worked on and improved by contact therapy. Marital disharmony can lead to avoidance of sexual contact and touch. Role-playing is a good way of exploring these attitudes. It is also a good idea to discuss the bad conditioning aspects of striving for orgasm. Some couples need to focus on becoming more sexually confident with each other. A useful reference is Heiman *et al* (1976).

Prior to *The Hite Report* (1976), 'no hands orgasms' were thought to be normal. However, Hite pointed out that only 30% of women were orgasmic during sexual intercourse as they needed additional clitoral stimulation. Women realised that the need for direct manual stimulation was not part of an abnormal classification. Indeed, in sex therapy the 'lateral position' is recommended to enable manual stimulation to take place during coitus. Kaplan (1974) has recommended methods to achieve coital orgasm.

Another method of helping such women is to give them permission to indulge in private sexual fantasies during intercourse; they do not need to share their erotica with their partner. High sexual arousal is also associated with women taking the sexual initiative.

In the US, Heiman *et al* (1976) described how excited men became when they heard stories about women taking the initiative and inviting a man to make love with them. They also reported that women had similarly high arousal when they listened to tapes of such stories as their vaginal blood flow increased. Sex therapists utilised this research and emphasis was put on the therapeutic benefit of the development of fantasies in which women took the sexual initiative.

Another method used for orgasmic problems is for the woman to exaggerate what she is afraid of; some women fear that they look repulsive and unattractive when they orgasm. The therapist teaches them to exaggerate this fear and then to do this in front of their partner, so they become desensitised to such anxiety.

Situational anorgasmia is more difficult to treat and partner involvement is often the problem. A woman can feel confident and sexy on her own, thinking of highly arousing fantasies, but when partner participation becomes a reality her behaviour changes, her fantasies fade and guilt ensues. Therapists encourage women with such problems to enjoy their fantasies with a partner.

Erectile dysfunction

The word 'impotence' carries a certain emotive association and therapists prefer to talk about erectile dysfunction. Few men suffer from primary impotence or erectile dysfunction, where they have never had an erection strong enough for penetration and sexual intercourse. Anxiety and fear can play a large part in this disorder. This is a rare problem which is difficult for therapists to treat. It could be due to organic problems. The most common form of erectile problem is that of secondary impotence in which the man shows a persistent inability to obtain and/or maintain an erection sufficient to penetrate the vagina and conclude sexual intercourse. The man might be perfectly potent with another partner. This disorder leads to partnership problems, as sometimes the female partner thinks he is seeking and enjoying sex elsewhere.

The modified Masters & Johnson programme is helpful; anxiety and low sex interest can be monitored during therapy. The therapist should also examine what the couple's relationship is like and how much pressure the woman is putting on the man to perform, or how stressed he feels himself over his 'potency'. We live in a society where men rarely mention their sexual inadequacy, whereas women more freely admit their sexual difficulties.

The Masters & Johnson 'teasing technique', of stopping stimulation and then starting again during the genital sensate focus stage, can be effective.

This is a positive technique for the relationship as the man can be desensitised into actually losing his erection and depend on his wife to stimulate him again. Masters & Johnson stress how performance anxiety can be fatal for erectile problems and that no man can 'will' an erection. Stimulation therapy can help men with low sex interest.

Ejaculatory disorders

Premature ejaculation is easy to treat, using the Masters & Johnson squeeze technique. In this condition orgasm and ejaculation persistently occur before or immediately after penetration. The partner relationship is often good for men with this disorder, but sometimes the partner will encourage him to 'come' quickly if she does not enjoy coitus or has problems herself. The therapist should focus on their interaction.

Delayed ejaculation

This is more difficult to treat and often the relationship has gone sour, as one woman complained: "I have had enough of him and his pushing and poking for hours on end, he makes me really sore, I'm fed up with sex". It is a similar problem to anorgasmia in women with a fear of losing control. Marital or contract therapy can improve the relationship. Often men with this condition are 'emotionally constipated' and role-playing can help them to express their emotions. The delayed ejaculator needs a lot of extra stimulation and often stimulation therapy devised by Gillan & Gillan (1976) can help.

Low sex interest

This is a common complaint shared by men and women. Maybe they have never been interested in sex, inhibited by anxiety and guilt. They need to talk and read about sex. Often a relationship has become "boring and burnt out" and "stale-mate" has ensued. Stimulation therapy is an effective way of increasing the libido. This therapy enables couples to increase their sex drive by: learning to appreciate their senses and the quality of their lives; communicating and establishing better contact with people by discerning and expressing their own emotions more clearly, thus becoming aware of other people's feelings; the use of audio-visual material; the recommendation of films; the development of fantasies. Disinhibition opens the door to enjoyment and sexual pleasure. Couples can be given reading lists of erotic literature. There are sex tapes available. All these techniques improve the relationship.

The modified Masters & Johnson basic sex therapy techniques, together with specific instructions for certain disorders combined with relationship/ contract therapy, give couples a good chance to make positive changes toward a happier relationship.

References

Bancroft, J. (1976) The behavioural approach to treatment. In *Handbook of Sexology* (eds J. Money & H. Musaph). Excerpta Medica

Barbach, L. G. (1975) *For Yourself. The Fulfilment of Female Sexuality*. New York: Doubleday.

Crowe, M. J., Gillan, P. W. & Golombok, S. (1981) Form and content in the conjoint treatment of sexual dysfunction, a controlled study. *Behaviour Research and Therapy*, 19, 47–54.

Gillan, P. (1987) *Sex Therapy Manual*. Oxford: Blackwell Scientific.

— & Gillan, R. (1976) *Sex Therapy Today*. Open Books.

Heiman, J., LoPiccolo, L. & LoPiccolo, J. (1976) *Becoming Orgasmic: Sexual Growth Program for Women*. New Jersey: Prentice-Hall.

Hite, S. (1976) *The Hite Report. A Nationwide Study of Female Sexuality*. New York: Dell.

Jones, E. (1955) *The Life and Work of Sigmund Freud*. London: Pergamon Press.

Kaplan, H. (1974) *The New Sex Therapy*. New York: Quadrangle.

Lobitz, C. & LoPiccolo, J. (1972) New methods in behavioural treatment of sexual dysfunction. *Journal of Behaviour Therapy and Experimental Psychiatry*, 3, 265–271.

Masters, W. H. & Johnson, V. E. (1966) *Human Sexual Response*. Boston: Little, Brown & Co.

— & — (1970) *Human Sexual Inadequacy*. London: Churchill Livingstone.

Wolpe, J. (1958) *Psychotherapy by Reciprocal Inhibition*. Stanford: Stanford University Press.

13 A counsellor's work with clients presenting with paraphilias

Christopher F. Headon

Whose sexuality is it anyway? • Attachments to paraphilias from childhood • Interest in paraphilias or people?

This chapter discusses issues raised during therapeutic work at the Albany Trust. These issues can be broadly described as psychosexual, ranging from sexual identity, orientation and preferences, to those of sexual dysfunction. The clinical approach is 'psychodynamic', but it also employs humanistic and behavioural insights and methods. The Albany Trust does take referrals from GPs and psychiatrists; however, most of our clients find their own way to us. If they have any experience of psychiatric intervention it is usually reported as negative and unhelpful. If they have not, they expect it to be negative and have a low opinion of their GP with regard to any possibility of help for their sexual problems.

Most clients with psychosexual issues are deeply ambivalent about the idea of being 'cured'. Some express the view that the cure will be to put an end to themselves. Few have an idea that they could ever be in a position to enjoy their sexual relationships. They are quite taken aback when it is put to them that they must get something out of their sexual activities to have "suffered for them" so much. Almost all have a sense that their sexuality is something they cannot help, although this can also accompany a feeling of self-disgust or guilt at their wickedness.

This type of sexual problem often engages the therapist in areas where they are vulnerable. It might be reassuring to reach for textbook psychiatric definitions at this point. We come across clients who have been referred to psychiatrists by their counsellors for treatment of 'their sexual side', which the counsellor feels at a loss to help them with. These kinds of clients often make any therapist feel at a loss. Fortunately, as counsellors we are not under quite the same pressure to come up with an instant cure, and if we are, we tell the clients quite simply that we cannot. Our instincts are then usually to re-examine our own sexualities and to face our own confusions and insecurities in order to help our clients understand theirs. As we engage with them in the therapeutic process we often do not feel very comfortable or as competent as we would want, but invariably we find we need to be in that particular place and sharing those difficult feelings in order to engage productively.

What is offered to trainee psychiatrists here, therefore, is perhaps not the usual approach with which they are familiar. The clinical examples that follow will point to the uncertainty of diagnosis, the anxious situation of the therapist, the lack of obvious 'medical cures' to suggest with any confidence to the client, and the very individual nature of the therapeutic relationship. None of these, we would suggest, are exclusive to treating psychosexual problems. However, if psychiatrists are to be in a position to offer help they must establish that they are approachable and open-minded towards these clients.

The clinical examples do not give names or details of actual clients. They are a composite of different client work to protect confidentiality.

Case 1

Several years ago a young man presented to me with a marked degree of gender dysphoria, being confused and unhappy about his inclinations to become female. Nine months of therapy led to his decision to attend a gender identity clinic where he was prescribed feminising hormones. He continued in therapy with me, and fairly rapidly over the next few months a young woman began to emerge. She did not wear dresses for sessions, although she enjoyed telling me about the black rubber one she wore to a night-club, but she did dress increasingly androgynously, grew her hair long, wore make-up and diamond earrings. She reported that people were clearly confused about her gender as she travelled and worked.

In the therapeutic exchange, I felt that my son had turned into a daughter, and that in a real sense she was entering a second puberty in her new gender role, learning how to appear and to be a woman. She undertook speech therapy in order to make her voice sound more feminine. If all of this was confusing for her, it certainly was for me. I asked her if in the sessions she wished me to use the female form of her name which she was increasingly employing outside, and my doing so was acknowledged by her to be powerfully validating. However, I noticed that when I spoke about her in supervision I would occasionally slip back into calling my client 'him' and using the masculine form of her name. Clearly I was reflecting her deep ambivalence about the course she was taking, and which was apparent in the incongruence of her dress style; a loose top being worn over her developing breasts while tight black jeans with a button-fly continued to direct my attention to a more male part which wished to engage with me homosexually and did not want to be cut off.

My client's mother increasingly seemed to be accepting that she had a daughter, but her father could not. Likewise in the therapeutic relationship there was a part of me that found it difficult to lose a son.

If there was something to be cut off as a result of the client's determination to change gender, it was still quite distressing to lose it. I tried to reassure myself that this uncomfortableness comes with the territory of gender reassignment. But I also wondered about the sexual aspects to 'her' problems of identity. My client was quite contemptuous of both her father and of me during the sessions. The picture painted, and which clearly applied to us both, was of a father both inept and stupid, who was repeatedly humiliated. In fact it appeared to me from her father's non-acceptance of 'her' that the father had a valuable insight into his son's condition. The portrait of shambling incompetence, which made excluding his opinions seem a sensible thing to do, was contrary to the strong sexual fantasies around the father: of being tightly held by him (as by the tight jeans) or else being alone with him at a romantic dinner in a restaurant, cross-dressed, where she was his intimate and exclusive partner. Such fantasies became distressing and were defended against by recurrent contempt. My client's contempt for me was shown through lateness, postponing sessions with me to visit the psychiatrist and psychologist, as well as dangling money or cheques above my head when paying me. These elements of strong sexual fantasies, humiliation and sexual sadism gave clues to an additional diagnosis of paraphilia, which accompanied the gender confusion.

Whose sexuality is it anyway?

The fourth edition of the American Psychiatric Association's (1994) *Diagnostic and Statistical Manual* describes the various 'paraphilias'. They are listed together with their codes as: 302.4 exhibitionism; 302.81 fetishism; 302.89 frotteurism; 302.2 paedophilia; 302.83 sexual masochism; 302.84 sexual sadism; 302.82 voyeurism; 302.3 transvestic fetishism; and 302.9 paraphilia not otherwise specified. In the latter category DSM–IV includes telephone scatologia (obscene telephone-calling), coprophilia (enjoyment of playing with faeces), and urophilia (similarly, with urine). DSM–IV includes seven examples but some other writers name considerably more, notably Malik (1973) who, in his numerous monographs, described dozens within this classification, linking many of them to various forms of scatological smearing.

Categories and labels are clearly useful to the clinician for finding one's way around and spotting the different exotic plants that fill the muddy and foetid paraphilic garden. Without some maps from previous explorers, it would be frightening to wander around its specimens of bizarre sexualities. However, the desire to label excessively also shows how much fear and anxiety paraphilias evoke in 20th century western culture. There is a long-established tradition of 'discovering' sexual diversity among foreigners or between remote native peoples. Their different sexual practices are 'objectively' documented by travellers and anthropologists. When sexual diversity is closer to home, however, scientific objectivity cannot conceal a considerable fearfulness about what these paraphilias are, or what they mean. This fear is experienced also by the clients presenting with paraphilias or their sexual partners.

It is important for the clinician to take a step back from labels and address the nature of the fear I am describing. Sexual difference, or deviance as it is sometimes called, seems to evoke powerful and primitive fears. Trainee psychiatrists should think carefully before attributing the fact of someone's difference to their personality being pathological. Just as female patients or patients from ethnic minorities are entitled not to be classified and treated for the fact of their gender or racial difference, so people with paraphilias should not automatically be assumed to be 'sick' because of the unusualness of their sexual activities. The element of fear and distress indicated by the client about their sexuality needs to be listened to carefully.

The basic fear centres on loss of control, and fear of behaviours that might very easily get out of hand unless firm measures are taken. This is also where the concept of paraphilia interfaces with that of criminality. Paedophilia, for example, according to the prevailing view needs to be punished as a crime, and the paedophile, if not cured, at least inhibited or curtailed through incarceration or chemical castration.

In the 19 February 1997 legal judgment of the European Court of Human Rights (case no. 109/1995/615/703–705, *Laskey, Jaggard and Brown v. United Kingdom*) concerning the appeal of some British adult gay men that their prosecution and conviction for S & M practices had violated their right to respect for their private life under Article 8 of the European Convention on Human Rights, it was ajudged that the interference of the state was "necessary in a democratic society" for the protection of health. The original conviction in the 'Spanner' case on 19 December 1990 and the failure of subsequent appeals (see *The Times*, 20 February 1997, 34, for details) had rested on the decision that informed adult consent to practices such as genital beating, piercing or abrasion did *not* make these sexual behaviours legal. The basic assumption is that it would be dangerous and socially unacceptable if people were given the unlimited legal right over their own bodies to use them for what they consider to be sexual pleasure. This raises the issue of whether psychiatrists are trying to help their patients or whether they are trying to protect society. Society justifies to itself a 'mediaeval' attitude towards sexual pervertsby convincing itself that both we (normal) and they (perverts) need to be kept as far apart as possible, in the matter of ordinary human rights for example.

Perhaps a useful analogy here is with the use of psychoactive drugs. Some clients regularly use 'ecstasy' or Prozac as part of their lifestyle choices. Despite the fact that this recreational use is also illegal, clinicians who are open-minded enough will be able to recognise an element of self-prescribing which might match what they would recommend if consulted. Of course, there are dangers in these behaviours, not least the uncertainty of what substances are being bought and sold. Even though the primary duty of psychiatrists, unlike the law, is one of care, the clinicians in these situations can often feel under pressure from two conflicting demands on their conscience. Each clinician will arrive at their own suloution, pragmatic or otherwise. It is more helpful if the problems of classification and definition of sexual problems, and diagnosis and prescription, are kept separate from judgements in the clinician's own mind which are moralistic. The more difficult task facing the clinician is in making interventions which can be received as caring and helpful by these clients who are often very sensitive to being judged.

It is important to keep in mind that most clients presenting with paraphilias will be suffering from fears around both having and losing control. It is as if their paraphilia comes to represent everything that is at stake. I shall provide some examples from my clinical practice which illustrate various dimensions of this battle around control.

Case 2

A young gay male client came to see me for the first time for an assessment session; he talked about his presenting problem, which was the fear of sexual intimacy. He would go to S & M bars where there was 'rough' sex engaged in. He spent much of his time watching other men have sex, and was ambivalent in his feelings about this, being sometimes highly aroused and at other times disgusted at what he witnessed. He said that he would sometimes engage in mutual masturbation with the various denim, leather or rubber clad men he fancied, but would never orgasm on the premises or pursue further sexual or emotional intimacy there. He would go home and then orgasm, using the images he recalled from the bars as masturbatory fantasy. While his public persona was that of a successful man who had achieved much professionally, his personal life remained stuck as that of a fearful little boy. He had in fact been abandoned at an early age by an abusive mother, and he described how he felt alienated from an emotionally unavailable father.

One thing struck me in this opening session and that was the way in which he conveyed to me the names of three S & M bars which he attended. My immediate sense was that at an unconscious level he suspected that I went to such places and was therefore saying to himself "I know your game and I can control you through this knowledge". Given this, a part of me immediately thought it extremely unwise that I work with him. On the other hand, I was concerned not to reject him, and I thought he was being genuine when he said that he liked me and wanted to work with me. I thought that what he presented was interesting and challenging, and I could empathise with him and take in his anxieties. My analyst wondered about what my gut feelings were as to whether I should or should not take him on as a client. My supervisor said that I would be mad to take him on as a client but she knew that I enjoyed a challenge and that she would still be there to offer supervision even if I did decide to work with him.

I followed my instinct and took him on as my client. Working with him proved extremely difficult but also rewarding and very interesting. The nature of our therapeutic relationship inevitably paralleled those relationships he forged in his social life, particularly in an S & M setting, and those he encountered in his family. Through my interpretations linking these three aspects he began to achieve a degree of insight.

Some particular points of the therapy highlighted certain aspects of sexual sadism and masochism. In the first few sessions he presented me with a written summary of the preceding session, as though he were in a sense the therapist taking the notes and one who might make a better job of them than I would. He clearly wanted to impress me with his competence, and to intimidate me about my own. Subsequently, he occasionally rushed to his chair ahead of me, and started the session as though he were the therapist. After five sessions he was again mentioning the names of the bars that he visited and I floated the observation that "I wonder if you might expect to find me there sometime". He smiled in agreement at this.

Some weeks later I went to a club to attend a discussion and demonstration of S & M with a group that he had never indicated that he attended, and there he was. I acknowledged him, spoke with him briefly, and was contemplating how I could stay at the event so as not to give him the impression that I had been inhibited or had left on account of him. However, I inevitably did feel inhibited when I left 45 minutes later. At the subsequent session we discussed the meeting and he said that it was perfectly fine for me to be there in my own personal time and that this was entirely separate from my professional capacity as a therapist. He had only gone there, his first visit, because a friend had taken him. I suspected that he was having to work quite hard to keep something 'unacceptable' (his S & M interests and mine) from something more 'acceptable' (innocent curiosity, friendship, our therapeutic meetings). The clue to his own deeper and repressed feelings towards me was evidenced, I felt, by his concern that I should not be worried or upset. Recalling his earlier attempts to take over from me as therapist, and trying to contain my own discomfort, I formed the view that he was defending against feelings which were quite murderous. I formulated an interpretation that he was frightened that what he might really desire was to murder me. The client agreed and said he felt relieved that I had recognised this.

In subsequent sessions he was quite passive, inviting me to put him right and give him homework to do so that he could learn and progress. This was in line with his expressed fantasy of being a subservient 'wife' to a dominant man who would display all the outward appearance of a fascist in uniform but without the unacceptable politics or personality of one. At other times he switched back and continued to try to control me, but the control was accompanied by destructive and vengeful impulses which increasingly brought out the 'fascist' in him, both in the sessions and outside. In clubs he would pick up and then drop quite ruthlessly anybody who showed an interest in him, telling them that they were only after one thing, his body, and that he found their treatment of him as an object to be quite disgusting. He felt that he had been let down by older sexual partners, as well as by his father. He recalled, for example, his father's oily overalls which aroused him by their smell when he was a small boy, although he also thought the overalls were 'revolting', like his father. Not until the small boy was in bed did father return from his work and he felt abandoned and furious about this. How could he get the closeness with his father that he wanted? What could he do with his early sexual feelings?

As the therapeutic relationship progressed these negative transferences became more projected on to me. He told me that the reason I followed him up the stairs to the consulting room was in order to ogle his bottom. He repeatedly denied any sexual interest in me while strenuously implying that I was sexually interested in him. I told him that I found him attractive but that I was not attracted to him (some therapists would question this kind of disclosure). The nature of his continued attacks on my professionalism made me wonder if he was attempting to destroy me and render me useless and in his power, by sustaining the excitement around a battle for sexual control between us. One story he recounted seemed to have me very much in mind. He had visited the club where he had seen me before and it was clearly his wish that he might find me there. He did not. It was, however, an S & M 'discovery night', on initiation. My client soon found a partner (a surrogate for me, it seemed to me in our session), whom he ordered to stand at the bar all evening without drinking, speaking to nobody and not moving until he was granted permission to do so. So now I interpreted silently that this was an acting-out of revenge against his father for not being there to put him to bed and kiss him good-night. This revenge was felt against me also for not being at the club that night. He was identified with his abusive mother.

I mentioned earlier that some of the dynamics of paraphilias have wider application. Most therapists will be familiar with issues of control around fees, for example (fees = faeces). Not unexpectedly, then, my client began to say that he could not afford to pay the full fee at the end of the month but would have to owe me a small bit. I was anxious in myself as to how the monthly deficits might soon add up to a considerable sum and that my own anger and resentment over this would enter into the therapeutic work. I asked him to reflect on what was going on, but I agreed to accommodate his request for deferred payment over several months. The withholding of fees confirmed for me my interpretation: that he was acting the role of an abusive, powerful and abandoning mother. At the same time he desperately wanted to tie me to him more closely, and he needed me to retain my own potency as a caring father-figure. The fees were a test: could he destroy me by turning me into the abusive mother? Bizarre though all this may sound to the student psychiatrist, I continued to put up with the shortfall in my fees, and I kept myself going with my silent interpretations.

Several months later he surprised me by paying me in full, including past sums owing. I thought that any enquiry as to his motives for this change might easily be construed as punitive and would detract from the power of his own ability to surprise me. The surprise 'presentation' had a more appreciative quality to it than when he had much earlier given me back my interpretations in the form of his improved notes.

The work with this client shows us something of the origins of paraphilic sexualisation in the traumatic experiences of childhood. My client needed to disentangle some of his sexualised feelings for me, perhaps partly through open acknowledgement, and through more primitive mechanisms where he was using me to contain certain aspects of his sexuality which he could not manage to reconcile within himself.

What was crucial was that I was able to respond with honesty while keeping my personal discomfort in check, and also remain concerned and involved with his conflicting and disturbing sexualisations of our relationship. I do not believe this would have been possible had I set out to 'cure' him of his sadism and masochism from the outset. I have used this case to emphasise, in fact, the reverse: my client needed his sexual encounters and desires in order to re-experience an intimacy which had become fused with overwhelming fears of abandonment, abuse and neglect. His need for murderous control was a serious problem, though. His sexual encounters were being used to justify the impossibility of sexual intimacy in his life. He needed me to remain open to the possibilities of something good being able to develop out of his conflicting sexual desires and needs.

Attachments to paraphilias from childhood

Thompson (1994) indicates that sadomasochism is not a distinct entity but a description of many sexual variations, desires and behaviours. Thompson's view is that the diverse elements of S & M came to be lumped together by the medical profession in order to establish a pathological condition in default of a proper explanation. He cites Magnus Hirschfeld (1868–1935) that pain in the masochist has nothing to do with sensations of discomfort but with those of pleasure. We should then be wary of interpreting sexual practices which look like cruelty but which may be understood by the participants as more to do with the giving and receiving of 'pain as pleasure', converted via endorphins and the neural pathways. What is more, we should be alert to the possibilities of diverse sexual activities leading to loving or mutually satisfying relationships, sometimes even where the practitioners are reluctant to acknowledge these more intimate aspects to themselves.

In my work with clients, and in informal interviews conducted with S & M practitioners, I see the associated paraphilias viewed as opportunities for enhancing personal freedom. This can embrace the paradox that sometimes people feel most free when they are in the confines of a particular role and can submit themselves to the behavioural constraints that it implies. In the categories for membership of a gay male skinhead club, for example, there are dominant and subordinate, active and passive, master, slave and novice. In practice, however, there is a significant switching in and out of various roles, according to the dictates and desires of the moment.

When I asked members of a fetish club why they enjoyed watersports and scat I received a variety of replies: "Piss, wonderful piss. I love it", responded one. Somebody who was getting into the 'brown' scat scene, as opposed to the 'yellow' piss one, spoke of it being in a different league. He liked to set the scene very carefully, and he clearly adopted a ritualistic approach to the action which raised the level of excitement and anticipation. He liked to watch a sexual partner defaecating, taking his time about this, and observed that the effect was rather like watching a birth. (One could theorise here a state of infantile omnipotent regression; the man is able magically to give birth from his anus.) He also liked the idea of dressing up as an infant, and relieving himself in his nappy. I have had several clients who said they did this, which seemed to go back to the infant state when they received attention and comfort, having soiled their nappies. Mainly, my interviewee said he enjoyed the act of watching (voyeurism or scopophilia) and he liked to make videos of what occurred in order to watch them later. He said that what he wanted was a "quality" experience. Another person I interviewed replied that he liked the outrageous and shocking element in coprophilia. After one session he had taken the train home with his boots covered in faeces. It was his fantasy to go to work one day covered in faeces; his work was that of a hospital nurse. Another interviewee had a deeper view as to why he enjoyed playing with faeces. It was to do with repeating difficult feelings around the anal stage. He recalled a sense of shame from soiling his underwear, which he thought from his own therapy had something to do with feelings concerning family shame that he had taken from his mother. He had been especially disturbed to recall his early burying of soiled underwear in the garden so that his mother would not discover it.

The common theme linking these different responses seems to involve a defiance, possibly a motivation to triumph over what is generally sexually acceptable, perhaps to replay and reverse a childhood defeat. The therapist's concerns should centre on the elements that simply repeat through sexualisation these childhood defeats, and which are either self-destructive or destructive to relationships with others. This is not an easy judgement to arrive at. Nor will the material be offered by clients straightforwardly or easily. Sometimes, the more bizarre the presenting sexual material the more mundane the frustrated needs it may represent.

I should like to propose a new formulation of an old therapeutic nostrum: the orgasm is the royal road to the unconscious. I appreciate this plays into the hands of those critics who dismiss Freud as only ever really being interested in sex but I think it reflects a truth about the clinical task which faces us into the 21st century. Psychosexual issues will need far more care and interest and respect than they have hitherto enjoyed.

Interest in paraphilias or people?

My final clinical examples concern the prospect for clients coming to terms in some way with their paraphilia. But first I want to re-emphasise some of the cautionary warnings about work in this field. When I read an article recently by Baddeley (1995) on the origins and nature of rubber fetishism, I was struck by how out of touch therapists can be with whole areas of the current scene which its inhabitants take for granted. The writer asserts that it is only men who are rubber fetishists. This is patently false. Pick up a *Skin Two* magazine or visit a 'Rubber Ball' and you will see equal numbers of women with a liking for rubber clothes, many of them taking a dominant attitude towards male partners. Counsellors also sometimes fall into the trap of making reductionist interpretations of their clients. In this case the writer posits a single cause for rubber fetishism, namely the desire of some men to recreate the sensations of having their penises rubbed and heads constricted when passing through the vaginal canal at birth. The picture presented is of sad men in masks and crotch-hugging gear, guilty about their fetish and loath to speak about it, who sometimes constrict their heads in a kind of umbilical auto-asphyxiation. Paraphilias, and sex in general, seem to inspire therapists to write speculative theoretical ideas, unaware that their readership might include the people they are writing about, often in a condescending or deprecating way, and betraying some basic ignorance of their subject. What prospects do people with paraphilias have when entering counselling or psychotherapy if the 'experts' are so remote from their lives and their feelings?

Case 3

One of my clients was a clergyman with a liking for rubber mackintoshes. His wife had withdrawn her cooperation from enjoying rubber with him sexually. He consequently admitted his fetish to a female parishioner who interpreted his needy embraces as sexual harassment and complained to the diocese. An inquiry was set up. Under this cloud my client arrived and was, perhaps understandably, both manipulative and intrusive as well as distressed in his early interviews with me. He was fearful of losing his parish, and demanded my collusion to help save him. He was chaotic, unable to contain his own anxieties, and attacking of me. I held my ground and the therapeutic space sufficiently for him to begin to do some work on his actual problem: the rubber fetish. It seemed to represent at one time 'the tent', in which he could be intimate with the women in his life. It was also "an exciting slippery skin", against which to masturbate and find comfort. It was the "magic garment" that protected him against both the loss of his father who had been away in the war during his early years, and the intrusion of his return. He was sad, rather than excited or guilty, when he realised he was searching for his father in the mackintosh. With me, now more trusting, he also strove to be the model client.

The importance of the therapeutic work with the clergyman was precisely creating enough space for more than one 'fixed' meaning to emerge. This is a warning which applies to psychiatrists as well as counsellors. In addition, because of their position of power, psychiatrists need to be careful not to seem over-rigid in their classification of patients' behaviours, or to be arrogant in their treatment prescriptions. Some of the treatments are abusive *per se*: aversive reconditioning, electric shocks and nausea-creating drugs, for those referred by the courts or confused by their own proclivities. Another example would be forms of so-called chemical castration for persistent sexual offenders, which eliminate the performance but do not always remove the troublesome desires. How much evidence really supports the idea that individuals of any sexual orientation can be 'cured' or changed to another?

Such attempts at behavioural conditioning are aiming unrealistically for a perfectly 'normal' world inhabited by perfectly 'normal' people and eliminating 'perverts'. The reality is that any treatment is only effective as long as the patient's ongoing motivation towards management and adjustment can remain positive. To do this becomes impossible if you are stuck with a label which can only be understood negatively, and a treatment which does not take into account the whole person.

Case 4

My final clinical vignette presents the case of a couple coming to see me in great distress. The female partner of a cross-dresser was unable to accept her husband's desire to dress up frequently, especially his wearing of female panties in which he would masturbate.

During the joint therapy the husband came to see that his wearing of female clothes represented an attack on his wife who had taken the place of his domineering mother, compounded by humiliation when she caught him in her underwear, as his mother had when he was five years old. Part of the wife's agreement involved attending a meeting at a cross-dressing club. There she talked with the members and wives present, who reported that while the frequency of dressing up increased over the years it did not form a compulsion that was uncontrollable. The group that my clients attended (the Beaumont Society) is one of an increasing number that cater for cross-dressers as well as a whole array of other fetishes. Here clients can explore, experiment in the management of their interests, and make the necessary adjustments and compromises to sustain their relationships.

One person's perversion, another person's nightmare

The final example suggests a model similar to that called 'coming out', which has been a phenomenon associated with lesbian and gay liberation. It is about self-acceptance and the concept of a new, more integrated identity. One could speculate that some of the paraphilias might follow the gay model. It was only in 1973, for example, that the American Psychiatric Association confirmed their decision that homosexuality be removed from the list of mental disorders. In this sense, sexual identities which are not 'normal' heterosexual ones are still quite young, as it were. As any parent knows, teenagers need *both* to find their own way in a new adult world *and* to be able to come back home. It is a sensitive balance. While changing social attitudes and sexual lifestyles are uncertain, I have emphasised throughout this paper the importance of treating the individual as a whole person. As a diagnostic category, paraphilia does not tell one much more than homosexual or heterosexual. If sexuality is sometimes a signal of distress, it is also the signpost towards the more intimate areas of human relationships, all of which is as good a reason for enjoying the work in this area as any other.

References

American Psychiatric Association (1994) *Diagnostic and Statistical Manual of Mental Disorders* (4th edn) (DSM–IV). Washington, DC: APA.

Baddeley, S. (1995) The birth of rubber fetishism. *Journal of the British Association for Counselling*, 6, 27.

Malik, S. M. A. (1973) *Sexual Disorders and Allied Conditions: The Psychopathology of Scatism*. Bristol: Roseneath.

Thompson, B. (1994) *Sadomasochism: Painful Perversion or Pleasurable Play*. London: Cassell.

Bibliography of further reading

P. De Silva

Psychosexual dysfunctions

Alexander, B. (1993) Disorders of sexual desire: diagnosis and treatment of decreased libido (Review). *American Family Physician*, 47, 832–838.

Balon, R., Yeragani, V. K., Pohl, R., *et al* (1993) Sexual dysfunction during antidepressant treatment. *Journal of Clinical Psychiatry*, 54, 209–212.

Bownes, I. T. & O'Gorman, E. C. (1991) Assailants' sexual dysfunction during rape reported by their victims. *Medicine, Science and the Law*, 31, 322–328.

Catalan, J., Hawton, K. & Day, A. (1990) Couples referred to a sexual dysfunction clinic – psychological and physical morbidity. *British Journal of Psychiatry*, 156, 61–67.

Coleman, E., Rosser, B. R. & Strapko, N. (1992) Sexual and intimacy dysfunction among homosexual men and women. *Psychiatric Medicine*, 10, 251–271.

Cull, A., Cowie, V. J., Farquharson, D. I., *et al* (1993) Early stage cervical cancer: psychosocial and sexual outcomes of treatment. *British Journal of Cancer*, 68, 1216–1620.

Jensen, P., Jensen, S. B., Sorensen, P. S., *et al* (1990) Sexual dysfunction in male and female patients with epilepsy: a study of 86 outpatients. *Archives of Sexual Behaviour*, 19, 1–14.

Kaplan, H. S. (1990) Sex, intimacy, and the ageing process. *Journal of the American Academy of Psychoanalysis*, 18, 185–205.

Koller, W. C., Vetere-Overfield, B., Williamson, A., *et al* (1990) Sexual dysfunction in Parkinson's disease. *Clinical Neuropharmacology*, 13, 461–463.

Lindal, E. & Stefansson, J. G. (1993) The lifetime prevalence of psychosexual dysfunction among 55–57 year olds in Iceland. *Social Psychiatry and Psychiatric Epidemiology*, 28, 91–95.

Mackey, T. F., Hacker, S. S., Weissfeld, L. A., *et al* (1991) Comparative effects of sexual assault on sexual functioning of child sexual abuse survivors and others. *Issues in Mental Health Nursing*, 12, 89–112.

McCarthy, B. W. (1993) Relapse prevention strategies and techniques in sex therapy. *Journal of Sex and Marital Therapy*, 19, 142–146.

—— (1990) Treating sexual dysfunction associated with prior sexual trauma. *Journal of Sex and Marital Therapy*, 16, 142–146.

Metz, M. E. & Dwyer, S. M. (1993) Relationship conflict management patterns among sex dysfunction, sex offender and satisfied couples. *Journal of Sex and Marital Therapy*, 19, 104–122.

Montgomery, J. C. & Studd, J. W. (1991) Psychological and sexual aspects of the menopause. *British Journal of Hospital Medicine*, 45, 300–302.

Palace, E. M. & Gorzalka, B. B. (1990) The enhancing effects of anxiety on arousal in sexually dysfunctional and functional women. *Journal of Abnormal Psychology*, 99, 403–411.

Ponticas, Y. (1992) Sexual aversion versus hypoactive sexual desire: a diagnostic challenge. *Psychiatric Medicine*, 10, 273–281.

Rowland, D. L., Haensel, S. M., Blom, J. H., *et al* (1993) Penile sensitivity in men with premature ejaculation and erectile dysfunction. *Journal of Sex and Marital Therapy*, 19, 189–197.

Russell, L. (1990) Sex and couples therapy: a method of treatment to enhance phsyical and emotional intimacy. *Journal of Sex and Marital Therapy*, 16, 111–120.

Segraves, R. T., Saran, A., Segraves, K., *et al* (1993) Clomipramine versus placebo in treatment of premature ejaculation: a pilot study. *Journal of Sex and Marital Therapy*, 19, 198–200.

Seidl, A., Bullough, B., Haughey, B., *et al* (1991) Understanding the effects of a myocardial infarction on sexual functioning : a basis for sexual counselling. *Rehabilitation Nursing*, 16, 255–264.

Spector, I. P. & Carey, M. P. (1990) Incidence and prevalence of the sexual dysfunctions – a critical review of the empirical literature. *Archives of Sexual Behaviour*, 19, 389–408.

St Lawrence, J. S. & Madakasira, S. (1992) Evaluation and treatment of premature ejaculation: a critical review. *International Journal of Psychiatry in Medicine*, 22, 77–87.

Paraphilias

Abel, G. G. & Osborn, C. (1992) The paraphilias. The extent and nature of sexually deviant and criminal behaviour (Review). *Psychiatric Clinics of North America*, 15, 675–687.

Blanchard, R. & Hucker, S. J. (1991) Age, transvestism, bondage and concurrent paraphilic activities in 117 fatal cases of autoerotic asphyxia. *British Journal of Psychiatry*, 159, 371–377.

Bradford, J. M. & Pawlak, A. (1993) Double blind placebo crossover study of cyproterone acetate in the treatment of the paraphilias. *Archives of Sexual Behaviour*, 22, 383–402.

Dickey, R. (1992) The management of a case of treatment-resistant paraphilia with a long acting LHRH agonist. *Canadian Journal of Psychiatry*, 37, 567–569.

Fagan, P. J., Wise, T. N., Schmidt, C. W. Jr, *et al* (1991) A comparison of five factor personality dimensions in males with sexual dysfuntion and males with paraphilia. *Journal of Personality Assessment*, 57, 434–448.

Gottesman, H. G. & Schubert, D. S. (1993) Low dose oral medroxy progesterone acetate in the management of paraphilias. *Journal of Clinical Psychiatry*, 54, 182–188.

Kafka, M. P. & Prentky, R. (1992) Fluoxetine treatment of non-paraphilic sexual addictions and paraphilias in men. *Journal of Clinical Psychiatry*, 53, 351–358.

Kaul, A. (1993) Sex offenders – cure or management? (Review). *Medicine, Science and the Law*, 33, 207–212.

Kiersch, T. A. (1990) Treatment of sex offenders with Depo-Provera. *Bulletin of the American Academy of Psychiatry and the Law*, 18, 179–187.

Kruesi, M. J., Fine, S., Valladares, L., *et al* (1992) Paraphilias: a double blind crossover comparison of clomipramine versus desipramine. *Archives of Sexual Behaviour*, 21, 587–593.

McConaghy, N. (1990) Assessment and treatment of sex offenders: the Prince of Wales Programme. *Australian and New Zealand Journal of Psychiatry,* 24, 175–181.

Miller, J. G. (1992) On mitigating professional arrogance in the treatment of sex offenders. *Medicine and Law,* 11, 485–491.

Moser, C.(1992) Lust, lack of desire and paraphilias: some thoughts and possible connections. *Journal of Sex and Marital Therapy,* 18, 65–69.

Myers, B. A. (1991) Treatment of sexual offenses by persons with developmental disabilities. *American Journal on Mental Retardation,* 95, 563–569.

Nutter, D. E. & Kearns, M. E.(1993) Patterns of exposure to sexually explicit material among sex offenders, child molesters, and controls. *Journal of Sex and Marital Therapy,* 19, 77–85.

Richer, M. & Crisman, M. L. (1993) Pharmacotherapy of sexual offenders (Review). *Annals of Pharmacotherapy,* 27, 316–320.

Simon, W. (1994) Deviance as history: the future of perversion. *Archives of Sexual Behaviour,* 23, 1–20.

—— & Schouten, P. G. (1991) Plethysmography in the assessment and treatment of sexual deviance: an overview (Review). *Archives of Sexual Behaviour,* 20, 75–91.

Stein, D. J., Hollander, E., Anthony, D. T., *et al* (1992) Serotonergic medications for sexual obsessions, sexual addictions, and paraphilias. *Journal of Clinical Psychiatry,* 53, 267–271.

Templeman, T. L. & Stinnett, R. D. (1991) Patterns of sexual arousal and history in a 'normal' sample of young men. *Archives of Sexual Behaviour,* 20, 137–150.

Thibaut, F., Cordier, B. & Kuhn, J. M. Effect of a long-lasting gonadotrophin releasing hormone in six cases of male paraphilia. *Acta Psychiatrica Scandinavica,* 87, 445–450.

Index

Compiled by Linda English

accommodation syndrome 108
acetylcholine 7, 9
acupuncture 94
adjustment disorders and HIV
  infection 115–116
AIDS dementia complex 117–118
alcohol 19, 93
alpha-adrenoceptors in penis 15, 85
alpha-antagonists 8, 18, 85
alprostadil 86–87, 88, 90
alternative levels of intervention
  (ALI) hierarchy in couple therapy
  68–69, 77–78
amantadine 15, 95
amitriptyline 85
amputations 151–152
amygdala 2, 17, 21–22
anal intercourse 127
androgenic progesterones 33
androgens 10–12, 20, 86, 95–96
  and gender development 30–34,
    39, 40
  prenatal androgenisation 31–34
  see also testosterone
animals
  aggression during mating 143
  bestiality and 150
  consumption of sexual parts of 47
  fetishistic behaviour in primates 147
  pheromones in 146–147
  studies on 3, 13, 15, 16, 21–22, 27
anorgasmia 9, 14, 15, 23, 73, 81–82,
  94–95, 189–190
anti-androgenic agents 20, 98
anticonvulsants 21
antidepressants, sexual side-effects
  of 14–16, 80, 85, 92–93, 95, 96
antihypertensives 17–19, 27, 93
antipsychotics and sexual
  dysfunction 13–14, 26, 92, 93
aphrodisiacs 46–47

apomorphine 13
apotemnophilia 151–152
appetite
  sexual see sexual appetite
  sexuality as 44, 46, 52
appetitive behaviour 2, 13
arguments in couple therapy 71, 75
arousal see sexual arousal
arterial insufficiency 7, 24, 25, 90
arterial surgery 79
Ashworth Inquiry (1992) 132
aspermia 14
assertiveness, inequality in couples 75
attachment theory 104, 175
autoerotic asphyxia 146
autonomic neuropathy 26

Beaumont Trust 162
behavioural-systems couple therapy
  (BSCT) 67–73, 75
behavioural theory
  and couple therapy 67–73, 177–178
  and fetishism 148
bendrofluazide 18
benzodiazepines 17, 93
bestiality 150
best interests criterion 137
beta-blockers 18, 93
bethanechol 95
bilateral anterolateral cordotomy 5–6
biology of sex 1–29
brain
  disease and HIV infection 117–120,
    121
  sexual 1–5
  sexual dimorphism in 3, 34, 52
  and variants in sexual behaviour
    142, 143
brain-stem 6, 10
brain workers 52
bulbocavernosus reflex 9

bupropion 93, 96
buserelin 20

calcium channel blockers 18–19
Carpenter, Edward 56
castration 11, 12, 20
castration anxiety 35
castration complex 148
caudal thalamic intralaminar nuclei 6
cavernosal fibrosis 88
cavernosography 25, 91
cavernosometry 25, 91
cerebellum 52
child abuse 101–113
  consequences 104–105
  definitions 101
  descriptions 102–103
  emotional 101, 102, 103, 104
  epidemiology 103, 107
  historical aspects 102
  intervention 105–106, 110
  neglect 101, 102–103
  physical 101, 102, 103, 104
  risk factors 103
  sexual 103, 106–112, 196
    consequences 108–111
    cultural issues 106
    definitions 106–107
    false memory syndrome 111–112
    intervention and treatment 110–111
    legal considerations 111
    presentation 108
    risk factors 107
child protection registers 102, 103, 105
chlordiazepoxide 17
cigarette smoking 19–20, 93
cimetidine 20
circular causation 63–64
clitoris 96, 186
clomipramine 15, 80, 94
clonidine 18
cognitive developmental theory 38–39
cognitive impairment and HIV
  infection 117–119, 121
colovaginoplasty 169
communication training in couple
  therapy 70
complete androgen insensitivity
  syndrome 31–32

congenital adrenal hyperplasia 31,
  32, 33, 34
consummatory behaviour 2, 3–5, 13
coprophilia 151, 195, 201–202
corpus spongiosum 23
counselling *see* paraphilias,
  counselling *and* relationship
  counselling
couple therapy *see* relationship
  counselling *and* sexual therapy
cross-dressing *see* transgenderism
cybersex 152–153
cyproheptadine 15, 95
cyproterone acetate 20, 98

Darwin, Charles 50
de-centreing in couple therapy 68
degeneration theory 45, 48, 49, 52–53
dementia and HIV infection
  117–119, 121
depression and HIV infection 116
desire *see* sexual appetite
detained patients 131–132
diabetic men 10, 21, 25–26, 85
diethylstilbestrol 31
differential reinforcement 36–37
digoxin 20, 93
dihydrotestosterone 12
L-dopa 14
dopamine 2, 12, 13–14, 26, 95
dopamine receptor antagonists 13
Doppler ultrasonography 24, 25, 90
dorsomedial nucleus of hypothalamus 3
drag artists 160
drive *see* sexual appetite
drug-induced sexual dysfunction
  12–20, 27, 92–93, 95, 96
drug treatment
  for disorders of desire 95–6
  for ejaculatory problems 80, 94
  for erectile dysfunction 78, 84–88,
    89–90
  in HIV infection 120–121
  for paraphilias 20, 98
dyspareunia 97

'ecstasy' 15
ejaculation 10
  and antipsychotics 14

delayed 14, 80, 94, 191
premature 64, 79–80, 90, 94, 179,
    188, 191
Ellis, Havelock 45, 46, 47, 51, 54
epilepsy 21–22, 148
erectile dysfunction 1, 8
and alcohol 19, 93
and antihypertensives 17–19, 93
and bulbocavernosus reflex 9
and couple therapy 61–62, 67, 73,
    77–79, 179–180, 190–191
and diabetes 10, 21, 25–26, 85
and hypertension 10, 17
medical/surgical causes 7, 10, 21,
    22, 23, 24–26
physical treatments 84–94
    intracavernosal injection (ICI)
        78–79, 86–88, 89–90
    oral medication 78, 85
    penile prostheses 92
    surgery 79, 90–91
    testosterone 85–86
    topical medications 84–85
    vacuum constriction devices
        (VCDs) 79, 88–90
and psychotropic drugs 13, 14, 15,
    16, 17, 92–93
and smoking 19–20, 93
erection
and androgens 11
cerebral localisation of 3, 5
nocturnal 11, 20, 24
and opiates 16, 17
and peripheral mechanisms 6–10
psychogenic 22–23, 89
reflex 5, 8, 16, 22–23
rigid 8, 9
and serotonin 14
and spinal mechanisms/pathways 5
see also erectile dysfunction
erotic piercing 145
eugenics 45, 50–51
external iliac steal syndrome 24

false memory syndrome 111–112
farinaceous foods 51
feel free position 187
fenofibrate 20

fetishism 146–150, 152, 161, 195, 201,
    202–203
fluoxetine 15, 93, 95
fluphenazine 14, 93
foetal abuse 102
follicle stimulating hormone 39
fountain of youth 46
Freud, Sigmund 34–36, 54–55

GABA 17
Galton, Francis 50–51
ganglion blocking drugs 18
gemfibrozil 20
gender constancy 38
gender consultants 167
gender development 30–43
gender dysphoria 164, 194
gender identity
    development of 30–39
    and transgenderism 156–157,
        160–161, 163–167
gender reassignment 98, 158, 164,
    167–170, 194–195
gender role 30–39, 156
gender schemas 38–39
gender stability 38
gender stereotypes 37, 38–39
genetic disorders 31–34
genital malformation 31
give-to-get tasks 185, 187–188
Graham, James: Temple of Health 47
gross indecency 127
'guevodoces' 32

haloperidol 13
Harry Benjamin Standards of Care 167
hebephrenia 50
heterocyclic antidepressants 15–16
historical attitudes to sexual
    behaviour 44–58, 159
homosexuality 151, 152
    attitudes towards 53, 56, 57
    in-patients and 127, 128
    in prisons and special hospitals
        137–138
    transgenderism and 158, 160–161, 165
homovestism 149
hormones 2, 10–12, 21, 96
    and gender development 30–34, 39

transsexualism and prescription of
98, 167–169, 170
see also androgens *and individual
names*
hospitals *see* mental health facilities
human immunodeficiency virus
(HIV) infection 114–123
and brain disease 117–120
non-organic psychiatric
manifestations 114–117
treatment of brain disease 121
treatment of related psychiatric
disorder 120–121
human rights issues 128–129,
136–137, 196
hyperprolactinaemia 26, 92
hypersexuality 52–53
hypertension 10, 17–19, 93
hypolipidaemic agents 20
hypothalamo-pituitary disease 22
hypothalamus 2, 3–4, 5, 11, 13, 22,
143, 147

imipramine 16
impotence *see* erectile dysfunction
indecent assault 126, 127, 157
individual psychological factors and
sexual dysfunction 63
informal patients 131
injecting drug-users 115
in-patients *see* mental health facilities
intergenerational transmission and
abuse 105
intracavernosal injection (ICI)
diagnostic 24, 25, 90
for erectile dysfunction 78–79,
86–88, 89–90
intracavernosal pressure 9

Kellogg, John Harvey 51
Kinsey, Alfred Charles 57
klismaphilia 51, 151
Krafft-Ebing, Richard von 45, 48, 53,
143–144, 146

learning disability patients and
problems of sexuality 135–137
Leriche syndrome 24
libido *see* sexual appetite

lithium 93
'lost manhood' 47–48
lower class male, hypersexuality of
52–53
'low sexual desire' 60, 74
luteinizing hormone 39
Lydston, Frank G. 52

male erectile disorder *see* erectile
dysfunction
male sexuality *see* sexology and
male sexuality
masochism *see* sadomasochism
massage 185
Masters, W. E. and Johnson, V. E. 40,
57, 59
masturbation 40–41, 128, 137
historical attitudes to 49–50, 51, 53,
159
sex therapy and 64, 186
maternalist movement 53–54
mechanistic solutions, reliance on 59
Medea 46
medial pre-optic area (MPOA) 2, 3,
12, 13
medical/surgical causes of sexual
dysfunction 20–26, 62
medicine and sexuality, history of
relationship 44–58
medroxyprogesterone acetate 20, 98
menstrual cycle 11, 39
Mental Health Act 1959: 124, 127
Mental Health Act 1983: 131
mental health facilities, problems of
sexuality in 124–141
control of offending (and case
example) 133–135
need for a sex policy 125–127
policy points to be considered
(and case example) 127–130
powers to discipline patients
(and case example) 131–132
prisons and special hospitals
137–140
problems of learning disability
135–137
methyldopa 18, 93
3,4-methylenedioxymethamphetamine
(MDMA; 'ecstasy') 15

metoclopramide 20
mixed wards 125, 130
moclobemide 96
modelling 36–37
monoamine oxidase inhibitors
  15–16, 92–93
monoamine reuptake inhibitors 15
moral defectives 124
moral hygiene 45, 47–48
Morel, B.-A.: theory of degeneration
  48
morphine 16
motivation *see* sexual appetite
multicultural society, awareness of 64
multiple sclerosis 22
muscarinic blockade 7, 16
muscle workers 52–53
myths and male sexuality 46–47, 64

naloxone 16–17
naltrexone 16
necrophilia 151
neostigmine 95
Nesbit's procedure 91
neurasthenia, sexual 51
neuroendocrine basis of sexuality
  1–29
  effects of drugs 12–20
  medical/surgical causes of
    dysfunction 20–26
  neurotransmitters 12–17
  peripheral mechanisms 6–10
  sex steroids 10–12
  sexual brain 1–5
  spinal mechanisms/pathways 5–6
neurological causes of sexual
  dysfunction 21–24
neurotransmitters and sexual
  physiology 12–17
nicotine 19–20, 93
nitric oxide 9–10
nocturnal penile tumescence 11, 20,
  24–25
non-androgenic progesterones 33, 34
non-oestrogen lubricants 97
noradrenaline 12, 15
normalisation concept 136
nucleus accumbens 13
nucleus of Onufrowicz 8

object relations theory 174–175
Oedipal theory 35, 175
oestradiol 12
oestrogen creams/pessaries 97
oestrogen receptor 12
oestrogens 11–12, 30–31, 39, 96
olfactory system 146–147
onanism 49–50
Onuf's nucleus 8
oophorectomy 11
opiates 16–17
opioid peptides 16–17
oral sex in couple therapy 186–187
organic sexual dysfunction 1–29, 62, 78
'organotherapy' 51–52
orgasm 4, 10, 40, 55–56, 144, 146,
  159, 202
  see also anorgasmia *and* ejaculation
orgasmic reconditioning 186
orgone box 55–56
ovulation 11
oxytocin 4–5, 17, 27

paedophilia *see* child abuse, sexual
  pain as pleasure 201
papaverine 19–20, 24, 78, 86, 87, 88, 90
paradox in couple therapy 72–73, 81
paragigantocellular reticular nucleus 6
parameter space concept 152
paraphilias
  counselling (and case examples)
    193–205
  drug treatments 20, 98
  evolutionary and developmental
    perspective 142–155
parasympathetic vascular mechanism
  and genital arousal 6–7
paraventricular nucleus (PVN) 3–4, 13
pelvic floor exercises 93–94, 98
pelvic plexus 23
pelvic surgery, effects of 23–24
penile prostheses 92
penile rings 93
penis envy 35
penis size dissatisfaction 98
peripheral mechanisms and sexual
  activity 6–10
peripheral nerve lesions 23–24
peripheral neuropathy 19, 25

permission-giving 66
Peyronie's disease 78, 79, 89, 91, 92
phallic stage 34–35
phallism 44
phalloarteriography 25
phenelzine 16
phenoxybenzamine 8
phentolamine 78, 86, 87
pheromones 146–147
Philips operation 169
photoplethysmography 6
physical treatments for sexual
    dysfunctions 84–100
pinacidil 19
police investigations in hospitals
    132, 134–135
pornography 127
postmenopausal women 11
premature ejaculation 64, 79–80, 90,
    94, 179, 188, 191
prenatal influences and gender
    development 30–34
priapism 15, 19, 78–79, 87–88, 93
primates, fetishistic behaviour in 147
prisons 137–140
progesterones 30–31, 33
prolactin 26, 92
propranolol 18, 93
prostacyclin 10, 19
prostaglandin E1: 10, 24, 78–79, 86–87
prostate surgery 23, 24
prostitution 127
pseudohermaphrodites 31–34
psychoanalytic theory 54–55
    and fetishism 148
    and gender development 34–36
    and relationship counselling 175
    and sadomasochism 143–144
'psychohermaphrodites' 56
psychosexual approach 60
psychosocial dwarfism 104
psychotic disorders and HIV
    infection 116–117
psychotropic drugs and sexual
    dysfunction 12–17, 27, 92–93
puberty 39–41
pygmalionism 149

rape 126
reactive attachment disorder 104–105

real life test 166, 167–168
reciprocity negotiation in couple
    therapy 69–70
reflex erection 5, 8, 16, 22–23
Reich, Wilhelm 55–56
rejuvenation and male sexuality
    46–47
relationship counselling/therapy
    172–183
    behavioural-systems couple
        therapy (BSCT) 67–73
    case examples 172–174, 176–177,
        180–182
    relationship causal factors and
        sexual dysfunction 63–65
    or sex therapy? 177, 180–183
    theoretical approaches 174–178
relaxation exercises 67
restraint and seclusion 132
rigid erection 8, 9
role-play in couple therapy 71, 188,
    189

sadistic murder 145–146
sadomasochism (S & M) 143–146,
    151, 195, 196, 197–201
selective serotonin reuptake
    inhibitors (SSRIs), sexual side-
    effects of 14–15, 80, 92–93, 94, 95, 98
semen, ingestion of 47
sensate focus approach 66, 77,
    178–179, 185, 186
septal area 3
serotonin 12, 14–15, 95
sex change 98, 158, 164, 167–170,
    194–195
sex and gender, confusion between
    156
sex offenders 20, 138–139, 145–146, 196
sexology and male sexuality 44–58
    control and continence 50–51
    from disease to desire 57–58
    hype, hyperidrosis and
        hypersexuality 51–53
    moral hygiene and 'lost manhood'
        47–48
    myth, magic and rejuvenation
        46–47
    sexual pathology 53–54
    sexual psychology 54–56

spermaticidal anxiety 49–50
third sex 56
sex steroids *see* hormones
sexual abuse 196
  and children 103, 106–112
  and couple therapy 81–82,
    173–174, 179, 180–181
  and learning disability patients 135
sexual appetite/desire/drive/
  motivation 2, 11, 13, 60, 74, 168
    disorders of 60, 74–77, 95–96, 192
    incompatible, and couple
      therapy 60, 74–77
sexual arousal 3–5, 16
  and fetishism 148
  and peripheral mechanisms 6–10
  problems in men *see* erectile
    dysfunction
  problems in women 81–82
  and sadomasochism 144, 146
  in women 4–5, 6, 11, 40, 81–82
sexual brain 1–5
sexual experience, gender
  differences in 40
sexual intercourse
  age of first 40, 106
  in couple therapy 187
sexualised behaviour in children
  108, 110
sexuality and reproduction,
  separation of 142–143
sexual relationships, development of
  39–41
sexual selection 50–51
sexual therapy for couples 57, 59–83,
  172–183, 184–192
  adjustment to symptom 73
  assessment 184–185
  and behavioural theory 177–178
  causal factors 61–65
  classification of problems 60–61
  delayed ejaculation 80, 191
  erectile problems 61–62, 67, 73,
    77–79, 179–180, 190–191
  female lack of arousal and
    anorgasmia 73, 81–82, 189–190
  general therapeutic principles
    65–67
  incompatible sexual drives 60,
    74–77

  partnership problems in 184–192
  premature ejaculation 64, 79–80,
    179, 188, 191
  or relationship counselling? 177,
    180–183
  sabotage of 187–188
  treatment of problems in couples
    65
  vaginismus 66, 81, 179, 187, 188–189
sexual variations
  attitudes towards 45, 48, 53–54,
    57–58, 195–196
  and continuum concept 54, 55, 57
  evolutionary perspective 142, 143, 152
sickle-cell anaemia 88
smoking 19–20, 93
snuff movies 151
social learning theory 36–37
social scientists, growth of interest in
  sex 54
socio-medical attitudes towards
  sexuality, history of 44–58
somatomotor mechanism and
  genital arousal 8–9
SPACE (single potential analysis of
  cavernosal electrical activity) 91
special hospitals 137–140
'spermatorrhoea' 49–50
spinal cord injury 5, 22–23
spinal mechanisms/pathways and
  sexual activity 5–6
split team message 73
squeeze technique 64, 191
staff and sexual misconduct 133
Stekel, Wilhelm 54–55
sterilisation 137
stimulation therapy 192
stop–start technique 64, 79–80
suicidal behaviour and HIV infection
  116
superstimulation 80, 94
surgery
  as cause of erectile dysfunction
    23–24
  for erectile dysfunction 79, 90–91
  penis enlargement 98
  and transsexualism 169–170
sympathetic inhibitory mechanism
  and genital arousal 8
systems theory 63–64, 67–73, 175–177

teasing technique 191
teflon implants 79
temporal lobe epilepsy 21, 148
testicles and 'organotherapy' 51–52
testosterone 10, 11, 12, 21, 39, 93
  supplementation 11, 85–86, 96
thiazide diuretics 18
thioridazine 14, 93
third sex 56
timetables and tasks in couple
  therapy 71–72, 75, 76, 178, 185
tomboyish behaviour 33, 34
total institutions 124–125
transdermal nitrate patches 84–85
transgenderism 148, 149, 156–171,
  176–177, 194–195, 204
    eroticism and sexual fantasy
      159–160
    and expression of personality
      161–163
    and gender identity 156–157,
      160–161, 163–167
    gender reassignment 98, 158,
      164, 167–170, 194–195
    and guilt about cross-dressing
      157–158
    and the law 157
    prescription of hormones 98,
      167–169, 170
    reasons for psychiatric
      involvement 157–158
    and sexual preference 160–161
    surgery 169–170
    transgender spectrum 158–167
transsexualism 98, 156–171, 194–195
  female-to-male 167, 169
transvestism 148, 149, 156–171
  closet transvestites 162
  counselling 176–177, 204
  dual role transvestites 161
  in women 163

traumagenic dynamics and child
  abuse 109
trazodone 16, 85, 93, 96

urbanisation, effects of 48, 52
urethralism 151
urethrogenital reflex 10
urinary incontinence 97–98
urophilia 151, 195, 201

vacuum constriction devices (VCDs)
  79, 88–90
vaginal cones 94–95
vaginal dilators 81, 97, 188–189
vaginismus 66, 81, 97, 179, 187,
  188–189
vascular disease 24–26, 90–91
vasoactive intestinal polypeptide
  (VIP) 7, 26, 78
veno-occlusive dysfunction 7, 25, 88,
  90, 91
venous leaks 25, 67, 91, 93–94
ventral striatum 2, 13
ventromedial hypothalamic nucleus 3
verapamil 18
vibrators 80, 81, 94
viloxazine 96
virtual reality 152–153
vocation and sexuality 55
Vogueing 149
vomeronasal organ 147

water, restorative powers of 46
woman above position 67, 81, 187
womb envy 36

yohimbine 17, 78, 80, 95, 96

zidovudine 118, 121
zinc deficiency 96
zoophilia 150

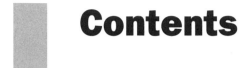

Contents

Foreword to the first edition   v

Foreword   vi

Preface   vii

About the author   viii

Acknowledgements   ix

Extracts from reviews of the first edition   x

Introduction   xiii

Part One: You can change your life
1 Life coaching and doctors   3
2 Are you ready?   8
3 Do you have a life?   13
4 Are you a square peg in a round hole?   19
5 How to change your life in seven easy steps   23
6 How will you respond to your wake up call   36

Part Two: Prescription for change
7 What would you do if you had the time?   43
8 No more procrastination   51
9 Looking after number one   55
10 What's draining you?   61
11 Living an abundant life   66
12 Relationship: what relationship?   70
13 Top ten tips for achieving your goals   74

Part Three: Medicine is more than a job: it's a lifestyle
14 Who heals the healers?   79
15 Wellbeing: reality or dream?   83

16 Do your colleagues understand? 89
17 How to see fewer patients in your clinic 97
18 The end of the road or a new beginning? 101

Part Four: Case studies
19 The overwhelmed GP 107
20 The disillusioned consultant 111
21 The doctor's other half 115
22 The independent soul, the sole doctor 118
23 The overstressed doctor 120
24 The mentor 123
25 The mentee 126
26 The enlightened doctor 128
27 The unsettled doctor 130
28 The doctor who has to re-take professional exams 132
29 A New Year story 134

Part Five: Life coaching for change
30 Let your heart sing 141
31 What on earth is life coaching? 145

And finally ... 149

Appendix 1: Frequently asked questions 151

Appendix 2: The International Coach Federation 154

Index 157

Foreword to first edition

It is hard to change. Often we get caught in a rut, existing rather than living in the mad 'hamster wheel' situation that many of us find ourselves in.

But is it enough to wait until you are at breaking point before you decide to do something about your crazy lifestyle?

I have been witness to many doctors at that breaking point. Some of them even cried uncontrollably when they suddenly realised that they were not in control of their lives. I didn't just want to pass them a tissue. I wanted to do something about it.

So, I commissioned Susan Kersley, to write a series of articles for Career Focus in BMJ Careers to help our readers realise that they could be in control of their lives and spiralling workload.

I received extreme reactions to some of her articles: some hated them, others loved them. Some saw them as glorified common sense and others as a prescription for change. As an editor, it is always satisfying to know that something you have published has caused a reaction. It means that your readers' apathy has turned into action. So I wasn't bothered about the negative feedback. I knew her articles were being read across the world. Every time I published one of Susan's articles, the number of web hits we had would soar.

Maybe it is uncomfortable to read something that makes you realise how miserable your life is. Maybe it is too unbearable to try and change. Susan certainly hits your vulnerable spot but also leads you through what practical things you can do to make a difference in your life.

So, take a deep breath, take courage and read on. You will not regret it.

Dr Rhona MacDonald
Former Editor
Career Focus
BMJ Careers

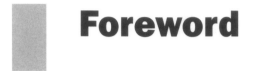

Foreword

It is difficult to be a consistently caring and compassionate doctor if you are not happy with your own lot. That's all day every day, throughout your career. Actually it's a difficult challenge even when you are happy with your lot – working in such a high-pressured environment as the NHS with a regular quota of emotionally draining work. You can lose perspective and get drawn into a way of life that is dominated by work. You're either at work or recovering from being at work, and so missing out on the out-of-work activities and fun that used to counterbalance work and worries.

Use this book as your personal guide to how to make changes to your working and home lives so that you can thrive – at work and in your well-being in general. When you have worked out what to do – perhaps with a mentor or life coach or your partner, as Susan Kersley recommends – you can plan goals that you'll actually achieve, you can have a life and be a doctor too. The working side of your life will be all the better for that.

Susan says 'This book is the catalyst for the life you want.' It is, so long as you read through it, reflect on what it means for you, and put your resolutions into practice in both the short and long term. That takes some doing, and Susan will give you the insights and framework you need to visualise your future and make it happen as you want it to. You can rediscover your old hobbies, work out a better balance of work and leisure, renew and strengthen your relationships with your partner and family, friends and colleagues. Sounds like a dream? Well make it come true by reading and working through this book.

Ruth Chambers
General Practitioner
Clinical Dean at Staffordshire University
Professor of Primary Care Development
at Stoke-on-Trent Teaching PCT
GP Adviser on GP Recruitment and Retention
to Shropshire and Staffordshire Strategic Health Authority
August 2005

Preface

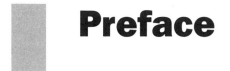

Since the first edition was published in 2003, there seems to be more recognition of doctors' needs to deal with the stress and overwhelm of their professional lives today and also their entitlement to a life outside medicine. This book gives gentle guidance and asks challenging questions to enable more doctors to have a life.

Those who experience the benefit of support from a mentor or a coach know how empowering this can be. However, there are still too many doctors reluctant to admit that they might gain benefit from engaging with this process. It is my sincere wish that this book will introduce those doctors to some of the tools offered by life coaching, so that they can use these to transform their lives.

You may find that the contents of this book is largely just 'common sense'. Perhaps it is, but common sense may be the forgotten ingredient in the lives of many busy professionals who don't stop to 'have a life'.

This edition has been revised where necessary and has some extra 'case studies'. I hope you find it a catalyst to transform your life.

Susan E Kersley
August 2005

Everybody gets so much information all day long that they lose their common sense.

Gertrude Stein

Common sense is not so common.

Voltaire

About the author

Susan Kersley has been a life coach since 1999.

Previously a medical practitioner and counsellor working in inner city Birmingham, she took early retirement in 1997 to live more creatively. A graduate of CoachU, she works with stressed and overworked doctors and others, on the telephone, wherever they live, to enable them to have a more fulfilled life both within and outside medicine. Her acclaimed articles about lifestyle and personal development, published regularly in the *British Medical Journal*, evolved to become 'Prescription for Change' to bring the message she is passionate about, 'You can be a doctor and have a life', to a wider audience.

To receive her ezine (email newsletter), find out more about her coaching, courses and other publications, please visit www.thedoctorscoach.co.uk.

Aims for 'Prescription for Change'

- To promote more self awareness by encouraging personal development.
- To educate doctors about the benefits of life coaching.
- To promote the more widespread use of life coaching amongst doctors at all stages of their career, both for themselves and their patients.

Acknowledgements

A very special thank you to Rhona MacDonald, former editor of *BMJ Careers*, who encouraged, motivated and coached me to produce my first published article, 'Striking the balance', in the *BMJ* in December 2001. Rhona recognised my potential as a writer and encouraged me to expand the original article into a series published in the *BMJ* during 2002.

This book stemmed from my desire to extend the message of the articles to a wider medical readership. Some of the chapters in this book are similar to the articles originally published in the *BMJ* and are included here with permission.

Supporting me during the gestation of the book have been my own coaches and also my husband Jonathan who, in spite of remaining somewhat bemused at my new identity, has given me steady support.

A huge thanks too, to all the doctors who contacted me after reading my articles in the *BMJ*. Most I have never met face to face. However, over several months of coaching conversations, I am delighted to have enabled them to transform their lives. I thank them for their trust in me and for sharing their life stories, which have informed the writing for this book.

To protect the confidentiality of the coaching sessions, the situations described do not refer to any particular individual but are a combination of several experiences.

Extracts from reviews of the first edition

Susan Kersley has written a very positive book which I'm sure will help doctor readers to get a grip on controlling their lives. This book should inspire doctors to see that they can change their work and home lives to do what they have always wanted to do – but haven't yet ...

Dr Ruth Chambers, Professor of Primary Care Development,
Staffordshire University

The quality of your life depends on the quality of the questions you ask. Taking even a small amount of advice on offer, asking even a few of the questions Susan poses, whilst acting on your answers will radically change the quality of your life, whether or not you decide to change direction. Reading this book will help reduce stress and mental ill health amongst doctors and that can only be good for the practice of medicine.

Lizzie Miller, Secretary, Doctors Support Network and
Occupational Health Physician

I am not a doctor, never have been and never will be ... but I experience similar problems with stress, overwork and frustration in my own career. Susan Kersley's brilliant and original advice on getting better harmony and more fulfilment in life is a terrific inspiration to us all – just what the (well-balanced) doctor ordered.

Mark Carwardine, best-selling and award-winning
writer and BBC Radio 4 presenter

'Just because you are a doctor, it doesn't mean you have to be one.' So advised a friend of mine, and I've never looked back. But there are lots of good things about medicine I miss, and if I'd had access to such inspirational, supportive, optimistic and insightful coaching as this, I might never have felt the need to leave. Thoroughly recommended, whatever you end up doing with your life.

Phil Hammond, writer, broadcaster, comedian and resting doctor

Susan Kersley is a doctor turned life coach, whose name is familiar to many who read BMJ Careers. *Now, her snippets of wisdom have been put together in a book.*

As doctors, we may find it easy to write prescriptions for our patients. But how

can we do the same for ourselves if our lives are not satisfactory? Change has to come from within – there is no-one else who will do it for us or give us a little pill to put things right.

Susan starts off by getting the reader to work out whether personal lifestyle improvements need to be made. Then she goes on to suggest how. A lot of it sounds like common sense, but if that is the case, why is it so difficult to implement? She advocates breaking tasks down into manageable chunks, rather than being daunted by something that is apparently impossible.

She comes up with some startling insights – for instance, 'The way you live now has some stability. Even if you aren't happy … you live in your comfort zone.' This description would be familiar to many.

The theory is interspersed with case studies about doctors, which make it more real. There is also a whole chapter devoted to detailed scenarios. The book is written in a conversational, down-to-earth style that is mostly easy to follow.

Overall, I would thoroughly recommend this book to doctors, to help themselves, their families or patients.

Dr Rachel Hooke, review published on www.doctors.net.uk website

Why did you choose medicine as a career? Was it because you wanted to use your knowledge to make people better? Or perhaps you felt the money was good? Or maybe you wanted the respect or the status? Whatever the reasons, over the years you may have come to regret your choice. You may be desperately wishing that you had done things differently and your dissatisfaction may be manifesting itself in a variety of different ways, e.g. an unhealthy lifestyle or a short temper. Susan Kersley's inspiring book illustrates just how it is possible to improve your life and lot by following some simple principles.

Changing your life can feel very uncomfortable and it is very easy to procrastinate. You need to set out your goals clearly – it's not helpful just to wish vaguely for an improvement in your life. Your goals must be realistic. For instance, dreaming of being a rock guitarist instead of a GP is unlikely to be achievable if you've never picked up a guitar in your life. But you could take up guitar lessons instead of crashing out every night in front of the TV! Bit by bit you can start to change things but it's up to you to start the ball rolling.

Read how to become more time aware and how to say no to tasks that you should not be doing. Doctors don't like to say no – by doing so, we feel uncaring and unreasonable. After all, aren't we supposed to help people all we can? A healthy body and mind are vitally important; we need to look after number one rather more. How many of us compound our problems by smoking, eating and drinking to excess? When we are ill, do we take time off and seek medical help or do we soldier on and self medicate, to the detriment of ourselves and our patients?

Although at first this book made me squirm as I drew parallels between the case studies in it and my own circumstances, it showed me the way to change my rather

blinkered thinking and will, I am confident, give many doctors the means to trans-
form their unhappy existences with sound advice and guidance. If you are not happy
with your career in medicine and you want to do something about it, I would
strongly suggest that you read this book.

Dr JM Sager, General Practitioner, Leeds

Introduction

A few years ago, frustrated by diminishing resources, unrealistic expectations from patients, managers, Government and the low morale of colleagues, I decided it was time to do something different.

My seven mile journey through the rush hour took nearly an hour. I stopped and started, edging forward through the underpasses of Birmingham, fed up with traffic jams and aware of the recurring thought, 'I don't want to do this any more...'.

Over several months this feeling spread from the car journey to issues about my work too. I was the senior family planning and women's health doctor for a community trust. Clinics were busier each week, staff morale was falling and patients' anger increasing. All this was happening against a background of budget cuts to reach targets to gain greater efficiency, allegedly. Since locums were no longer available, return from holidays meant a greater workload. I knew I wanted to change my life but wasn't clear about the details: the 'how', 'what', 'when' or even the 'why', I began to ask the question, 'Who am I, apart from a doctor?'.

I talked to various people about my wish for a different sort of life but my ideas were dismissed. Colleagues and friends showed their concern. They said 'You'll miss it', and 'You'll long to deal with patients.' They tried some emotional blackmail too: 'You are so good at what you do', 'The patients always ask for you when you are away.' There was no encouragement to do what I truly wanted. With hindsight, what I desperately needed was someone, anyone, prepared to listen, challenge and support without judgement. What I heard instead were comments based on the listener's personal reaction to me, a doctor, who wanted to leave medicine, after more than 30 years, to change my life.

If only I had known about coaching then, my transition could have been much easier. A life coach might have said, 'go for it', and encouraged me with, 'whatever you want in your life is what is right for you'. This would have validated, valued and motivated me to achieve more quickly. However, at the time, I'd never heard of coaching and how useful it might be. On my own I found it easier to remain in a situation with which I was familiar, even though I knew very strongly I wanted something else. I was comfortable in my discomfort, at least for the time being. Nevertheless, the feeling stayed with me until, at last, I had to answer the call.

So what did I do? Eventually, I found the courage to write my letter of resignation and take early retirement. It was a very difficult and somewhat scary decision to make.

At last, I knew I had done the right thing because something magical happened. Although people kept telling me that 'I could always do some locums', I knew it intellectually, but emotionally I was convinced that this was it, the start of a new journey. Since then I've enjoyed travelling from Alaska to Antarctica, reading and writing novels, and discovering who I am without the doctor label. I've trained and now practise as a life coach, enabling and encouraging stressed and overworked doctors and others to become more fulfilled in their professional roles while achieving a better balance between their work and the rest of life.

This has been a time for me to re-invent myself and find a new way of life, another way of fulfilment. Since leaving medicine I've learned new ways to use my life experiences as a doctor, a professional and as a person.

Now I'm passionate about working with doctors and enabling them to improve their lives. I *know* doctors can be happier and more fulfilled by applying coaching techniques. You *can* improve not only your working and personal relationships but also have a better work–life balance, look after yourself more and have fun.

Although, for me, the way forward was to leave medicine, I truly believe that doctors can improve their lives while remaining in the profession.

Change has a considerable psychological impact on the human mind. To the fearful it is threatening because it means that things may get worse. To the hopeful it is encouraging because things may get better. To the confident it is inspiring because the challenge exists to make things better.

King Whitney

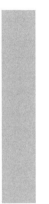

Part One

You can change your life

What we call the beginning is often the end. And to make an end is to make a beginning. The end is where we start from.

TS Eliot

1 Life coaching and doctors

What would make your life better?

Could it be any or all of the following:

- improved communication skills
- better relationships
- a more effective use of time
- better self-care
- a clear focus on what is important for you
- an understanding and application of boundaries
- giving and receiving support
- more balance between work and home life
- happiness
- feeling valued.

If you know something is missing in your life and want the opportunity to reflect on your medical career and change the way you deal with challenges, then life coaching, which is for successful people, may be for you.[1] Like many doctors you may be unhappy, especially if you believe you are over-worked, underpaid, inadequately supported, have falling status, are worn out by change, have less control over what you do and are increasingly accountable.[2,3]

The Health Service is deteriorating as politicians raise patients' expectations of what is possible.[4] As you become more harassed the quality of your patient care might be affected.[5]

Does life as a doctor have to be like this?

Life coaching offers you support, discussion, encouragement and motivation, enabling you to deal better with the strain of being a doctor. By developing enhanced relationship and communication skills, the way you deal with difficult colleagues or patients can be improved.[6]

Coaching provides you with the chance to re-think what you value in your life. A life coach is there for you, encourages you to follow your own agenda and gives you the opportunity to talk to someone who listens fully. This can provide a new perspective on a situation. A challenging question or two may strike a chord, help you recognise patterns in your life and decide how to change them. The process can empower and motivate you. When you recognise and satisfy your own needs you become even better at what you do, which is important for coping with the ups and downs of life.[7]

Coaching opens your eyes to parts of life which you have neglected and encourages you to introduce new habits to improve your fulfilment in areas unconnected with work.

If you are experiencing the frustration, stress, low morale, disempowerment and overwork of being a doctor, this may become detrimental to you, your wellbeing and the health of your patients.[8,9] When you are fit emotionally and physically, you and also your patients benefit.

A life coach listens, reflects and encourages you to set and reach your goals, by helping you to focus on specific actions and steps. Rather like a sports trainer to a champion, a life coach encourages you to go that little bit further than you would on your own.

How does life coaching differ from counselling?

Life coaching is a forward looking, active process, whereas counselling tends to deal with and explore emotional issues from the past and cope with crises.

Life coaching is about improving the quality of your life and creating what you want in it now and for the future. It enables you to close the gap between how your life is and how you would like it to be. It encompasses all areas of life, not only your career.

The medical model

You are used to patients with unrealistic expectations of what you can do. The traditional model is of the doctor with all the answers, able to cure everyone and everything. This misconception by your patients, and possibly believed by you too, includes the belief that you are superhuman and cannot possibly have any health problems yourself. Sadly this is not the case and you, like many doctors, may find it difficult to deal with your own mental or physical illnesses and recognise your own needs.[10,11]

As a frustrated general practitioner (GP) or doctor working in hospital or the community, you are likely to be part of a multidisciplinary healthcare team so the way patients are treated is often arranged to fit around reaching the latest government targets (such as reduction of numbers on the waiting list), which may or may not be related to clinical need. Managers have the final say about much of what you do, and you might not have been part of the decision-making process.[12] You may be fed up about being at the mercy of a system which you believe you have to put up with because it can't be changed.

The coaching model

In an ideal world you would work and cooperate well with colleagues and managers, listen to each other and recognise that everyone involved has something to contribute. Every member of the team would respect and value each other. Your medical skills would be used appropriately and non-medical tasks delegated correctly to others trained to do them efficiently. You would learn new skills regularly to keep up to date and work even more professionally. Moreover, you would have the time and energy to have a happy and fulfilling life outside work, since you are clear about setting and maintaining boundaries and have excellent communication skills with patients, colleagues and managers.

Women doctors

Women doctors have twice the rate of suicide of other women.[13] In spite of opportunities for job sharing and part-time appointments, full-time colleagues may resent this.[14]

There are now more women than men qualifying in medicine. The culture of the medical profession is slowly recognising this. However, if you are a female doctor you have added stress possibly in relation to:

- a desire to succeed in your chosen specialty while being aware of your biological clock and worrying about the ideal time to have children[15]
- coming to terms with not having any children
- if you have children – concerns about adequate childcare.

However well organised you are, there may be problems, such as having to stay with a patient, knowing that your child is waiting to be collected from school or wondering if your child minder will be able to comfort your sick child.

Medicine, like being a parent, can be an all-encompassing way of life, not just a job. As a doctor, you are involved in looking after everyone else's needs while, perhaps, neglecting your own.

Life coaching: is it for doctors?

It is widely known that there is low morale and frustration amongst doctors in the NHS. The word 'doctor' seems to be permanently linked to the word 'stress'. There are harassed consultants and GPs buckling under the strain.[16]

Life coaches encourage you to consider the advantages of looking after your physical and emotional needs. They encourage you to have better balance and fulfilment in all areas of your life. When you work with a coach you learn to say 'no' more often and set clearer boundaries, both physical and emotional. In this way you gradually rid your life of whatever drains your energy and increase the things which give you more 'get-up-and-go', so that your life as a doctor can be much improved.[17]

What would make your life as a doctor more bearable?

- Being valued more.
- More money.
- A professional support network.
- More time.
- Less paperwork.
- Less isolation.
- Being able to express early grievances.
- Constructive peer review.
- More sleep.
- An opportunity to express and deal with anger.
- The collaboration and communication of team members.[18]

Coaching is your *prescription for change* to achieve all of these.

References

1   Atik Y (2000) Personal coaching for senior doctors. *BMJ Career Focus*. **320**:S2.
2   Smith R (2001) Why are doctors so unhappy? *BMJ*. **322**:1073–4.
3   Ferriman A (2001) Doctors explain their unhappiness. *BMJ*. **322**:1073.
4   Kmietowicz Z (2001) GP dossier. *BMJ*. **322**:1197.
5   Firth-Cozens J (1998) Hours, sleep, teamwork and stress. *BMJ*. **317**:1335.
6   Camm J (2001) Why bad teams make you ill. *Hospital Doctor*. 24 May, p. 11.
7   Stewart-Brown S (1998) Emotional well-being and its relation to health. *BMJ*. **317**:1608.
8   Wafer A (2001)Waiting list pressures put doctors health in danger. *BMA News*. 19 May.
9   Williams K (1998) Coping with work stress. *BMA News*. 11 April.
10   Baron S (2001) Doctors who have chronic illnesses. *BMJ Career Focus*. **322**:S2.

11   Ahuja A (2000) Doctors in despair. *The Times*. 6 July.

12   Bratby L (2001) Survey shows pressure A&E doctors are under. *Hospital Doctor*. 5 May.

13   Harper V (2001) Operating under pressure. *The Independent on Sunday*. 13 May.

14   Grant S (2001) The battle for flexible work. *Hospital Doctor*. 19 April.

15   Thompson A (2001)When is the best time to have children? *Hospital Doctor*. 5 April.

16   Clews G (2001) BMA dossier paints a stark picture of overworked GPs. *BMA News*. 19 May.

17   Building Healthy Attitudes and Coping Strategies, 12 Steps for Health Professionals. Physician Health program (administered by the Ontario Medical Association). www.phpoma.org/php/export/sites/default/Resources/pdf/12_steps_04_text.pdf

18   Luck C (2000) Reducing stress among junior doctors. *BMJ Career Focus*. **321**:S2.

2 Are you ready?

Life is what happens to you while you're busy making other plans.

John Lennon

Have a life and be a doctor too

How would you like to lead a happy and fulfilled life with plenty of time for everything? Can you imagine what it would be like to:

- be naturally tired after a satisfactory day's work,
- have enough energy when you go home
- spend quality time with your family
- look after your body, mind and spirit on a regular and enjoyable basis.

Is this an impossible dream?

Here are some questions for you to consider especially when you find yourself on the treadmill of unrelenting work from demanding patients and government quotas.

- How you will get through not only another day, but every day for the next however many years?
- What happened to your golden dream of life as a doctor?
- How can you stop it becoming more tarnished?
- Have you resigned yourself to the never ending pressure of being a doctor?
- Have you decided to put up with the erosion of work into your personal life?
- Did you work hard for so many years for this?
- Are you now ready to do something to change your life?

What is so special about being a doctor?

There is no doubt that medicine is a very fulfilling and satisfying profession. But does being a doctor inevitably mean you are prevented from fully enjoying your family or your partner and taking an active part in your community?

Does being part of the medical profession stop you looking beyond your role and realising that you, like everyone else, have your own personal, emotional and spiritual needs, too? Does your inability to 'switch off' relate to a desire in you to feel wanted and important?

Does the challenge of sorting out problems, making decisions, arranging appropriate investigations and initiating the right treatment blur the reality of many doctors' experience of:

- not being valued
- lack of personal choice
- long hours of work and frustration.

As a doctor, you spend most of your time caring for others and may neglect looking after your own general health and wellbeing. Your physical or emotional health suffer as a result of the demands made of you.

You know, deep down, if only you had the courage to say 'enough is enough', you would be able to live a better life. You may be anxious about the possible response of others, so you carry on doing things you no longer want to do.

If you hope for *someone else* to initiate change, you may wait a long time. Sometimes the only way things can be different is for you, yes *you*, as an individual, to take action.

Prescription for change

Now is the time for you to find your own *prescription for change* to be a doctor and have a life. You won't find what you are looking for on a pharmacy shelf but, if you are ready to change your life, this book will guide you with signposts and tools. If you read it with a receptive mind and be open to new possibilities then you will discover what you seek.

Teachers open the door. You enter by yourself.

Chinese proverb

What's stopping you from doing what you want?

It may be fear, lack of clarity about your desired outcome, or not knowing how to convert your dreams into achievable goals. Be prepared to look at your beliefs objectively and be creative in your thinking. It's called 'getting out of the box'. The instructions for getting out of the box are written on the outside. In other words when you look at your world from another perspective, you will know what you have to do.

This book is the catalyst for the life you want

If you are clear about what you want to achieve then you will be looking for the right map to reach your destination.

You have a choice right now. You can continue on the way you are and be fulfilled medically while you neglect the rest. However, if you dream of a better life then this book could be the beginning of a new journey. You can choose to take action or do nothing. What will you do?

This book will start you thinking about your life. Some of the questions may challenge you. Some will have an obvious answer, others may take a while for you to consider. The questions are there to encourage you to reflect on your life, how you'd like it to be and how making changes in the way you deal with a situation can make a difference, not only to you but also to others around you.

It's very easy to sit back and resign yourself to what is, rather than what could be, the 'I've made my bed, now I have to sleep in it' mentality. Instead of complaining about the 'system' you could start to believe that you can make a difference.

Recording your journey

Buy yourself a special notebook or a journal to keep a personal record of the ups and downs of your life's journey. Over the next few weeks there will be times which seem very difficult, when you feel as though you are being tossed about in a storm and wonder if you've made a big mistake to even think about making changes. Writing your own account, and reflecting on what's happening to you, will help to keep your focus on your ultimate destination and guide you into calmer waters to carry on towards it.

Are you ready to start?

The first step to getting the things you want out of life is this: decide what you want.

Ben Stein

Take a moment to think about and imagine your ideal life. Consider the sights, the smells, the sounds, and how you feel. Close your eyes and see it all in glorious technicolor.

Would you like to be there instead of here? Don't worry if you have no idea at this stage how you can reach this life; you are on your way. If you have a vision or some ideas then the next thing is to get on to the right path. Break big goals into smaller steps that you can begin today. You've already taken the first step by recognising that you would like things to be different and imagining specifically what it is you want instead.

Well done! Too many people put up with an unsatisfactory life, believing it is their 'lot', and their fleeting ideas are dismissed as impossible or ridiculous.

> Dr A would like to be a photographer instead of a GP. He wants to gain a professional qualification. He must find out what courses are available, so the very first step is to make a phone call to the local college. He does this and asks for an application form. He's on his way towards his goal!

Life has its ups and downs

Not everything is the way you want it to be. There is always a lesson to be learned from adversity. Try it. If you have a particularly difficult day, ask yourself the following.

- What have I learned from this experience?
- What positive can I find amongst the negative?
- If I were ever to find myself in the same situation, what would I do differently?

Foster a more positive mindset

> Dr B was exhausted because of visiting his dying father each week. The positive outcomes were that he spent more quality time with his mother than he had for years and was happy to be able to give her the support she needed. He also realised how nice it was to have a few hours each week to catch up on some medical journal reading on the train journey to London and back.

As you explore the various options to find your own *prescription for change* take time to think about anything which resonates with you. There may be a reason for the 'gut feeling' you get from a particular example or quotation. Explore those things more fully and let the thoughts lead you wherever they do. Don't forget to write down your reflections on what happens.

However brilliant your ideas, your life will not change unless you do something you are not doing now. It's a well-known adage that if you continue to do what you've always done you will continue to get what you've always got.

I encourage you to find someone to support you – a mentor, coach, friend or colleague – someone who inspires and motivates you to continue when you feel stuck and be a sounding board. Who is there for you?

Your journey

Like any expedition, life's journey is not always plain sailing or comfortable. There may be times when you are filled with doubt and wonder whether you've made a big mistake. Keep your mind open to different possibilities and take advantage of the opportunities you find, even though you may have a bit of a rough crossing with pressure from friends, family or colleagues who don't understand, or think you have lost your way and try to get you back on the track you were on before.

If you hang on and keep your ultimate goal clearly in your mind, then eventually the storm will settle and you will reach your destination. Be aware of possible hazards so you can ride the storm. Remember there is likely to be some sense of chaos on the way to your ideal life.

Are you ready?

There is no such thing as a long piece of work, except one that you dare not start.

Charles Baudelaire

3 Do you have a life?

Doctors' lives

Several doctors talked to me about their lives. To my surprise there were two distinct responses.

There were those who were angry because they felt:

- undervalued
- overworked
- underpaid.

They complained bitterly about:

- not having enough time
- working with colleagues and partners with whom they found it difficult to communicate.

They were frustrated by:

- lack of understanding of their role
- unsatisfactory working relationships.

They found it difficult to maintain a happy home life when demands of their patients had to be dealt with as a priority.[1]

Many of the doctors told me they neglected their own health and well-being and were unable to follow the advice they would give their patients.

Do you recognise yourself?

A female GP knows her children are waiting to be collected from school while she deals with a suspected heart attack in the surgery.

Another GP continues seeing patients when she is ill herself because there is no one else to do the work. She is frustrated when a large proportion of the patients come for non-medical reasons. Perhaps, as a result of not looking after herself and taking time off when she is ill, she feels unwell and tired for several weeks afterwards.

A hospital consultant is irritated because he is unable to maintain his high standards when he has to see too many patients during an outpatient clinic in order to reach government targets.

Medical way of life

As a result of the lifestyle of many doctors and the unrealistic expectations patients have of them, there is a high level of stress in the profession and doctors' health is suffering.[2]

When you arrive at your clinic or surgery, do you inwardly groan when you pick up the notes and recognise another of your 'heart-sink' patients waiting to see you?

You know you have to reach certain targets each month and find it frustrating when many of these are unrelated to clinical need.

Both your physical and emotional health are affected by your lifestyle. If you were your own doctor you would say it can't go on like this, the time has come to take yourself in hand, pull yourself together and make some changes.

So why do you continue to put up with the way things are?[3] Perhaps it's because making changes seems so difficult to do and you may believe it's easier to keep the status quo rather than rock the boat.

Is this a life?

- Is your life balanced when work is the only thing which is important?
- Being a doctor takes all your time and energy.
- You find it difficult to come to terms with the demands of patients and the reality of working for the NHS.
- You would like to connect again with your values.

The other side of the picture is that there are some doctors who aren't fed up. If you are one of these, you are content, fulfilled, lead a happy life and may be wondering what this chapter is about. Even when you are busy, you are able and know how to 'switch off' in order to relax, have fun and plenty of time with your family and friends. You also find time to pursue your own interests and hobbies.

Congratulations! Please support your colleagues and show them how to live the same way.

Differences between the two groups

Members of the second group of doctors manage to have a good quality of life. What they do eludes the first group. Their secret is that they:

- are very clear about boundaries, particularly between work and leisure
- work hard and when they go home, they switch off
- have an interest or hobby – creative or sports-oriented
- are excellent time managers
- are clear about how they spend their day
- know what to do themselves and what to delegate
- don't waste time
- have outstanding communication skills
- look after themselves physically and emotionally.[4]

Is it difficult to change?

It's not that some people have willpower and some don't. It's that some people are ready to change and others are not.

James Gordon

The way you live now probably has some stability. Even if you aren't happy, you know the rules and you live in your comfort zone. To introduce new habits in to your life may take a few weeks of self-discipline before they become automatic.

The first time you try something different you may feel your actions are contrived and uncomfortable, but eventually they become a habit and your comfort zone increases. It's worth enduring a little awkwardness to make a big difference to the rest of your life.

Do you recall how ill at ease you were and how difficult it was to remember all the actions needed to drive a car? It's the same with life. At first making changes seems easier said than done until eventually you get into your 'autopilot' mode and make them almost without thinking.

It's easy to stay in an unsatisfactory situation unless you have the strong desire to get out of it and are prepared to do something.

How do you change the system?

By changing what you do. You can't transform other people, only yourself.

Because everything is interconnected, when you do something different, others will modify their behaviour too. Don't wait for them. Be proactive and take the first step.[5]

Making a start

Decide what you want to achieve, your desired outcome. *Begin with the end in mind.*[5]

Be very specific about your goal. For example, 'I want to feel less stressed' is vague. A specific goal could be, 'I want to see a maximum of 15 patients in my outpatient clinic by the end of December'.

At first, your goal may seem to be totally unachievable. Ask yourself, if it is theoretically possible. Decide on the date by which you want to reach your goal, and write it in your diary.

Take the first step. Make a definite commitment, an undertaking to yourself, to do something that you are not doing now. What will you commit to doing by the end of this month? By the end of this week? By the end of today? For example, if you want to see fewer patients and you put up with overbooking week after week, ask the appointments clerk to book one less patient per clinic each week. That would be four less per month, each month. In nine months you could go from 48 patients to 12 per clinic. Unbelievable? It could happen!

What's stopping you?

Fear is the most common reason for not doing something; fear it might not work; fear of what other people will say about you; fear about making a fool of yourself.

The thought of challenging the system is scary. If you are worried your manager would lose their job, think instead about how you are perpetuating an unsatisfactory system. If the system needs to be changed it can be done by individuals making their own small changes.

If you are letting fear stop you making progress, would you prefer to continue as you are because of it? Consider what might be the worst thing to happen if your fear materialised compared with what will happen if you continue as before. List the advantages and disadvantages, for you, of making the changes you want.

Top ten benefits from making changes

1   When you start to change one part of your life other parts change too.
2   You have more time.

3   You stop procrastinating.
4   You spend some time each day doing something for yourself.
5   You get rid of things which drain energy.
6   You enjoy more satisfactory relationships.
7   You understand and create your boundaries.
8   You look after yourself.
9   You know what really matters in your life.
10   You take action, instead of waiting for others.

Moving forward

Some people have their own reasons for keeping things as they are and they enjoy telling you all the negative outcomes, as they see them, of what you plan to do. Once you've made a start it's easier to continue. So, having made the decision to change it's important that you:

- do something
- start with a small step
- find someone to motivate and encourage you.

The best time

The optimal time is now. It's easy to think of reasons why it would be better to postpone the decision. Do a reality check to make sure there are genuine reasons for delaying or whether your own beliefs are stopping you. Too often you have good ideas and you even tell others what you've decided and then do nothing. Don't procrastinate any longer. It's making a start that's so important. You don't have to wait for a whole day to complete the task. There is something empowering about making a start and doing a little bit each day.

Is there a need for change?

Many doctors believe they have to deal with whatever the system throws at them. Some leave medicine entirely, a few seek part-time jobs, others continue until they reach breaking point, overdose with alcohol or tablets, or take time off for stress-related illnesses.

   If you want your life to be better, happier and less stressful, it's a sign of your strength not weakness to talk about and get support to achieve what you want. Don't wait until you can't cope any more. You need lots of energy to make changes.

But nothing changes

Unless you take personal responsibility then nothing may change. If you wait for someone else then you may be disappointed. The system takes many years to alter but you can begin to enjoy your own life much, much more if you decide what you'd like and take action sooner rather than later.

Imagine a miracle

Close your eyes for a moment and see yourself in your ideal life. How do you feel? What do you see, hear, smell and taste? From your vision for the future decide on something you can do now to move you nearer towards what you want. Then start with the first step. *Today.*

> *Know the true value of time; snatch, seize, and enjoy every moment of it. No idleness; no laziness; no procrastination; never put off till tomorrow what you can do today.*
>
> Lord Chesterfield

References

1   Smith R (2001) Why are doctors so unhappy? *BMJ.* **322**:1073.
2   Stewart-Brown S (1998) Emotional well-being and its relation to health. *BMJ.* **317**:1608.
3   Clark S (2000) Why do people become doctors and what can go wrong? *BMJ Career Focus.* **320**:S2.
4   Gray C (1997) Life, your career and the pursuit of happiness. *BMJ Career Focus.* **315**:S2.
5   Covey S (1989) *The Seven Habits of Highly Effective People.* Simon & Schuster, New York.

4 Are you a square peg in a round hole?

This above all: to thine own self be true.

William Shakespeare

How can it be different?

If the thought of the day ahead fills you with dread and you have the 'Monday morning feeling' every day, then, even though you are a doctor, a pillar of the community, following a worthy profession, you may not be living the life you want. You may wonder how or why you are so disheartened and unhappy about the decision you made to become a doctor. Thoughts about whether you've picked the right specialty or even career can make you insecure and anxious.[1]

Did you make the wrong choice?

Studying medicine and becoming a doctor was a major decision in your life. Were your motives for entering the profession misguided? Do you regret your chosen career, wish you were happier with it but believe that there's nothing you could change?

What can you do?

Take an objective look at where you are. Don't linger too long in misgivings or examining what might have been. The past can't be changed, it made you the person you are today. You may have already spent a lot of time going over and over what happened, the how and the why of it all. But eventually the time comes when you have to look to your future. Will it be the opportunity you want? If you are prepared to do something to alter the course you are on, you can look forward to a better life.

Dr A did medicine to spite a teacher who said he wasn't clever.

> Dr B chose radiology, which she doesn't enjoy, instead of her passion orthopaedics, because she was told surgery would be too difficult.

Then what?

Turn your mind's eye to what is yet to come and create a mental picture of how your life could be. See yourself in the image. Be very clear about what is important to you.[2]

Think about when you last felt that everything was going well for you, when life seemed effortless, when you were confident and going with the flow. Then explore how you can have more of those feelings brought into your life again, both in and out of work.

Who are you?

You are a doctor, but what or who else are you without the 'doctor' label? Take a look at what's left without it. Is anyone there, or has the rest of you disintegrated like the wicked witch in *The Wizard of Oz*?

Recognise what is unique and special about you. Your medical hat may have become so much part of you that you may not be able to take it off very often. It's as if it is stuck with superglue.

Since working is such an important part of your life it's vital to find ways to combine it with your hopes and values so you are content, happy and fulfilled both inside and outside your job.

You are so busy with your work-related activities, you have no time for anything else in your already stressful life. Your colleagues are little help as there is a culture of 'grin and bear it' and 'why worry about things which may never happen'.

But you do worry and a major concern is the answer to the question: 'Who am I?'. You might wonder who you would be if a decision to leave medicine was forced on you, if you had to take early retirement on the grounds of ill health, for example.

What do you need in your life now to complete your personal jigsaw? Have you forgotten who you really are? You are a doctor, full stop. Is that truly all? Sometimes you might find yourself wondering who you are without the label, and who you would be if you decided to leave medicine. Perhaps there are times when you feel almost invisible, as though others only see your white coat and stethoscope.

Do you need to find the missing pieces before you reveal yourself more fully? Where do they fit? Where are they hidden? When you introduce yourself to someone you've just met, what do you tell them and what do you leave out? What does this say about you? Is there something important about you that you hide, ration the truth about, or choose to keep as a secret?

> Dr C entered the same specialty as her father but found it almost impossible to live up to his expectations.

> Dr D never told his colleagues that he used to be a priest.

> Dr E avoided telling his colleagues about his episodes of mental health problems.

> Dr F dreaded anyone finding out that he had a partner of the same sex.

What are you ready to tell?

Do you have a lack of clarity about your personal identity? Does what you say about yourself give a sense of your values, of what you feel passionately about, or what you love to do? If you are in the wrong specialty or profession, if you are a square peg in a round hole, how can you ever be true to yourself?

- What's stopping you being honest, first with yourself and then with others?
- What do you fear?
- What's the worst thing which could happen?
- Whose life are you living?
- What do you need to do to make yourself more comfortable with your life?
- Is it time to let your true self shine through?

Being seen

In parts of West Africa people greet and respond to each other by saying 'I am here' to which the response is 'I see you'.

Notice the effect of someone saying they see you, and how much more powerful it is than 'How do you do?'. It's rather like the greeting used in Nepal, 'Namaste', meaning 'the divine in me recognises the divine in you'.

Do you recognise the person beyond the job, beyond the stereotype? When you see them as they really are, they will begin to see the authentic you too.

Is it too late?

Yes or no. Whatever you believe is true. But if you are unhappy then any change, however small, will begin to make a difference to what you believe about yourself and to your life.

When others perceive you differently, then they may change the way they behave towards you too (for better or worse).

Like a garden, what you want is unlikely to bloom overnight (unless it's artificial). You have to plant lots of seeds, tend them, and then be patient until eventually some of them blossom.

> Dr G wonders about giving up medicine as he's always wanted to be an artist. He decides to continue to work as a locum GP to earn enough while pursuing an art degree. He becomes happier and more self-confident as he takes some positive steps. An unexpected outcome is that he enjoys the medical work much more and decides to do both in parallel.

Here is a challenge. The next time someone says to you, 'Tell me a bit about yourself', avoid saying, 'I'm a doctor' as the first thing. Instead, start with telling them what you value, what the most important thing is for you. Perhaps this will lead you towards a renewed sense of personal worth and heightened self-esteem.

What seeds for change will you plant this week?

He who knows others is wise. He who knows himself is enlightened.

Lao Tzu

References

1   Dosani S (2002) Stop the rotation I want to get off. *BMJ Career Focus*. **324**:S125.
2   Houghton A (2002) Values? What values? *BMJ Career Focus*. **324**:S59.

5 How to change your life in seven easy steps

If you don't like something, change it. If you can't change it, change your attitude. Don't complain.

Maya Angelou

Step one: Do you want change?

If you've had enough of being overworked, undervalued and not doing things you really would like to do, then you can choose what to do. You *can* choose to make the decision to change your life especially if any of the following resonate with you.

- Perhaps you are fed up trying to reach unrealistic targets and you find yourself wondering if there is more to life.
- You regularly wish you had more time to do things outside of medicine, but there don't seem to be enough hours in the day.
- You suspect, or know for sure, your emotional or physical health is suffering.

Instead of a life governed by meeting objectives which don't relate to your values, if you would love to have more autonomy and be able to make more decisions in your life then you *do* want to change.

If you spend so much time at work so you hardly ever see your partner or children, then it *is* time to change. If you missed your child's first steps, first words or other milestones, or haven't had the time to find your life's partner, then it *is* time for you to change.

If you want to be much better organised, so you can look after your own needs then it *is* the moment to make a start.

Become aware of how, when you change your thoughts, your behaviour changes too.

How do you answer the question Do you want to change, now? If your answer is yes then continue with Step two.

Step two: How would you like it to be?

You are ready to take the next step. You've decided you really do want to make some changes but are not sure how to start. Stephen Covey says in his book *The Seven Habits of Highly Effective People*, 'Begin with the end in mind'. If you want to change your life, you have to develop a clear vision of how life would be if everything was as you want.

Visualise

Sit quietly and close your eyes. Starting with your feet, relax your lower limbs. Then working your way through your body, relax your abdomen and your arms. Finally, let your face and your head settle down. Your breathing will become slow and shallow. Then imagine opening a door into a wonderful place. Keep your eyes closed, take a look around and using all your senses, in your mind's eye, look and hear, smell and touch your surroundings. Be aware of your emotions. Once you are sure you have explored as much as you can of your vision, take a few deep breaths, and slowly open your eyes. Have a good stretch. Then take your notebook or journal and write about what you saw, heard, smelled, tasted and felt.

Visualisation is an important tool to assist change because it helps you know what you want. If you regularly say 'I can't stand this any longer' but fail to think what you want instead, it is much less likely that anything will change. It's as though you went into a shop and asked for a map, any map. You would be confused if you were given a map of Birmingham when you were exploring Glasgow.

Getting what you want is to know specifically what you would like. It's not enough to say 'No more of this'. You have to be able to state positively what you wish for: 'What I want now is…'.

If you could be transported into your vision, how would you behave? What would be different about you? What about the expression on your face, your posture and the way you move about? How would others realise that you were having the time of your life? What can you start doing now? How would your behaviour or your body language be if you were already living your ideal life?

Another way to define what you want is to ask yourself the questions which follow and reflect on your answers in your journal.

- What is most important to you?
- What do you value in life?
- How can you live in a way that recognises your values?

A consultant in an inner city hospital would love to live by the sea so he can sail regularly. Although he says this often to his colleagues and family over many years, he takes no action.

- Does he really want to change?
- What scares him?
- Is he clear about the vision?

What could he do? He has various choices.

- Continue as now. What would life be like if he stays put and doesn't make any change? How will he feel when he retires and realises he is no longer well enough to do what he wants?
- Fit the things he wants into his current lifestyle. Perhaps he can't move to the sea but he could go sailing on one of the big reservoirs, or take regular holidays by the sea.
- Decide to make a big change in his life and move to live on the coast. When he looks at the job adverts he finds there are suitable jobs available in coastal towns.

The last option might seem so big and so scary, he ends up doing nothing. He may, on the other hand decide to follow his dream and take a first step by making some enquiries to find out if it would be practical to pursue it. Something like this might happen: he contacts various hospitals to enquire about job vacancies and looks in the *BMJ* each week for adverts for posts in areas he is interested in. He and his wife spend a weekend driving around the area and they talk about schools and house prices and what a move might mean for all of the family. With this knowledge he can begin to make an informed choice.

Things happen when you have a clear vision.

Here are more examples of what some doctors discuss with their life coach.

A GP would like to work part time so that he can present television programmes. He hasn't done this yet because he thinks he is too old and would have to do a course for presenters too. So, he does nothing and life goes on as before. His beliefs stop him taking any action. His coach challenges him to make enquiries to find out some facts, about possible age barriers and qualifications needed. After he talks to some people he has greater clarity about the situation and applies to become a news reader on local radio. This is the first step towards the vision.

A pathologist always wanted to join a choir. He hasn't done so because he's much too busy. During coaching he is challenged about what he could do to create more time in order to join a choir. He thinks about what doesn't have to be done by him (things that he can delegate). He realises that filing patients' notes is the clerical officer's task, not his. He also devises a more efficient system of dictating notes as he goes along. As a result he finishes on time and is able to go to the choir rehearsal.

That's the crux of it. You have to become clear about your vision for your future, be creative and let your ideas flow.

If you are a doctor there is nothing, except your own beliefs, stopping you from finding time for whatever you are passionate about. There is plenty of room in your life to do more than you could possibly imagine. You might even find you begin to enjoy the medical work much more when you take some time out, regularly, to do something which gives you joy.

What do you regret giving up?

Do you tell people about hobbies or activities you used to do before you got so busy? Wouldn't you like to do those things again and regain some balance in your life, and look after your physical, mental and emotional health much more? Do you love dancing, yoga, painting or playing the violin? Is it ages since you did any of these?

Stop talking and start doing. Start by day dreaming, thinking vividly about how it would be if you did some of the things you have given up or put on hold for the time being. It's time to work out ways to do them again. With your vision in mind, you can start behaving 'as if' what you want is already in your life.

Change your body language

If you want more confidence you can walk with your head held up high. If you want to be happy, have a broad smile on your face.

Imagine feeling sad and depressed. Put your head downwards, round your shoulders, look to the ground. Does that make you feel even sadder? Then, stand up straight, with a big smile, shoulders back and striding out confidently. How do you feel now? Still feel depressed?

So this is Step two. How would you like it to be? Have you got your vision clear? Are you ready to move on to Step three?

Step three: What's stopping you?

How is your life now compared with how you would like it to be? Take a look at the possible obstacles in the way of having the life you want. It's easy to find excuses for not doing anything.

What's stopped you in the past? Is that a valid reason? Really? Does your fear of what people might say or think of you stop you from doing something beneficial for yourself?

Beliefs

If you are certain that jobs for doctors by the sea are oversubscribed then you don't send an application form.

Unproven assumptions

If you do something different it would upset other people. Are you so sure of what others would think or say if you did what you want to do? These ideas actually stop you from doing what you want.

Communication

Ask for what you want. If the other person says 'Oh no you can't do that', ask yourself 'What's the worst thing that can happen?'. Someone may react negatively to what you ask. They may be angry or jealous or sad. But it's their responsibility, not yours. Are you really not doing what you want because you worry that another person may be angry?

Take a risk every now and again.

A consultant gynaecologist, who lives in a large house and whose children go to a private school, is worried what his colleagues would think if he moved away to live in the country and work in a district general hospital. He realises he would lose most of his private practice income and his wife wouldn't be able to wear designer clothes any more. But he's always wanted to live away from the city and own a smallholding. Suddenly he understands it doesn't matter what his colleagues think of him and his children will be fine in the local school. His wife doesn't care if she wears jeans and a fleece as she plans to write a novel.

You may have a whole script of what various friends or colleagues would say or think about you if you did something they might find extra-ordinary.

But if there is something which you long to do, is it really out of character?

Could you believe, instead, that what you truly desire is absolutely in character, in contrast to the rest of the stuff, which bores you or causes your stress levels to rise.

Making changes is often scary. You may have reassured yourself for years with phrases such as:

- when the children have left home I'll…
- when I've lost weight I'll…
- when I get the job I'll….

What delaying tactics do you use? List them in your journal and decide how you will deal with them in the future. There is no need to wait. Wouldn't it be much more fun to start the life you want now rather than at some undefined time in the future? What else is stopping you? Is it:

- deciding how to do it
- needing to learn some new skills
- wanting to gather more information before you proceed
- making a commitment to when you will do it.

Now you've found out what may be stopping you, move on to Step four.

Step four: Make a start

Be truthful. What small change do you need to introduce into your life, your week or your day to improve your health and wellbeing? Even though there may not be an instant result, you have to start somewhere, with something.

Consider the future, your future. Do you stay stuck because you might upset someone by your action? Do you prefer to stay unhappy?

Is the change you are thinking about something that you really want? Are you listening to your own voice? Or is it someone else's plan for your life? Is your desire for change coming from your own enthusiasm or because of internal messages from a parent, partner, teacher or someone else? Are the ideas in your head from someone who told you the 'rules' for life from their perspective? Your circumstances have changed since then. Perhaps you are no longer single or have become so again. You may now have a young family or your children have grown up and moved away. Life changes. It's important to recognise what your life is like now. Is what you want a 'choice' or is it a 'should'?

Sometimes it's easier to stay in your everyday discomfort than to move into 'new waters'. For example it is well known that some people become chronic invalids until the court case to grant them compensation is complete. Recognise and reflect on the 'pay-off' from not changing.

Are you a bit of a 'control freak' and find it difficult to let people make their own decisions? Let go of trying to control others. Trust them to do whatever they need to do. This allows you more energy to do what you want.

What scares you?

Do you really know how others will react? Are you stopping yourself doing what you want because you are convinced that so and so would be upset or offended? Ask yourself 'If that person behaves as you believe, what would be the worst thing that could happen as a result?'.

Reflect on this – you are responsible for yourself. You can decide how to respond to your experiences. You always have a choice. You can choose whether to be angry or sad, happy or indifferent.

How do you feel if you look out of the window and it 's raining? Are you sad as you wanted to do some gardening or happy because you have the opportunity to go to a museum? Notice your reactions

If you are at a social event and moan that you have better things to do, notice what happens when you tell yourself you are enjoying yourself, how great it is to have the opportunity to meet such interesting people.

However wonderful your plans and intentions, nothing will be different in your life unless you take some action. Think back to all the times you've decided something without doing anything. It doesn't get done, does it?

Are you making excuses, valid reasons to justify staying where you are? Do you believe that you can't do anything until:

- a new consultant is appointed
- another year or two
- the new ward has been built
- you are less busy.

To make something happen, you have to make a start. Begin by letting the idea of change permeate inside you. Jot down as many ways you can think of as steps towards your goal. Some examples follow.

- Make a telephone call to someone who may know the answers you seek.

> Dr X wonders how many nights on-call he will have in a particular job, so he phones the person currently doing the work. He is pleased to hear there is a night on-call service.

- Look at job adverts.

> Dr Y assumes that jobs by the sea 'never come up', but when she starts to look through the BMJ each week there are suitable vacancies.

- Use local facilities.

> Dr Z has always wanted to join a band but has no idea if there is one nearby. He buys the local paper and looks at notices in the library, until he finds one not far away.

> Dr A wants to meet people to form a walking group. She puts a card in the corner shop and soon finds some like-minded people to walk with each weekend.

- Make enquiries.

> Dr B has put off learning Spanish because he's too busy. However, he finds that the adult education college has a course that he can attend during his free afternoon.

> Dr G looks up Alaska on the internet and books the trip she's always wanted to do.

What will be your first step?

It could be something very small, such as:

- making a few phone calls
- writing a letter
- arranging to talk to someone who can give you an insight into what you want to do.

But be wary: the other person has come from a different life experience. Listen and discuss with them but in the end the decision has to be yours, based on what you have found out about the subject and your own feelings.

Are you prepared to make a start? Then it's time to move to Step five.

Step five: Decision time

Action

So, you've thought about what you could do, now decide what you will do. It's time to make a plan. Write down a list of the various stages you need to complete before you can get to where you want to go. For example, if you would love to do a part-time course then until you find out where to do it, when the next course starts, how much it will cost and when you have to apply, then you will remain stuck.

Is what you want to do possible? Make an informed decision. It's easy to dismiss something by saying 'I'm too old to apply for that' or 'I wouldn't have the time for that'. When you have the facts, you have a basis to know if your idea is feasible or not. If you really want something, don't give up at the first hurdle, work out ways to overcome the challenges.

Presuppose change is always possible

Question your personal practice and consider if you are doing what you've always done without any good reason for continuing in the same way. You may have done something for years and realise you waste time and energy on a procedure which has a dubious outcome, or which doesn't produce any worthwhile results.

> Should doctors wear white coats or not? Are the arguments for and against valid today? If not then consider other ways to achieve the same desired outcome.

Perhaps rather than a possibly dirty white coat, either a uniform or clean plastic aprons and antiseptic hand wash might be more effective in preventing cross-infection.

> Do you advise patients to return for follow-up appointments, without considering whether you really need to see them regularly, or could you ask them, instead, to contact you if certain signs or symptoms develop?

There are routines for follow-up appointments which are based on habit and have little basis on the patient's need or the doctor's time.

You may need to change your schedule, if you really want something that isn't in your life right now. Be open minded about what is flexible, what can be stopped to free up time and facilitate the change you want.

Dr C decides to give up one hospital practitioner session. He never enjoyed doing it and he knows he will have a more enjoyable time attending a ceramics class.

Dr D finds a trombone teacher for a weekly lesson instead of going to a boring meeting.

Don't limit yourself

Be open to other possibilities and consider all the other options.

Dr E buys a set of oil paints and an easel. She finds a distance learning course and starts painting beautiful pictures.

How much will it cost?

If money or your perceived lack of it stops you from doing something, you may be listening to your inner voices rather than taking a realistic view of the value you might have from spending. How do you measure value of doing what you love?

Dr F knows that flying lessons are expensive, but he wants to indulge himself and can afford to pay for them. The joy he gets as a result is immeasurable in monetary terms.

Who can support you?

It's tremendously useful to have someone to talk to regularly while you are making changes in your life. Especially during times when progress seems slow, it's good to have someone to help you realise the progress you have already made. And when things go well, it's motivating to have someone to say, 'Well done'.

Dr H wants to make changes and knows it will be easier to keep to his plan with the support of his colleagues. They arrange to be regularly accountable to each other.

Have you ever considered that there may be others in your network who want to make changes and you might find you could form a supportive group.

Who do you have in your network to encourage you? Beware of people, with their own agenda, who don't want you to change because you might upset their lives.

In an ideal supportive relationship you have someone who listens, motivates and challenges you to explore your options, persuades you to take action and celebrates your achievements. This is more helpful than the person who tells you what to do, or is upset if you decide to do something different from their suggestion. Hiring a life coach is one way to have objective support.

You've made your decision to start and made a plan but still feel uncertain. Move on to Step six.

Step six: Indecision time

Suppose you are sure you've had enough of things as they are now but have not been able to visualise an alternative. What can you do? There are ways to make some space for the new ideas to flood in.

Take time to sit quietly, meditate, listen to music or go for a walk. Don't talk. Just allow whatever is in your subconscious to come into your conscious mind. Notice your thoughts. Don't edit anything but record your ideas in a notebook or on a tape recorder. Be patient. The whole picture may be shortened or dismissed too quickly. However ridiculous, there could be something useful.

Maybe you need to have a bit of a 'clear out' both mentally and physically. They say that nature abhors a vacuum and so it seems to be. When you start to clear away your clutter, take it to the dump or put it into your 'mental shredder', there will be a space for new ideas and opportunities.

Make a list of everything that gets on your nerves, preferably 50 or even 100 items. Start with the easy things, and eliminate them one by one. It's a great feeling when you can cross things off from your long list. Get them done; or ask someone else to do it, for pay, or as a favour, or as an exchange. As you do this, you may realise that some of the nagging things don't need to be done at all. Have you been keeping a broken toaster for years and know that it's cheaper to buy a new one rather than have it repaired?

Stop putting things off. Just do them as you see they need doing. Throw away old journals and out-of-date invitations to meetings. Do you ever get around to reading the editions you missed? Be honest with yourself. What can you get rid of? Just do it!

> Dr J throws away old medical journals and newspapers.
> Dr K gets rid of out-of-date pharmaceutical samples.
> Dr L arranges for a carpenter to build the shelves he needs.
> Dr M asks the receptionist with the loud voice to speak more quietly.
> Dr N asks that all patient files are put away at the end of the day.

Taking action in areas unrelated directly to your goal provides space and energy for other things to change.

Move on now to Step seven.

Step seven: Do something for yourself

You are important – very important. And sometimes it's good to do something special just for you. Reward yourself for what you've achieved this week. Celebrate the changes you've already begun to make. A special indulgence can be an incentive to get things done.

How will you treat yourself? Here are some ideas:

- go for a walk
- have a relaxing bath
- go to the gym
- go out to a restaurant
- cook yourself a special meal
- see a good film
- buy a new outfit in a different colour
- change your hairstyle
- sit quietly.

What other ideas can you think of?

Doing something special for yourself is important to raise your self-esteem, to value yourself and recognise that you've achieved something. It's easy to do things for other people most of the time and forget about your own needs. Now is the time to ask for what you want. Are you ready for the challenge?

Make a list of treats and incentives. Make a commitment to nurture yourself.

The bonus

Life is like an ever-shifting kaleidoscope – a slight change, and all patterns alter.
Sharon Salzberg

Everything is interconnected, so whatever changes you make will result in other things and people changing, too. You will be different and so will those around you. You can live a better life in which you are happy and fulfilled.

Never believe that a few caring people can't change the world. For, indeed, that's all who ever have.

Margaret Mead

6 How will you respond to your wake up call?

Opportunity is missed by most people because it is dressed in overalls and looks like work.

Thomas A Edison

Thinking about life

If you've had one of those landmark birthdays recently, the sort which makes you reflect on your life, then maybe you looked back over the years and wondered where they'd gone.

As you get older you become more conscious of your own mortality and realise you are not as young as you thought you were. The shock from recognising time passing and opportunities lost is a considerable one.

Life is for living

However, when you are part of a profession which encourages total immersion in work, so much so that medicine can be more a lifestyle as much as a profession, you may have put off doing things 'until you are not so busy'.

If you are waiting for some mythical time in the future for this to happen, then get real. It's unlikely, unless you make some changes to your way of life. Only then can you start to do what you want to achieve during your lifetime.

Wake up

One day something happens to spur you into action. Something which is totally unexpected and possibly rather sudden gives you a jolt and makes you decide the time has come to get moving on the things you plan to do with your life.

A middle-aged GP is overworked and stressed and would like to spend less hours in his practice. He recently found he has hypertension, and started treatment. He would dearly like to move to a smaller house and drive a less expensive car but his wife won't agree to the changes. So he is committed to staying in the practice until he is 65 years old because of his heavy financial commitments. He wishes he had done things differently. However after working with a life coach he explores ways to change. He involves his wife in planning their future together.

Have you had a 'wake up call'?

Just like the shrill call of your alarm clock signalling the start of another day of overwork and stress, this is a 'get up and get going' type of call. A persistent call that shakes your thoughts, resonates your conscience and asks the question, '... if not now, when...'.

Perhaps you've had symptoms which mean you aren't quite as well as you thought you were. Maybe a friend or relative has a serious illness or died suddenly. Possibly you've discovered you have a disease you were unaware of until recently. Realistically you know that something has to change, things have to be different.

If so, then this is the time to rouse yourself, look at where you are in life and decide how you would really like it to be; not only deciding but also working out how to do what you've made your mind up to do.

Whose life is it anyway?

You may be living the life that someone else has decided is 'best' for you. However well-intentioned this may be, other people may not really understand what matters to you. Sometimes your parents, your partner or your boss may have aspirations which don't seem right to you and yet there is a persistent inner voice telling you what you 'should' or 'shouldn't' do.

Are you following someone else's path or one they wish they had followed?

Dr B never wanted to do medicine. She only did it to please her father who was a well-known surgeon. She found the stress of living up to his reputation very difficult and in the end decided that the only way to cope was to limit the times she saw her father. Following some coaching she realised that she could begin to communicate more effectively with him and make it clear that she was following her own path.

Look at your limiting beliefs

Consider what your reasons are for doing or not doing something. When you say you want a different life, yet you never do anything about it ask, 'What is the worst thing that could happen if I did?'. Listen to your answer and then ask again, 'So what if it happened … what is the worst thing which could happen as a result?'. If you limit yourself by a belief you can't do something, ask 'Why?'. Whatever your answer, keep asking yourself 'Why?'. After about five 'whys' you will realise the only thing stopping you is you.

Get out of your comfort zone

There are things you feel secure about doing. In order to do something different you often have to step out of that comfort zone into a distinctly uncomfortable one. Don't expect that it will feel easy. You have to be prepared for some feelings of unease as you make changes. However, what happens as a result of taking a risk and doing something you expect to be difficult is that after a while the discomfort becomes less, your comfort zone increases in size and you have succeeded in making the changes you want.

How can you actually get on and do those things?

- Become clear about what you will or won't put up with any more.
- Say 'no' more often. When you say 'no' what are you are saying 'yes' to?

> Dr A says 'no' to seeing any pharmaceutical reps after 12 noon, so she says 'yes' to meeting a friend for lunch once a week.
>
> Dr B says 'no' to meetings in the evening, so he says 'yes' to communicating with his colleagues when he is less tired.

Look at the positives

A wake up call can be depressing and distressing. It may take over your life for a while. When you are in the midst of the crisis it can be difficult or even impossible to recognise anything positive from the experience. However, when the time is right for you and the clouds become less heavy, it may be useful to jot down your thoughts about the experience and what you have learned from it.

- What might be worse than what happened?
- What is better as a result?
- What insights have you had as a result of this experience about you and your life?
- What will you do differently as a result of your wake up call?
- When will you start?
- What are you waiting for?

You *can* make a choice

There is always a choice. You can choose to recognise the benefit of what happened for what it is – the chance to make a start, without further delay, to do what you want. Or you can ignore it completely. You can switch off the metaphorical buzzer in your head and heart. That's fine. The next call may be much louder and more insistent.

Have you ever set your clock and then felt cross when you found that you set it for the wrong time? It's difficult to go back to sleep when that happens, isn't it? Just like that, life's alarm bell tends to ring at what may seem to be the wrong time. However, instead of being cross about it, you can decide to recognise the opportunity it brings you to get things done, to try something new, or to complete something started but never finished.

A journey

If you imagine your life as a journey, your wake up call may be telling you it's time to change direction, change your plans too and head off to a different destination.

Even with these insights if you would like to benefit from your wake up call, the secret is to take action. Unless you do something differently then the opportunity passes by and nothing much changes.

Look forward to what you can realistically achieve if you are aware that something major has changed in your life. Where would you like to go? What have you always wanted to try? There may be difficult times ahead. Unless you do something now then you won't even begin. It will happen if you are willing.

Keep your ears, eyes and mind open and look and listen for opportunities and ideas. Jot down every idea you think of, however weird or wonderful, and pick one which appeals to you most. Think about it. Picture yourself achieving it. Imagine how you would feel. Then draw a mind-map, flow-chart or list with small achievable steps you need to do to make the progress you want. Decide what you will do this month, this week, today. And then do it!

A remarkable opportunity

If you have responded to your wake up call and recognised it for what it is, don't let the possibility for change pass you by.

The Chinese use two brush strokes to write the word 'crisis'. One brush stroke stands for danger; the other for opportunity. In a crisis, be aware of the danger – but recognize the opportunity.

Richard M Nixon

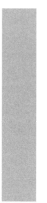

Part Two

Prescription for change

Change your thoughts and you change your world.

Norman Vincent Peale

7 What would you do if you had the time?

Time is the coin of your life. It is the only coin you have, and only you can determine how it will be spent. Be careful lest you let other people spend it for you.

Carl Sandburg

You know that time is finite and you cannot have any more than 24 hours each day. Each week there are 168 hours for you. If you deduct 10 hours each day for sleeping and eating there are still 98 hours left! You *can* make a difference in your life; changes *will* happen if you are willing to consider ways to do things differently and are prepared to take some action and shift some energy!

Dr A leaves his busy surgery and wonders where another day has gone. When he arrived the appointment list was already full and so was the waiting room. Before half an hour had passed, the receptionist brought in more sets of notes, and he felt a tension headache develop, which lasted until every patient had left. The list of visits had grown by then. The woman who lives over the road won't have anything much wrong with her except a hangover. Meanwhile his own children are asleep in bed, and his wife is furious with him for being late again. He would dearly love to have more time for his family and for himself too. He would like to play squash again, but each day is the same. Whatever plans he makes have to be abandoned because he is so exhausted by the time he eventually gets home.

If you are frustrated about not getting things done and find that weeks go by when you never manage to find extra time for the things you used to love to do before you got on the unending treadmill of overwork, then you need to manage your time differently.

You may not recall when you last said, 'That was a fantastic day', and realise there has been something lacking in your life over the last few years.

It's important to be clear about what you would do if you had extra time.

Knowing this gives you an added incentive to free up time. By planning to do something very specific you will have a measure of whether or not you've been successful. What would you like to do again without feeling the pressure? Would you like to spend more hours with your partner, family and friends? Are you keen to be more involved in your community?

Make a list of all the things you want to do

Write a date next to each item by when you want to have done it. Month by month write what you need to do in order to reach your goal for the end of the year. For example, you've decided that you want to complete a certain project. That's fine. It's a good idea which is specific, measurable, achievable and realistic. But it's no good saying to yourself 'Well that's OK then, I don't need to worry about doing that until November'. No, that's no good at all. What you have to do now is to divide the big project into 12 tasks which you can set yourself to complete by the end of each month. You could then divide each of these into four weekly tasks. By doing that you will ensure that the whole project is completed by the end of the year.

Stop wasting time

People find life entirely too time-consuming.

Stanislaw J Lec

How do you spend your day? Do you know specifically? How long do you speak on the telephone, answer emails, drink coffee, talk to colleagues, watch television, and eat?

Become more time aware

Keep a log of everything you do over 24 hours. Jot down what you are doing every quarter of an hour and make a note every time you change activity.
   Notice how long you take for:

- each phone call
- a cup of coffee
- chatting to a colleague about nothing in particular
- your lunch
- sitting and staring into space
- commuting
- exercising.

Keep a note of all your activities for a day or two. What do you notice? When you discover some of the time wasters, decide what you can do differently to free up some time.

Dr B realises that he has long telephone conversations during the day. He decides to preface any future calls with 'I have five minutes available'. He keeps an eye on the clock and then at the end of that time concludes with 'Sorry, but I have to go now'.

Dr C takes much longer than the other doctors to see his patients. He lets them 'ramble on' and as he sorts out one thing for them they get into the 'while I'm here doctor…' scenario. He comes to terms with the 10 minutes he has allotted for each person and has a large clock on his desk so he can keep an eye on it. As the patient starts to talk about other things he learns techniques for getting them back on track. 'OK then, so is the bottom line that you have a new pain in your shoulder you are worried about … let's arrange to have it X-rayed and in the meantime take these tablets and see if they help.' He hands over the form and the prescription while standing up and going to the door.

Delegate

You have identified time wasters and are beginning to eliminate these. Now, look again at how you spend your day, notice what you are doing and if it is actually your job? Are you spending time doing tasks which someone else could or should be doing?

If you are a doctor and spend time filing patient notes, ask yourself if this is your job. Even if there is a staff shortage, it is still not your job. You may believe you are helping a colleague but in fact you are masking a problem. If you were too busy, would the clerical staff do your clinic or surgery for you? Why not? *Because it's not their job.* You have very specialised skills and experience. Using them is what you are paid to do.

So, make a list of tasks you actually do, and note who *should* or *could* be doing them, instead. Tell your colleagues that you will no longer be doing those things. Scary? Yes of course it is.

It's time to change

Perhaps you offered to help out one day when things were busy and what started as a gesture of kindness has become an expectation and even an obligation.

It's difficult to say 'no'

Saying 'no' more often, will have a huge impact on the time you have available to do what *you* want.

- What is the worst thing which could happen if you say 'no'?
- What is the best thing that can happen if you say 'no'?
- When you say 'no' what are you saying 'yes' to?

How come you do someone else's work? Did you say yes for the sake of a quiet life? A quiet life for whom? A quiet external life maybe, but what about the turmoil and frustration you feel inside? Are you someone who agrees to do whatever you are asked? Do people say 'Oh she'll do it' or 'He'll do it'?

Challenge your beliefs

Consider what is it about saying no you find difficult. It may be you feel guilty about something when you say no, and come up with a lot of 'shoulds' to justify what you do.

Complete the phrase: 'I should…'. These will be some of your internal rules of life (your beliefs). How many 'shoulds' are on your list? Ask yourself after each statement 'Why?' until you can't answer it any more.

Where do those beliefs come from? If they came from your parents, think about their situation, their childhood and how different it was from yours. Most parents do the best they can for their children. But they are influenced by what they learned from *their* parents and so on, *ad infinitum*. Their rules do not need to be your rules today. You are an adult and can change the way you do things.

See what happens when you adapt your list of 'I should' statements to a list of your 'I choose (if I want)' statements. How does reading from the 'I choose' compared with the 'I should' seem? It's about choice. You do have a choice (you really do). You can choose the way you do this or do that, with a smile or with a frown. For example, 'I should invite so and so over to dinner next week', becomes 'I choose (if I want) to invite so and so for dinner next week'.

What can you delegate to someone else?

- Tasks that you don't enjoy.
- Things that it is not your job to do.
- Routine tasks that you can train someone else to do.

A few suggestions for you follow. You can add lots more.

> Dr C is increasingly frustrated by sorting through thick files whilst listening to her patients. She persuades her partners that the practice would benefit by employing a filing clerk who systematically tidies up the files.

> In an effort to delegate tasks, Dr D does all the smears for the practice while Dr E sees all the patients with diabetes.

What can you delegate to someone else?

Stop completely

What could you avoid or stop doing altogether? They may be things which do not need to be delegated because they don't need to be done at all.

When you've been through the 'why' questioning suggested, you may have identified some tasks which you realise are on your 'to do' list because they are things which 'have always been done', rather than things which need to be done today in today's circumstances. Take them off your list and reduce your stress.

> The GP who retired used to see pharmaceutical representatives whenever they chose to come into the surgery. Even though they had to wait until he had seen some patients, he always spent time with them. This irritated the new partner Dr F, who didn't like the interruption. He decided to only see the reps between 9 and 10 am on Wednesdays. Once they knew the changed routine the reps cooperated and Dr F managed to leave the surgery on time regularly.

Stop procrastinating

Procrastination is the thief of time.

Edward Young

Just get on and do the things you absolutely have to do. Why don't you? If you don't have the skills you need for the task, then acquire them. Find someone to help.

> Dr G isn't very good with computers, so he asks his teenage son to help him.

Sometimes a task seems so big its very size is off-putting. Break the task into bite-sized chunks so that you make a start, however small. For example, you need to clear the clutter of a lifetime and you realise this may take several weeks or more to complete. As you haven't got this time to spare you end up not even starting because of time limitations. However, if you recognise that even though you don't have some weeks or even a whole day to spend on the project, you do have an hour tomorrow morning. If you decide to look, you can find the odd five minutes during the day when you could sort through a file or two.

Thinking of the big project, what could you complete in an hour? Perhaps you could clear one quarter of your desk. So do it. And another quarter the next day and so on. You are getting it done. Chunk by chunk, some progress is being made!

Say 'no' more often

Have you been asked to do something you don't really want to do? Sometimes it's difficult to say 'no'. You may feel guilty, especially if someone is asking you for help. Saying 'no' is a vital skill to develop if you want more time. Just say it, and try not to get into a discussion about why. This is about you recognising your own needs and keeping within your personal boundaries. When you look at how you spend your day, if you find that a considerable amount of work is unplanned, and consists of doing extras for others, then saying 'no' is an important skill to acquire urgently.

> When asked if he could 'just fill in this market research form', Dr I replies he doesn't want to do that.
>
> Asked if she would mind 'reading through this report and telling me what you think of it', Dr J says she will do it later.

Streamline your tasks

So you've freed up time, delegated some things, got rid of others, decided not to procrastinate any more and learned how to say 'no'. However, there are still some tasks that have to be done by you. What else can you do?

Have you reached your 'enough is enough' time?

Has your partner or spouse told you things will have to change otherwise you can't stay together? Do you fear the break up of your partnership, your life, your world? Do you try to please all of the people all of the time and now realise you are desperately unhappy and near to breaking point?

Go back through the suggestions in this chapter and decide on one thing you can change this week.

Devise systems for doing regular tasks

You can decide what to delegate and what to dump, but you might not be as efficient as you could be for the tasks you have to do. Have you ever watched yourself and notice how streamlined you are in the way you do your tasks? You need to improve and streamline your systems.

> Dr K realises that every time he wants to look up something in the *British National Formulary* he has to get out of his chair to reach it. He puts some bookends on his desk and keeps it within easy reach.

> Dr L designates half an hour (timed) at the start and end of each day to read and answer emails.

> Dr M decides the amount of time each day that she will use to sign prescriptions, the day of the month that she will check her credit card receipts, and the day and time each week when she will go to the gym.

What steps can you take this week to free up some time? Be specific about what you will do. Ask or tell the appropriate people about the changes you decide to make.

Who can support you?

> Drs N, O and P decide to support each other to make life better for them all. There is some resistance at first, but eventually their colleagues find the new way of running the practice works well and has the bonus of a much happier atmosphere between them.

Stephen Covey suggests drawing a grid labelled as follows.[1]

1 *Urgent and important* e.g. medical crises, pressing problems, deadline-driven projects, meetings, preparations.
2 *Not urgent and important* e.g. preparation, prevention, values

clarification, planning, relationship building, empowerment, true recreation.

3   *Urgent and not important*   e.g. interruptions, some phone calls, some mail, some reports, some meetings.

4   *Not urgent and not important*   e.g. trivia, busy work, junk mail, some phone calls, time wasters, 'escape' activities.

Many doctors spend their time doing things which are both 'urgent and important'. However, if you plan more carefully, it's possible to do more in the 'important but not urgent' segment; eliminate, by delegating, most of the 'urgent and not important' tasks; and eliminate completely most of the 'non-urgent/non-important' things (the time wasters).

So … what will you do now? Remember, nothing changes until you take some action.

Reference

1   Covey S (1994) *First Things First*. Simon & Schuster UK Ltd, London.

8 No more procrastination

Procrastination is the art of keeping up with yesterday.

Don Marquis

Excuses

You decide to change yet nothing happens because you don't actually put your ideas into practice. How come you are so good at delaying? What is it about you or your personality that means, in spite of all your good intentions, your ideas stay on the back burner? They simmer away, draining your energy and yet are never cooked enough to make a difference.

Is it because you are so busy each day that some things never get done, even when they reach the top of your 'to do' list? If so, perhaps you need to look at your time management skills. Do you regularly find a reason not to do what you promise? Are you angry when someone asks, 'Haven't you done that yet?', because they don't understand how difficult life is for you? Some make excuses such as the following.

- There's no point in starting to clear the cupboard in my surgery desk as I haven't the time to finish it this afternoon.
- I can't use the new software as I'm not sure how to apply it to my practice.
- I don't have time to finish dictating letters because the patients talked too much.

Do you start each day putting aside tasks which have been in your head for days, weeks or months, because something more urgent has come to the top of your list? When will you actually do what you plan? The things which don't get done stay waiting, the thought of them lurking in the back of your mind, draining your energy.

What can you do?

You will have the jobs you've been putting off for ages done in record time.

Sometimes, when you are stuck in one task, everything else is forgotten. Unfortunately there are always the urgent and important tasks which have to be dealt with under pressure. However, if you've made an effort to put a routine in place for daily tasks which help you cope with it all, then you will be able to get back on track again quickly.

- Stop wasting time on non-urgent and non-important tasks.
- Plan your day more effectively.
- Write down what you want to do each day.
- Break the tasks into much smaller chunks.
- Get the file out.
- Develop efficient systems to be more efficient.

Decide on a set of daily tasks and set yourself a time for each. Then move on to the next task even if you haven't finished the first one.[1]

Change your routine

A very important part of time management is to stop doing the things which you don't need to be doing. When thinking about getting things done consider whether what you are attempting to do is really on your own agenda or if it's because you are under pressure from someone else.

You may be doing things for no other reason except that 'it's the way it's always been done in this department'. Is there another way to do it more efficiently or could some of the things be dropped as not being relevant any more?

> Dr P knows he spends too much time on the internet or answering emails instead of getting more important tasks done. He sets a limit for emails and internet surfing to half an hour morning and evening.

What do you have to learn?

Do you need to acquire new skills to be more efficient? If you are finding it difficult to keep up with information and ways of doing things, then admit this to yourself and tell your colleagues that you would like some assistance or support for some specific training, instead of struggling to do it all.

Ways to learn

There are many different ways you might do this:

- read journals and textbooks
- go on a course
- find support from others
- learn from the internet
- view an educational video or television programme
- discussion with colleagues
- the 'hands on' approach of someone talking you through a procedure.

> Dr C, whose keyboard skills are not very good, feels frustrated until he signs on for a course to learn to touch type and subsequently becomes less stressed.

Who can you ask?

It's OK to ask for assistance. You believe that you have to do it all and would appear incompetent if you ask for help. Talk about what you find stressful or difficult. Let go of your fear that others will see you as lacking ability if you admit that something is challenging. Ask yourself, 'What is the worst thing that could happen to me if I called for some support?'. You may be surprised at how ready people are to lend a hand when you ask and find they understand your difficulty. If they are not able or willing to assist you themselves they may suggest someone else who can. Wouldn't you do the same for them if they were struggling with something that was easy for you?

Just do it

You've delegated everything you can, you've surprised yourself and said 'no' more times than you thought possible without the world falling apart as a result, you've set up efficient systems and acquired all the skills you need to do the tasks without feeling incompetent. You've eliminated as much as possible after asking the question, 'Does this actually need to be done by me or indeed by anyone, or has it become a routine with no rationale?'.

So there's no basis to procrastinate any longer. When will you take action? Make up your mind about what you are going to get done this week and 'just do it'.

No more excuses

If you are extremely clear about what you want to achieve then it is more likely you will succeed. Break huge tasks into 'bite-sized pieces' and make a start. Don't wait any longer.

Dr R wanted to get up to date with reading through the pile of medical journals but never got around to it. He decided to look through this week's *BMJ* for an hour on Friday afternoon, and takes those older than one month, read or unread, for recycling.

What happens next?

You will get on with your life and do whatever you really want to do.

'Off days' are a part of life, I guess, whether you're a cartoonist, a neurosurgeon, or an air-traffic controller.

Gary Larson

Know the true value of time; snatch, seize, and enjoy every moment of it. No idleness; no laziness; no procrastination; never put off till tomorrow what you can do today.

Lord Chesterfield

Reference

1   Forster M (2000) *Get Everything Done*. Hodder and Stoughton, London.

9 Looking after number one

Equipped for life

Your life in and out of medicine is full of gadgets and equipment all of which need regular servicing, maintenance and care. You may have been persuaded to take out a contract to cover every possibility. You are clear that disaster would strike if such and such didn't function the way it should, so you sign on the dotted line. You have covered yourself for all eventualities. This gives you some sort of satisfaction, since you know what you would miss most if it broke down and could no longer be mended.

What is the most vital piece of equipment for your medical practice? Is it your computer, your car or your mobile phone? How would you manage without one of them? Maybe you have some spares, or an older model kept in a cupboard, although it may need repairing, ready for any possibility. Perhaps colleagues would be willing to lend you theirs (for a while at least).

You live in a world dependent on technology working well and being available.

Dr A has his computer operating system upgraded to the latest version. The newest practice management software is installed. Anti-virus software scans regularly. Everything should be working well but it isn't. One day he has to delay starting the surgery because the computer has crashed so he has no access to patient records or prescriptions.

Dr B is annoyed when the local garage tells him it will take three days to repair his car. He has to employ a driver at great expense to take him on his visits (even more frustrating because most of them could have come to the surgery).

When Dr C arrives at her outpatient clinic on the other side of the city she finds it has been cancelled because of a shortage of nursing staff. No one has been able to contact her as her mobile phone was switched off.

These examples remind you how much modern medical practice depends on equipment working well. If you keep up to date and all your equipment is serviced and upgraded regularly, then your life may run pretty smoothly. Or are there several outstanding jobs that you have in this area of your life?

What do you need to look after above all else?[1]

However careful you are, you may be neglecting the most important piece of technology in your life. Yourself. Do you fully take care of your most essential tool? Do you do the things that you know are good for your health and wellbeing? Do you service yourself regularly and check that you work properly? Is your energy generated from the best source? Do you provide yourself with the most efficient fuel or do you poison yourself with alcohol, drugs, unhealthy food or nicotine?

Take a moment to think about yourself – your body, mind and spirit. Consider these as your own, your very own 'personal operating system', which needs as much or even more care and attention as all your other equipment put together. This is the most important machine you have and you know, better than most, that it cannot be replaced if and when it fails.

Does your system need optimising?

Are you functioning as well as you can? You may believe you are fighting fit and can do as much as you always could, yet somehow you don't feel the same as you did years ago and the sparkle isn't there as often. You want to get it back again but feel you have lost your enthusiasm for life. When your *BMJ* arrives do you go to the Obituaries first? Does that make you aware of your own mortality?

You don't want your colleagues to see you as weak and unable to cope, of course you don't. The culture still persists among the medical profession that doctors don't get ill and can cope with everything. Perhaps this is the reason you carry on bravely and tell people everything is fine, even though you know it isn't. You may be tempted to self-medicate or talk to a colleague about your 'friend' who has certain symptoms, instead of arranging a pro-fessional consultation. Your colleagues probably know that you are not man-aging. They may talk about you behind your back and yet not give you the support you would like.

Pause for a moment. Take a look in the mirror. What do you see? Does your face show the strain of the last few years?

Glance around at your colleagues. Are they happy at the thought of another day in the outpatient clinic, or are they fed up too? Are their faces tense and do they look tired? Of course it isn't right to make instant judgements about someone's appearance; however, looking at yourself and the way you've changed over the years may be helpful.

During your working week you advise many of your patients about ways to look after themselves better. You may tell them to give up smoking, to take more exercise and to eat a more healthy diet. Do you walk your talk? Do you follow the guidelines yourself or is it a case of 'Do as I say not as I do'?

Think about yourself

How can you make positive improvements in your life? Start with your diet. What can you do to improve this? How do you boost your energy when you are exhausted?

Are you poisoning yourself with excessive sugar, too much food, caffeine, junk food, tobacco, alcohol or drugs, prescribed or otherwise? Can you think of other ways to feel more energetic, for example, taking a walk at lunch time, eating more fruit or vegetables? Is your diet as nutritious and healthy as it could be?

When you look after yourself everything else works well and life becomes easier. The clinics may still have too many attending, but you won't feel quite so stressed. The patients may be as demanding and rude, but you will be able to cope much better.

Upgrade the way you look after yourself this week and notice how much better you feel.

Dr B is too busy to eat anything at lunchtime and keeps herself going with cups of black coffee. She is exhausted at the end of the day. She decides to bring a sandwich and go over to the park to eat it quietly away from the hospital.

Mr C arrives on the ward out of breath. His only exercise is from the car to the clinic, the clinic to the ward, the ward to the car. He is putting on weight and has no energy. He decides enough is enough and it's time to do something for himself. He realises that it is only five miles to the hospital. He buys himself a new bike and uses the cycle route to and from work each day. He's surprised how quickly he gets there after the first week which is a bit of a struggle. He gets used to the jokes from his colleagues and begins to feel more alert and energetic.

Are you muttering 'Oh, I'll do something when I'm not so busy' under your breath as you read this? Are you thinking something along the lines of the following:

- It's no good expecting me to make big changes when things are completely overwhelming.
- Yes, I know what to do and I'll do it one of these days. Just stop putting pressure on me to do it right now.

That's not good enough. If you want to change, that is not a valid excuse. Do you really believe that you'll wake up one day and say 'I'm not busy today'. This is a delaying tactic. You can make a very small change today, if you decide to do so. Small changes grow into bigger changes. What very small change could you commit to making every day this week? If you really want things to improve you have to find the time you need. How much time does it take to choose a healthy dessert instead of a pudding, or have a piece of fruit instead of a bar of chocolate? Of course you can do it, even if you are busy. The only thing that stops you is your own mental attitude. Change from saying to yourself, 'I don't have time' to 'I have all the time I need to make a small change today'. Do it now before it's too late.

Now is the time to take stock, to change things, step by small step, even while you are busy. Suppose you realise you don't eat enough fruit each day. To eat five portions may seem impossible so how about starting with one piece? Instead of dismissing the big change as not possible, do a bite-sized version of it. Commit yourself to introducing your new habit, however small that may be, on a daily basis from today.

Imagine your working day as enjoyable, stress-free and with everything going smoothly, and at last you have the time to start looking after yourself more. What would you do? How could you improve yourself? Would you start with your mind, your body or your spirit? Just one new habit this week. Make the commitment. It's often motivating to have someone to be answerable to. Is there a friend or colleague who could encourage and inspire you to keep going for the first few days when it may seem an impossible prospect to change the routine of many years?

> Drs X and Y who live near each other and not too far from the surgery decide to meet at the end of the road and walk together to and from work.

> Drs P and Q realise how unhealthy their diet is and so they decide to take it in turns to bring a healthy packed lunch.

It's time to listen to yourself and take the advice you already know and regularly give to your patients. These headings serve as reminders.

For a healthy body
- Eat a balanced diet.
- Reduce the amount of caffeine, sugar and fat in your diet.
- Eat plenty of fresh fruit and vegetables.
- Don't smoke.
- Exercise regularly – walking is as good as anything.
- Stretch with yoga or pilates.
- Aerobic exercise – running, dancing, cycling.
- Drink alcohol in moderation only.
- Avoid unnecessary medication.
- Seek advice rather than self-prescribe.

For a healthy mind
- Be curious.
- Ask questions.
- Take chances.
- Recognise your needs and satisfy them.
- Don't expect your nearest and dearest to be all things to you.
- Learn new things.
- Be dedicated to lifelong learning (and not just medicine!).
- Be open to possibilities.
- Get out of your rut and follow wherever your spirit leads you.

For a healthy spirit[2]
- Take time for yourself: meditate or sit quietly away from others; spend time in nature; by water or whatever puts your inner self at peace for a few minutes each day.
- Spend time with your family. Maintain your priorities: if you have small children, they only take their first step once.
- Be involved in your community.
- Do what you are passionate about: a feeling of joy and wellbeing comes from doing something you really love to do.
- Be at peace: let go of anger, frustration and fear.

Whatever is happening is what is perfect for you at this time. Find the positive amongst the negative and relax. However much people irritate or anger you, be more accepting. Whatever will be is for the best. It's time to let go of your wish to be in control and trust that others will do whatever needs to be done.

You can do it

Start, step by step. Introduce the changes you want to make one by one, week by week. Some people find it helps to make a list of 'daily habits'. These could start with one or two small things you could easily introduce into your routine. Week by week add another new habit. Do these regularly each week until after about a month they become automatic.

Go on, give yourself the greatest chance to live the best life you possibly can. Don't make any more excuses. Start today with one or two small changes. It won't take long for you to understand how much better your life can be.

Five ways to survive as a doctor[3]

1   Make sure you do things other than work.
2   Create your dream work schedule.
3   Learn to say 'no', without feeling guilty.
4   If you need help, ask for it.
5   Seek peer support.

References

1   Clark S (2000) Why do people become doctors and what can go wrong? *BMJ Career Focus*. **320**:S2.
2   Elliston P (2001) Mindfulness in medicine and everyday life. *BMJ Career Focus*. **323**:S2.
3   Berger A (2000) Surviving (and even enjoying) medicine. *BMJ Career Focus*. **320**:S2.

10 What's draining you?

Every time you don't follow your inner guidance, you feel a loss of energy, loss of power, a sense of spiritual deadness.

Shakti Gawain

Here you are

You wonder if anything can ever change. You resign yourself to feeling like you do, for the rest of your life, even though that makes you feel very unhappy. What else can you possibly do? You've done all the things the personal development books tell you to do. You've perfected your time management skills, looked after your mind, body and spirit until they are all shining beacons to anyone who wants to look, and yet you still feel drained at the end of the day. You wonder if things will ever be better and if you can be 'full of the joys of spring' again; or even the joys of autumn.

As you sit down at your untidy desk you dread the thought of putting it in order. The task would take days to complete and there never seems to be a spare moment, let alone a spare day to do that. You shy away from throwing out your piles of old medical journals until you've sat down and read them all, or at least skimmed through them. You might chuck away an important article.

Clear the clutter

The 'clutter-clearing' scenario is something you've studiously avoided. Perhaps you've read about how clearing out your unwanted junk can be useful to create a vacuum and so clear a space for other things to happen. But you're always too tired to start doing any of that. Have you been amazed at those television programme participants who allow someone to clear everything out of their house and then put up with the ritual humiliation of having all their possessions scrutinised on air?

Maybe you've wondered how a few tidy drawers can help to find the right job. How indeed? There's something going on, no one understands what it is, but it works. Some call it synchronicity or serendipity, others call it good luck or fate or random chance. But whatever it is, it happens. Whether you like it or not, changing one thing in your life enables other things to happen. No doubt, like most of us, you have cupboards and drawers full of old clothes and shoes which you know you will never wear again, or that you'll be slim enough to fit into once more. Dream on!

Life is like a spreadsheet

When you alter one element, everything else automatically adjusts. Be more aware and notice what happens, what starts to come into your life when you create the space. Try clearing a few drawers and watch out for the opportunities which come your way. Hocus pocus? Or metaphysics? Do we have to know how or why something occurs?

If you really want to attract things into your life to be happy and more content, here is the simple formula:

Get rid of what drains you and **Do more of what energises you.**

Your environment

Home
Consider what you will do now to make it the way you want it. You could start by unpacking and sorting out all the boxes in the attic.

If the furniture is not to your taste, but more what friends and family offloaded on to you, and the lighting isn't in the right place for what you want to do, then it's time to make some changes. If the temperature is a too hot or too cold, or the colour scheme doesn't make your heart sing, and there is too much clutter lying around, do something about these things.

- How much more can you tolerate?
- How much time can you commit to clearing some papers each day?
- What do you need to do to stop more mess accumulating?

Geographical
Do you live and work where you want to be? If not, have you thought about your ideal environment?

The first step to making any change is imagining what it is that you want. Once you can see it in your mind's eye then it will begin to happen. Involve all your senses. Is your current situation too noisy or too quiet, too urban or too rural? Thinking about where you are, and where you want to be, is a small step you can make now.

> Dr D wants to live by the sea, so in the meantime he makes sure he goes there at least once a month.

Your relationships

Work
- Do you get on well with your colleagues?
- Do you communicate with them regularly and talk and listen to each other?

If you want something at work can you explain, listen and be heard, and be prepared to try other options.

Personal
- Do you have a happy close relationship?
- Do you listen and talk?
- Do you seek to understand and then be understood?[1]
- Do you have friends who nurture rather than drain you?

Community
- Are you part of a supportive community of people who share your interests?
- Do you give and receive support from those who are part of it?

You, the person
- Who are you without the professional label?

Your needs
- What are they?
- Are they being met?

Your values
- Are you living by yours?[2]

Your body
- Look after yourself[3]

Money
- Are you earning enough?
- Are you saving for the future?

- Are you wasting money?
- Can you afford your lifestyle?

Make a list

Note everything you can think of which is draining you. Start with ten things. Expand each by making them very specific. If you have written a person's name establish specifically what it is about that person that annoys you (and use the opportunity to reflect whether what really annoys you about others is actually something in you). Keep adding to your list until you have at least a hundred things on it. Then get rid of everything on the list.

Start with the easy things

For example, you could:

- throw away the broken printer that you know will never get mended
- take all your old medical journals to be recycled
- buy the extra gadget or pair of scissors or screwdriver, so you don't have to spend time looking and trying to remember where you last put it down
- go through your credit card receipts or bank statements regularly
- repair the dripping tap or call a plumber to do it
- pay someone to do the housework
- clear your clutter bit by bit, piece by piece.

Let your heart sing

What would do it for you? Could it be:

- a place you love to go
- music you adore
- friends you haven't seen for ages
- being alone in nature
- special people
- walking in the countryside.

Whatever is your passion, bring it back into your life. You've made excuses long enough. Make time for whatever energises you. Even an hour a week is enough to get you off the treadmill of life to recharge your batteries. Find time to be creative, to be in touch again with who you are and to gain a new perspective on your life.

The outcome will be:

- space for everything
- more energy
- more fun.

Don't wait any longer.

When you have confidence, you can have a lot of fun. And when you have fun, you can do amazing things.

Joe Namath

References

1   Covey S (1989) *The Seven Habits of Highly Effective People*. Simon & Schuster, New York.
2   Houghton A (2002) Values? What values? *BMJ Career Focus*. **324**:S59.
3   Kersley S (2002) Looking after number one. *BMJ Career Focus*. **324**:S85.

11 Living an abundant life

Abundance is, in large part, an attitude.

Sue Patton Thoele

Abundance and you

Do you think about your life as half empty or half full? Perhaps you are you stuck in 'scarcity mode' and avoid making changes in case the barrel of life has no more to offer, If so, you may be nervous about 'letting go' in case you never get a refill.

On the other hand, if you are confident there will always be more than enough to go round, and that closing one door allows others to open, then you appreciate abundance already.

If not, then imagine what it would be like to have a cup of life so full it runs over with contentment, confidence and satisfaction.

What does it mean to live abundantly?

The important parts of your life can be represented on a 'life's wheel'.[1] This is a pie chart divided into equal segments, each representing an area of life that is important for a fulfilled and balanced life.[2]

Which part of your life has a very low score? Which one takes too much of your energy from the others? What can you do to address this and improve that part of your life that you neglect at present?

It *is* possible to make a shift from a negative view of the world to a more positive attitude. If you can do this, your 'glass' becomes not only full but overflows and it is possible to have more than you could possibly need.

Are you ready for the challenge?

Start by picturing your ideal circumstances. Imagine someone looking at you living that life. What would they see?

Time

Is finding more time a priority? What can you stop doing to free up time to do something you love? What can you say 'no' to? Do you recognise the bonus of extra time if a meeting or trip is cancelled?

> Dr A is disappointed at first when she fails to get the consultant job she wants. However, she decides to use the time to travel for a few months instead.

> Dr B is ambivalent about whether or not to attend a conference in her own time. She realises that instead of jet lag and exhausting flights she could tidy her office and paint some pictures in the time available.

Money

> *Money is better than poverty, if only for financial reasons.*
>
> Woody Allen

Is more money the answer? It certainly helps. Do you need to make external or internal changes around money? If you never have enough is this a result of spending beyond your means or buying unnecessarily? Do you make your money work for you or do you work for your money?

The state of your financial health may derive from your family and their way of life. Are their beliefs relevant to you and your life today? If they feed your feeling of never having enough, how can you change these beliefs? How about making a subtle shift and putting yourself first for a change; each month decide how much is for you to save and how much to spend. Look at what's left and decide which expenses to reduce.[3]

> *Money is like a sixth sense without which you cannot make a complete use of the other five.*
>
> W Somerset Maugham

Stock up on everything

Start with something easy and useful, for example, household goods (and I'm not joking). Even something as simple as knowing you don't have to buy these items for ages can begin to ease the pressure of thinking about mundane tasks and give you the sense of abundance.[4]

What else do you have to keep on replacing? Would having more of whatever it is relieve some of the drain on your energy? You see, abundance is about having plenty of energy, space, light, health and friends, as well as time and money. You can work towards having enough of everything. Maybe you need to look at what is 'enough'. Are there adjustments you can make to your lifestyle to allow you to have more of the life you really want? Thinking about what motivates you may help with this.

Give something away

What can you be generous with apart from money? What can you give away – time, love, expertise or friendship? What else? Some people say that what you give returns to you eventually, in some way or another. So by giving, your reserves will grow.

I'd rather have roses on my table than diamonds on my neck.

Emma Goldman

What else?

An abundant life means having more than you need in every aspect of your life. It doesn't depend on the amount of money in the bank. It relies on building resources of everything when you can, so that in lean times you will have stores not only of money but also of time, love, learning, ideas and fun. If you do, you will have the following to look forward to:

- a fulfilled life in and out of medical practice
- money to live the life you want
- time for friends, family, yourself and your community
- love
- learning
- fun and laughter.

Do you want a more abundant life? How are you improving your life today?

To love what you do and feel that it matters – how could anything be more fun?

Katharine Graham

References

1   Cameron J (1995) *The Artist's Way*. Pan Books, London.
2   Kersley S (2001) Striking the balance. *BMJ Career Focus*. **323**:S2.

3   Kiyosaki RT (2002) *Rich Dad Poor Dad*. Time Warner Books, London.

4   Leonard TJ (1998) *The Portable Coach*. Scribner, New York.

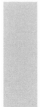

12 Relationship: what relationship?

The easiest kind of relationship for me is with ten thousand people. The hardest is with one.

Joan Baez

Perhaps there is something about close personal relationships that is particularly difficult for doctors. If you and your partner are both medics, you share an understanding of the reality of working in the medical profession. Your similar education and background may lead to frustration and resentment if one of you is more successful than the other.

Connections

What we're all striving for is authenticity, a spirit-to-spirit connection.

Oprah Winfrey

You might have met when you were both students, two like-minded people who formed, potentially, an ideal partnership. You might both have been working in the same specialty, which sparked your interest in each other. This may have been ideal at that time, although sometimes you may wonder whether it would have been better to have partnered instead with someone as far removed from the medical world as possible.

Coping

If a problem has no solution, it may not be a problem, but a fact – not to be solved, but to be coped with over time.

Shimon Peres

How do you cope with on-call responsibilities, especially when you have young children?

Dr A, a GP, and her husband Mr B, a surgeon, paid for a babysitter even though one or other of them was usually in the house, in case they were both called out at the same time.

Dr C, another GP, arranged to be on call on different days from her husband Dr D, an anaesthetist, so that one of them could look after the children. This resulted in them never having time together, free from the persistent phone.

Compromise

Relationships of trust depend on our willingness to look not only to our own interests, but also the interests of others.

Peter Farquharson

If you find yourself wondering what happened to the person you fell for when you were both students, or worked in the same hospital as junior doctors, and you wonder whether he or she fancies the night sister or charge nurse more than you, then it's time to talk more to each other and work on your relationship.

If your social life is virtually non-existent because one of you has a medical emergency to deal with at the time you were supposed to be going out, or you come home too tired to do anything, maybe it's the moment to have some give and take in both your lifestyles.

If you both expect everything to be organised around you and really wish you had a support team so that life at home would be as straightforward as going into theatre to do an operation, then decide what help you need and organise it or make adjustments to your working hours.

If you are so used to telling others what to do and having your requests carried out without question, and find it exasperating when they refuse to do something at home and regret how quickly you lose your temper, then, maybe, you are bringing home too much of the tension of your day, and you need to find ways to stop doing this.

When you notice how many of your friends and colleagues in similar circumstances have separated or divorced, you realise that unless you both do something soon your relationship may be doomed too.

Consideration

A little Consideration, a little Thought for Others, makes all the difference.
Pooh's Little Instruction Book, inspired by AA Milne

Accept that home is different from work. Doctors are used to advising people what to do, but they often don't like others directing them. As a doctor you have excellent communication skills. Start to use these to exchange a few words with your partner, rather than being too busy looking after others to make time for your own relationship.

Cooperation

You have both moved on, your career aspirations may not be the same as they were several years ago. Whether or not to have a career break in order to have children may be an issue. Perhaps you have children now and one of you may or may not want to put their career on hold in order to look after them. This is a crunch point – whether being around when your children are small is worth progressing more slowly along your professional path for. You need to cooperate with each other and live to your true values. It's difficult to make up for the years at work which happen when children are small.

> Dr Y was so keen on reaching the top of her specialty that she forgot about relationships and having children. When she decided it was the right time she realised her biological clock had been ticking and it was possibly already too late.

Perhaps it's now the moment to make some changes in the way you live. Reflect on your life, think about and try to understand what life is like for your partner.

Think about what the most important thing is for you, whether it is progressing in your career or being with your partner and children. If you've been delaying starting a family until you reach a certain stage, or worrying that you are getting older, then you know it's time to make different decisions.

Whatever has happened in the past has contributed and enriched your life in one way or another. There is always something positive to learn from every experience, however negative it seems at the time. If you've been unlucky in your close relationships, please take a moment to consider what you have learned to help you do better next time.

Communication

The most important thing in communication is to hear what isn't being said.

Peter Drucker

It's important for better communication to listen twice as much as to talk to your partner and recall when you last had a fun time together. Successful relationships depend on a number of things:

- being clear about boundaries
- letting go of trying to control someone else
- respecting your needs may be different from theirs
- realising that you are a worthwhile person in your own right – your partner is too
- finding areas of common interest
- doing what you love to do and letting your partner do whatever gives them joy
- saying no this week to things you no longer want to do
- taking time to do something with your partner that you both enjoy.

> Dr X realised that he and his wife, Dr Y, only ever spoke to each other about domestic matters. He remembered how much they used to enjoy walking in the countryside together near their home. He made a decision to ask her to have a long walk with him at the weekend. She was very pleased to do that and it was an opportunity to talk again.

Take time also to do something you really enjoy, without your partner. Remember what life was like before you were a 'doctor's partner' and try to recapture that feeling again. Go on, indulge yourself! Don't make any more excuses about why you can't do this. Make a start today with something, however small.

What you risk reveals what you value.

Jeanette Winterson

13 Top ten tips for achieving your goals

To will is to select a goal, determine a course of action that will bring one to that goal, and then hold to that action till the goal is reached. The key is action.

Michael Hanson

1 Make your goal SPECIFIC

If your goals are too vague, it's difficult to know what you are trying to achieve. Some amazing goals aren't reachable because they are too vague. If your goal, for example, is 'I want to be happier', ask yourself the following questions.

- Happier than what?
- What does being happier mean to you?
- What will you be doing when you are happier?
- How will you recognise yourself as happier?

It's a great goal but not specific enough. If you connect being happier with, let's say, spending time with your family, then a specific goal from this might be 'I want to spend an afternoon each week with my family'.

If you are happy when you go to the cinema then you might say to yourself, 'My goal is to go to the cinema once each week'.

2 Make your goal MEASURABLE

How will you know when you've achieved your goal? This follows from making your goal specific. If you decide to get a new job, then you either have or haven't got a new job. It's 'measurable'. If you decide to run in a marathon next year, then you will know when you've done it. If however you decide to be happier it's more difficult to measure 'happier' or to know if you've achieved it.

3 Make your goal ACHIEVABLE

Is your goal something that you are capable of doing? For example, if you are an overweight, unfit 80-year-old and you decide your goal is to win a gold medal for running at the next Olympics, then perhaps that is not an achievable goal.

4 Make your goal REALISTIC

If you are a lightweight woman and your goal is to lift a bus on to your shoulders, then your goal is not realistic.

5 Give your goal a TIME-SCALE

It is very important for your goal to be timed. You may decide that by the end of the year you want to lose a certain amount of weight. So decide on a date by which time you will achieve this.

6 Write down your goals

There is a story about a group of college students who were asked, when they graduated, to write down what they wanted to achieve in their lives. It is said that when they were contacted some years later those that had clear goals were more likely to have achieved them. Whether this is true or not, keeping a written record of your goals gives you something to refer to in the future, and a way to assess how your life is going and whether you still want the same as you did years ago. It's OK to make changes as you grow and your life evolves!

7 Decide the first steps

Work out what you want to achieve in the next six months, the next three months, the next month, the next week, in order to get to the goal in, for example, a year's time.

8 Keep a journal

Write something each day. Write your thoughts and feelings. Just let your hand move across the page (flow of consciousness writing). Don't censor what you write and don't re-read it immediately or correct it. As time goes by you will learn how this process frees up your mind to be much more creative and you may find that you have ideas about how to progress or how to move out of a stuck situation.

9 Do something, however small, each day

The way to get things done is to make a start and take action. Even five or ten minutes a day contributes to the whole and is a better technique than waiting for some 'never to arrive day' when you might have plenty of time.

10 Celebrate your achievement

If you follow these tips, you will achieve your goals. Tell yourself how well you've done and do something special to celebrate your success.

YOU CAN DO IT!!

Part Three

Medicine is more than a job: it's a lifestyle

When making a decision of minor importance, I have always found it advantageous to consider all the pros and cons. In vital matters, however, such as the choice of a mate or a profession, the decision should come from the unconscious, from somewhere within ourselves. In the important decisions of personal life, we should be governed, I think, by the deep inner needs of our nature.

Sigmund Freud

The tragedy of life is not that it ends so soon, but that we wait so long to begin it.

WM Lewis

14 Who heals the healers?

As I see it every day you do one of two things: build health or produce disease in yourself.

Adelle Davis

Expectations

I am not in this world to live up to other people's expectations, nor do I feel that the world must live up to mine.

Fritz Perls

Being a doctor may be a difficult role since there are all sorts of expectations placed on you. These go beyond your working day and may permeate your very being. Wherever and whenever someone knows you are medically qualified, you are expected to be able to deal with an emergency anywhere, anytime, any place. You have to know the answer about what to do and not show any weakness. Your colleagues, or so you strongly believe, know it all and you don't want to be shown up when you are amongst them. So it goes on. Some of this is a perpetuating myth. Of course, as a doctor, you are vulnerable, you do get upset, there are times when you don't know what to do and times when you feel emotional or unable to cope. Who can you turn to? Who can you share your emotions with? Very often the answer is no one and so these feelings are ignored for a long time.

Support

Who do you turn to when you begin to wonder how you'll get through the next few years, or even the next few hours or days? Ideally, the answer is someone in whom you can confide who will listen to you without judgement and accepts you as you are, with only your agenda. If you ask for help and support will this will be seen as your Achilles' heel? Some doctors, build a sort of protective outer skin around their emotional self, so that it's impossible or very difficult for people to make contact or connections with them.

Do you do this when you are feeling vulnerable and frightened and so stop yourself seeking help because you think you have to cope on your own?

It's difficult sometimes to admit you don't know all the answers, especially if you believe others will think less of you if you admit ignorance. To avoid this:

- stop putting obstacles between you and other people
- don't put up barriers to communication
- hold back from jumping to conclusions.

If you give someone your absolutely full attention, truly listening to what the person is saying, then it is more likely that they will do it for you too. Once you experience another person really hearing you, you'll appreciate that what we give out, we get back. If you want someone to hear you then it's important to be a much, much better listener to others.

Find someone who you would feel comfortable to talk to and make a request of them. Tell them that you want them to truly listen to what you say. Ask them not to tell you what to do, only to reflect back to you to indicate that they have really heard you.

If you have the habit of jumping to conclusions when someone starts to tell you something, it may be valuable for you to attend a basic counselling course to improve your listening skills, to be aware of the power of being truly listened to, yourself.

As an alternative, ask someone to be a listening partner, in order to give and experience this – no comments, no advice, just unadulterated listening for a set time each, with feedback at the end ('what I hear is ...'). This technique is used in co-counselling.

Don't wait until you are at crisis point. Who can support you now? Who can be there for you and accept you and who you are?[1]

Without more ado

We never live; we are always in the expectation of living.

Voltaire

Now is the right time to improve the quality of your life so that you have time for family as well as patients. Make time for more opportunities to enjoy being away from work doing things which you haven't done for years, such as going for a walk, a cycle ride, reading a book, painting, writing, any other almost forgotten hobby or whatever you've been saying to yourself, 'one day I'll have time for such and such'. Now is the time to get more balance between your medical work and the rest of your life, connecting with the part of you which has been denied for years.

Don't wait until you're well and truly 'burnt out'. Re-discover who you are now. Start today to make small changes. Be clear about what you have to do against what you 'should' do.

Self-care

You may believe that you are indispensable, but you might, one day, become too ill to work. What then? Become more 'selfish'. The word 'selfish' may have bad connotations for you. Think about it meaning 'self-care'.

When you take more care of yourself and your own needs, you will cope much more effortlessly with those of your patients. Don't wait to find solace in drink or drugs, or until you reach crisis point. Find someone to encourage and support you unconditionally. Talk to them about your frustrations and the difficulties of overwork in an environment of feeling undervalued and where endless demands are made of you.

Supervision

Counsellors are always supported by regular supervision from someone there to help them to sort out what issues are the client's and what are their own. Once you experience this support, it is difficult to know how you managed before. It is not to do with your standard of practice but about having someone to offload on to, without the fear of recrimination, from a person with whom you don't have to keep up the front of perfection. Some doctors are beginning to recognise its value.[2] Perhaps it would be more acceptable for doctors if it had a different name.

When you experience the power of support and encouragement rather than demands and intimidation you will be more able to coach your patients to do whatever they need to do, rather than reaching for the prescription pad or becoming exasperated with them. When someone listens to your concerns and acknowledges them as legitimate, you will become a better listener to your patients and hear more of their underlying issues and be able to empower them too. You will be able to convey to them that they can make a difference to their own lives when they take responsibility for it. Every small change you as an individual make will eventually help to change the system. Take courage and start to care for yourself, much more.

We deceive ourselves when we fancy that only weakness needs support. Strength needs it far more.

Madame Swetchine

References

1 Miller L (2002) The doctor's support line. *BMJ Career Focus*. **325**:S117.
2 Wilson H (2000) Self-care for GPs; the role of supervision. *New Zealand Family Physician*. **27(5):** 51.

15 Wellbeing: reality or dream?

The best six doctors anywhere
And no one can deny it
Are sunshine, water, rest, and air
Exercise and diet.
These six will gladly you attend
If only you are willing
Your mind they'll ease
Your will they'll mend
And charge you not a shilling.

Nursery rhyme quoted by Wayne Fields

Wellbeing

Wellbeing is:

- a state of 'being well, healthy, contented etc.'[1]
- 'the state of feeling healthy and happy'[2]
- about the connection between your mind, body and spirit.[3,4]

It's easy to become so engulfed in work issues that you are too tired to enjoy yourself away from the hospital or your practice. Is this how you are?

Do you have a dim and distant memory of how you used to be? Do you look back with longing to a time when you really enjoyed seeing your patients and greeted each day with excitement? What's changed? How can you get the sparkle back?

Balance

Imagine a wooden beam steady on a narrow fulcrum. It moves to one side and then to the other. Over all, however, it maintains its equilibrium. I'd like to invite you to think of this balance as a metaphor. At one end is you and your life, at the other the patient and theirs.

As you deal with each patient, even though you try to keep the sense of balance fairly steady, sometimes you tip too far over on the patient's side and you feel tired and drained. At other times, you move more to your side and you are energised, happy and satisfied with the outcome of your work. If, day after day, week after week, you find that you are giving out far more than you get back and the balance of your life is almost perpetually tilted away from your own needs and values, then perhaps it's time to redress the situation.

What can tip the balance one way or the other? How can you maintain more equilibrium in your life? What can you do to get back or maintain the wellbeing, the quality of life you so want?

Put yourself first

Being selfish is not always considered to be an enviable trait. But why not? Surely your own needs are of paramount importance? It's OK to look after yourself, physically, mentally and spiritually. Do you have a mentor, partner or close friend who will listen to your concerns and acknowledge them as legitimate?

Take a break

When was the last time you felt uplifted? Moved? Energised? Quite simply, when did you take some time out for yourself? Do you know that even five or ten minutes each day just for you, can make a profound difference?

> Dr A walks out of the hospital door each day at lunchtime and goes to a nearby park to eat his sandwiches and breathe some fresh air.

> Dr B packs her swimming things in her car and goes home via the swimming pool. After swimming a number of lengths she feels ready to deal with her domestic commitments and her family.

> Dr C walks her dog each evening for half an hour.

> Dr D meditates regularly.

When did you last have a holiday? How about being a tourist for a day and visiting somewhere locally? Is your life in tune with your values?[5] Are you nourishing your body, mind and spirit?

Big changes start with very small steps

Do you hear yourself saying 'One day I'll have time for such and such'. What are you waiting for? Find time this week to re-connect with yourself. You could enjoy again doing things you haven't done for years.

Re-discover who you are

Don't wait until you're 'burnt out'. Be clear what you have to do against what you 'should' do. Teach others your skills so that you can delegate more. Do you think that you are indispensable and that no one else can do what you do?

Have you ever had to take time away from work and noticed that somehow or other they have managed without you?

Life has its ebbs and flows

Even if you are the most positive person you may have some days when you are a bit down. Try to remember that without the off days you may not appreciate so much the good times. Who can you talk to?[6]

Body, mind and spirit are interconnected

If you are lacking in one area and don't know how to improve things, concentrate on nurturing another of them. Notice how when you do that, other parts of your life improve too.[7]

Keep a journal

Are you in the midst of a major transition at work or at home? It's easy to believe that things can't improve. Some people find it useful to track their moods and become aware of circumstances or situations which make them better or worse. You may find that the process brings the insight you seek.

Become more aware

Laughter is said to be the best medicine. What makes you happy and feel on top of the world? Notice what you are doing when you feel great. Keep a 'treasure store' of things to do for days when you feel that things could be better. This could include, for example, ideas about places to visit, people to call, music to listen to, something to create, exercises to do, inspiring books to read or tapes to listen to, something delicious to eat. What would be on your list?

Develop a positive mental attitude

This is probably the most important shift you can make to improve the way you are and your feeling of wellbeing. Your attitude affects the way you are and that affects the way others are towards you.

> Dr D feels annoyed about some of the practice staff who seem unfriendly. He hasn't realised that they are reacting to his scowls, until he greets them with 'Good morning, how are you today?' with a big smile. To his amazement they suddenly become friendly and quite human!

What we give out we get back. If you are unhappy in a situation think about what signals are coming from your verbal or body language, reflected in the way that person reacts to you. Become more aware of the words you use. Do you tend to moan about how awful things are? Do you use words like battle or struggle? You can change the way you regard a situation.

Live in the present

Enjoy whatever is happening in your life now. What are you learning? What will you do differently next time? What can you do to improve things? Who do you need to have a conversation with? Who can you encourage and validate today? Here's a challenge for you. Think of someone who you don't like or who irritates you and tell them something you admire about them.

Nurture your supportive networks

Have you considered being part of a support group? Be there for others and they will be there for you when you need them. Share and celebrate your good times.

Take regular time out

Arrange outings, holidays, time away from work. Reading is good too, so make time for books apart from medical textbooks and journals. Refresh you body, mind and spirit and notice the effect on your whole life.

Remind yourself of things going well

Keep thank-you letters from grateful patients. They are a wonderful morale booster to read if you feel low.

Create the future you want

To do this successfully it helps if you can:

- picture it in your mind
- feel, hear and smell it
- believe in yourself
- repeat positive affirmations each day as though what you want is already happening, for example, 'I am happy and content in my work and at home'.

What is a doctor to do?

The following is a summary of an informal survey I conducted amongst a few doctors.[8]

To maintain general wellbeing, they:
See friends and family; sleep; exercise; play music and sing; pray; eat; cook; walk the dog; go to the cinema; practise photography; laugh; swim; scuba dive; go to the gym; have a hot bath; take vitamins and other dietary supplements; designate time for self; count blessings; maintain a life outside medicine; have glass of red wine; enjoy their partner and children; practise yoga; take a holiday.

To maintain the wellbeing of their body, they:
Walk to work; walk the dog; do aqua-aerobics; have enough sleep and rest; eat a decent diet; exercise regularly; play tennis; wear nice clothes; practise yoga; cycle; swim; go to a steam room, sauna and Jacuzzi; practise martial arts; run.

To maintain the wellbeing of their mind, they:
Have a range of interests; get a balance between work and life; are spiritual; maintain family life; get plenty of sleep; eat good food; exercise and have fun; keep a sense of humour; look at the BIG picture of life; read; spend time praying; write morning pages (see p. 143); practise their hobbies; drink wine; cook; attend courses; travel; remember the good times; laugh, spend time with friends; listen to music; go to the theatre; paint; sculpt; seek creative challenges; acquire new knowledge.

For the wellbeing of their spirit, they:
Spend time with friends and family; take holidays, look at art; attend mass; meditate; sing in church choir; pray; go to church; count their blessings; live

for the moment; watch the sun, sky, sea; read inspiring books; read poetry; involve themselves in freemasonry; listen to classical music; look after personal relationships; visit a temple; practise yoga.

How about you?

How do you, or will you, maintain your wellbeing now?

The patient's treatment begins with the doctor, so to speak. Only if the doctor knows how to cope with himself and his own problems will he be able to teach the patient to do the same.

CG Jung

References

1   Pearsall J and Trumble B (1996) *Oxford English Reference Dictionary*. Oxford University Press, Oxford.

2   Procter P (2002) *Cambridge International Dictionary of English*. Cambridge University Press, Cambridge.

3   Chopra D (1989) *Quantum Healing*. Bantam Books, London.

4   Siegel B (1986) *Love Medicine and Miracles*. Harper Perennial, New York.

5   Houghton A (2002) Values? What values? *BMJ Career Focus*. **324**:S59.

6   Miller L (2002)The doctors support line. *BMJ Career Focus*. **325**:S117.

7   Yamey G and Wilkes M (2001) Promoting wellbeing among doctors. *BMJ*. **322**:252.

8   Kersley S (2003) *Doctors talking* www.thedoctorscoach.co.uk/doctorstalking.htm

16 Do your colleagues understand?

Communication is a skill that you can learn. It's like riding a bicycle or typing. If you're willing to work at it, you can rapidly improve the quality of every part of your life.

Brian Tracy

Viewpoint

You may make assumptions about how another person understands what you say, without taking into account how their view of the world is likely to be very different from yours. Not only that but you may also be inhibited in what you say because you are sure they will think this, or that, as a result, about you.

Inhibition

You may not actually say what you really mean to say. Instead you wait silently wishing you had the courage to speak up, to say what is in your head, which you would dearly like to tell them.

Maybe you wish you knew more, scared to admit to gaps in your knowledge, with the realisation you don't know everything there is to know about the subject. You may be racking your brain, desperately searching for the right words which you think are required, and, not finding what you search for, ending up not saying much. Then you realise that the moment to say something has passed, again.

You might remain silent, so at least no one can know or hear how little you know.

Are you stupid?

Perhaps, in the past, you may have said something, and the response from the consultant or trainer was to ridicule you in front of your colleagues. This is not an ideal culture for learning; what they said was their opinion at the time. It doesn't have to be the way you are at other times with other people.

More useful

How much more helpful it is when your answer is acknowledged and accepted. After you have studied for years and you are expressing what you know, there is no need to belittle your opinion. There may be more you might have said. There may be extra examples you could have given. Instead of humiliating you, your questioner could have thanked you for your answer and asked, 'What else is there?', or added 'There are a few other things you might want to mention next time...'. Finally, you could be thanked again for your contribution.

> As a medical student I was the sole female on my medical team (at that time there was a quota of 10% for female students!). I have a vivid memory of the consultant who rarely looked at or acknowledged me unless it was to put me down with his endless questioning and there was no acknowledgment of any correct answers given.

Communication is very important

You probably think you are pretty good at communicating. After all you spend a lot of your time with patients, don't you? But do you *really* connect with them or, as you hear certain clues, or certain symptoms, is your finger poised over the modern equivalent of the prescription pad, the computer key, ready to print out the appropriate pills or potion?

In a busy surgery or clinic this might be entirely appropriate, the way you've adapted to the limited time available to see the maximum number of patients, but, in an ideal world, communication is more than that isn't it? It's about interaction, an exchange of ideas, a two-way process of listening and talking. Improving your communication skills can benefit the way that you relate with both medical colleagues and other health professionals.

Good communication is about recognising the other person. It's about realising the other person has something valuable to say as well as you. You learn from them as much as they do from you. It's about realising that you don't know everything and every individual may have something useful to contribute.

Think about it

Mull over how you get on with others at work, and whether you are irritated by people who either never say much, or who don't cooperate. Consider how this may be because they feel their input is unimportant, or not worth much.

Perhaps this is because of the way you've spoken to them and dismissed what they say, or made a judgement based on scanty evidence that they wouldn't have anything to contribute to a discussion about such and such.

If you are annoyed by something about them, you could try showing your appreciation of something they do correctly before launching into an attack about what you consider is incorrect. They, like you, don't like to be told that everything they do is wrong. By hearing that something is correct and being told 'well done', they are more receptive to the learning which they need to do.

Improvements

Think about how to improve your ongoing communication with your practice partners, fellow consultants, registrars and colleagues you work with regularly. Start by thinking about the different opportunities there are for exchanging information. You probably have several ways for regular contact with colleagues.

Formal departmental meetings

Decide what your role is in the communication. Are you the leader or a participant?

If you are chairing a meeting:

- allow time for everyone present to have their say
- if someone is dominating the meeting, ask them to wait for a moment to let some of the quieter people have their say too
- when someone contributes, always thank them for their input rather than being too quick to tell them that their idea couldn't work or is wrong
- make sure you have you a clear agenda
- be specific about the length of the meeting, its purpose and the expected outcome.

Make sure you avoid a possible tendency to ramble on for ages with people closing their eyes, or leaving because they thought the meeting would be shorter and they have other commitments.

If you are a participant, decide why you are attending, what outcome you want as a result and what contribution you will make.

If you feel you don't usually have the opportunity to say what you want or if the meeting is dominated by one or two outspoken members, give the chairperson constructive feedback.

Informal meetings

You may find these are easier opportunities in which to have your say. Perhaps you chat with colleagues over a quick lunch to sort something out. There are likely to be constant interruptions by mobile phones and others coming to your table with 'Can I have a quick word with you about so and so?'.

It's not an ideal situation, is it? These circumstances are not best if you want to discuss any deeper issues. Instead of casual, chance meetings with the person you want to talk to, make an arrangement to talk at a definite time, for example, 'Can I speak to you for about 20 minutes later today? When would be best for you?'.

Notice boards

Do you read them? Do others? Are they so crowded with old notices that no one sees the flyer you put up for a meeting, or the notice about the information you want? Does someone take away out-of-date notices? How can you make your notice eye-catching so that it will be read? What do you want from your notice? If you are calling a meeting make sure you have all the details of the time and venue correct. Do you want people to sign up, call or email you?

Email

This may or may not be an effective way to discuss an issue with a colleague. Some people reply quickly and relevantly while others ignore your email completely, so if you want a quick reply this can be frustrating.

However, although it's a good way to communicate information without disturbing someone too much, it can also be a big timewaster. It's easy to start the day by downloading emails which you answer straight away. It's easy to be distracted from what you're doing with the beep of new mail arriving. Emails are handy when you organise using them in such a way as to benefit from their convenience, while not letting them take up too much of your time.

Good communication is vitally important in the workplace

Unless you communicate clearly with colleagues, patients and their relatives, part of your effectiveness is diminished considerably. How well do you really connect with others? Have you ever asked for feedback? It is often assumed that doctors have a good 'bedside manner' naturally.

Improving communication skills

The first step is to become aware of yourself and how you communicate. Communication is a two way process.

- It's about giving out and receiving.
- It's about listening and about talking.
- It's about understanding and accepting. It's about acknowledging and valuing.
- It's about being in rapport.

If you are frustrated by colleagues who don't understand you, it may be you, as much as them, who is lacking in communication skills.

Listen more intently to what they actually say and really hear and understand their concerns. When you do this you will begin to notice how often you jump to a conclusion when someone has just started to speak to you. If you want others to understand your point of view then the first step is to start to understand theirs much better. When you do that, you will find that they hear yours more clearly too.

A big step forward in improving your communication skills is being able to explain to others what's bothering you. So often you may assume that the other person is able to read your mind. Unless you describe clearly what you want to tell them, they may not be able to guess what you are concerned about. Perhaps you find it difficult talking about yourself. If so listen more intently to them and notice that they may have a similar challenge.

Deep listening

Deep listening means listening for what is not said as well as what is said. You can listen for emotions too. The more you become interested in them, their lives and their problems, the more they will tell you about themselves and the more likely it is they will eventually listen to you too.

Obstacles

What stops you from doing whatever would be the greatest help to you? Perhaps you avoid the conversation you need to have, about finding it difficult to cope, because you are anxious about the reaction it will have. You might worry that you will be considered useless if you admit to some vulnerability, or that others will wonder about your references if you complain about the situation or say that you are not prepared to put up with it any more.

If you have felt for a long time that your situation is intolerable and yet you continue to tolerate it, ask yourself what's stopping you making the changes you want. If you believe you can't alter the system, that may be true, but you can make the system more bearable. Don't wait for others to make the first move; you can make it.

For things to change you have to do something differently yourself, by making a decision, then and there, to take some action. One of the most effective ways to start the process of change is by having a conversation with the people involved. You have to listen as well as to talk. You have to understand others as well as yourself and to explore creative ways to do things differently.

Communicating more effectively

Is there a way that you can meet with your colleagues, if you have concerns about the running of the department, or have suggestions for ways to improve it? Call a meeting. You could ask for an item to be on the agenda to bring the matter to the others' attention.

Have your say and make sure your opinion is acknowledged and considered. Notice if there is a hierarchy in your department. If so and you are senior, listen to the views of the juniors instead of dismissing them. If you are junior make sure your opinions are heard. We have two ears and one mouth to listen twice as much as talk!

If you have an issue for discussion about a change or improvement, how quickly can you consult your colleagues? Are they open to different ideas? Are you?

Dr X, a specialist registrar, dreads outpatient days. The list is always twice as long as the optimum length as recommended by the College. She finishes the clinic exhausted and frustrated because there is seemingly nothing she can do about the situation. She starts to think about how the outpatient list is filled. She hands a slip which says 'six weeks' to the patient. The booking clerk books the patient for the appropriate clinic however many names are already on the list. What is the basis of the decision to see the patient after six weeks? Why not 12 weeks, or 24 weeks? Do they actually need a follow-up appointment, or is this 'the routine'? Could they be given guidelines and asked to call in for an appointment if certain symptoms occur? (The responsibility of care is handed to the patient.) With some trepidation, Dr X brings this topic to the next departmental meeting.

To her surprise there is unanimous agreement from the consultants and registrars that the situation is intolerable for them too. The outcome of the discussion is that the clerks are told to inform the doctor when the clinic is fully booked so that a decision about when the patient will be seen can then be made.

Dr X looks forward to her clinic and her colleagues thank her for initiating this simple change in procedure.

(See Chapter 17 for further discussion.)

Clarity

Be clear about:

- what you are prepared to do
- what you are not prepared to do
- what your colleagues expect of you
- what your specific role is
- how flexible you are prepared to be
- when you will say 'no'.

Maintain standards

Decide how you want your department or practice to run, and what your standards are for this. Think about what is important to you in your working environment, whether there is something that your colleagues do or don't do which irritates you. Have you discussed this with them? (Communication again!)

Dr A believes his partner, Dr B, isn't doing her fair share of the work in the practice. He resents her being part time. He thinks she should be doing more on-call work. He doesn't discuss this with her and is very irritable whenever he speaks to her. Because they are so busy they only talk to each other when they pass in the corridor at the surgery.

Dr B finds the situation unbearable. She wants to leave the practice but her husband encourages her to stay because it is convenient for where they live and there are no vacancies advertised locally. She tries to be all things to all people, a perfect doctor, mother and wife, but the strain is beginning to show.

She asks Dr A to set aside an hour for a meeting to discuss these issues. She decides what she wants to achieve from their meeting. She wants to be clear about what he expects from her in terms of on-call work and time in the surgery. She wants him to understand that she would like to leave on time at the end of the day so that she can pick up her child from school. She suggests several options to enable this to happen and to do her full share of the work. She writes this down and gives it to him to consider, before they meet. The outcome is that they understand each other much more. They come to an amicable agreement and their working relationship improves.

You can make a difference. Have a conversation.

Good communication is as stimulating as black coffee and just as hard to sleep after.

Anne Morrow Lindbergh

17 How to see fewer patients in your clinic

We're so engaged in doing things to achieve purposes of outer value
that we forget that the inner value, the rapture that is associated with
being alive, is what it's all about.

Joseph Campbell

A clinic day

It's another day. Your heart sinks. You dread finding out how many patients
are waiting to see you. You know the day is totally unpredictable and you
will be handed a fully booked list with another name or two squeezed in.
This probably won't represent who actually attends the clinic because some
will fail to arrive at all and others will be added as last minute emergencies.
Some will come who have nothing at all wrong with them because 'they
don't want to let you down'.

How are you?

You feel your blood pressure rise as you walk towards the outpatients clinic or into your surgery and the beginning of a stress-related headache, as
you say to yourself yet again, 'I can't stand this situation much longer'.

You are fed up complaining and grumbling bitterly to anyone who will
listen. There is no way you will put up with yet another busy clinic. You've
definitely decided enough is enough and you know you can't carry on with
the stress, so something or someone will have to give. And it could be you.

It's always the same

Nothing changes, unless it's for the worse. You get there, take one look at the
list on your desk, groan inwardly and wonder how you'll ever get through
them all. 'It's the system', you say, and 'I can't change the system'.

You are you relieved when several patients fail to arrive, although you
dread the possibility of the day when everyone turns up and you wonder

how you would cope. You know the system is near breaking point but believe you are powerless to do anything about it.

But is this true?

Can you do something to improve this state of affairs? Everyone you speak to shrugs their shoulders and tells you not to complain, because that's the way it is. You wonder if you ought to stop making a fuss. Nevertheless, you count yourself lucky you're not working in the hospital on the other side of town. The doctors there have to see twice as many patients as you. So, you take a deep breath, swallow a paracetamol or two and push the buzzer for the first demanding patient who storms in complaining that she has been waiting for over an hour.

Ask yourself

Ask yourself the following questions.

- Why is every clinic overbooked?
- Who decides it's OK to go over the designated limit?
- Who actually makes the appointments?
- How are the appointments made?
- How many are new patients, how many are follow-ups?
- What is the time interval before seeing a patient again?
- What is achieved from seeing a patient at an arbitrary fixed time interval?
- Whose needs are satisfied?
- What is the rationale for the time interval between visits?

If you are doing what you've always done, don't be surprised that you get what you've always got. Perhaps now is the time to start to think about the situation differently. Can you picture a clinic which begins and finishes on time? What options have you got for this to happen in your clinic?

An ideal clinic

To achieve your perfect clinic situation, you need to clearly define the following.

- The number of patients you would like per session.
- The amount of time designated for each patient.
- Ways to ensure that booked appointments are kept.
- The criteria for follow-up visits.

- Emergency provision without disrupting everything.
- Ways to lessen the number of emergency visits.

In your mind's eye, start by imagining what an ideal clinic would be. See yourself there now. Picture it. Listen to it. Hear the calm voices. Feel the relaxed atmosphere. (Difficult, but keep trying!) Imagine yourself, with a smile on your face. You are unruffled and stress-free. You arrive at your bright and airy consulting room filled with sunshine and fresh flowers to find a neat list with exactly the number of patients booked which your College recommends. There are a couple of vacant appointment times for any emergencies or for patients anxious about symptoms they have.

Smiling patients are seen at the correct time of their appointments. They too are tranquil and serene. They discuss with you and are fully involved in their treatment options and each patient fully understands both your role and theirs in the management of their medical condition. All patients leave your consulting room pleased and are heard to say something along the lines of, 'Thank-you doctor. I will do whatever I need to do so that the treatment you've prescribed will work in the very best way for me'.

At the end of the clinic, you do a ward round and complete your correspondence before having a delicious healthy lunch in the beautiful hospital restaurant. You are happy and know you have done a good morning's work.

Then the alarm goes off and you wake up. It was all a dream. But does it have to be? What can you do right now which will help towards making this dream a reality? Write down the answers to the questions below, brainstorm, draw a mind map, decide to take some action and then you may find that the action of one or two people can make a difference.

- How can your patients be more involved and responsible for their treatment and wellbeing? There is a subtle difference between telling someone they have to give up smoking and asking them, 'What do you need to do differently to help you recover?'.
- Do your patients know and understand their illness so that they recognise which symptoms to look out for?
- Do you provide a telephone number and a time they can call to talk to you if they are concerned about their condition? A few minutes on the phone to you may relieve their anxiety and prevent another appointment being used.
- When you've finished with someone in your outpatient clinic, you hand them a piece of paper to take to the desk to book their next appointment. Ask yourself, do they need to be seen again as a routine?

Review

Have you reviewed with your colleagues the reasons for seeing patients as follow-ups? What is an optimum time? Why six weeks? Why not four weeks, eight weeks or six months? Do you want to know if they have developed signs or symptoms? Do you need to see them if they feel well? Could any tests be done without taking up clinic time? Could they be told the result by telephone, email or even via the Internet?

Talk to your colleagues about the routines in the department? Have a creative discussion to explore other ways of practice.

Be prepared to listen twice as much as to talk, to find imaginative solutions.

Draw up new guidelines

When you change things you and your colleagues arrive for the outpatient clinic, look at the patient list and feel relaxed about the hours ahead. What will you do now to take more responsibility for a lasting change in the system, to make the dream a reality?

Assumptions allow the best in life to pass you by.

John Sales

18 The end of the road or a new beginning?

When I retire I'm going to spend my evenings by the fireplace going through those boxes. There are things in there that ought to be burned.
Richard Nixon

How do you feel about reaching the official end of your everyday life as a doctor? Perhaps you've been considering ways of staying in medical employment after retirement.[1] But how do you view the idea of giving up medical work? Do you see it as the end of the road or a chance to do something entirely different? Will it be a time for closing down or opening up for you? Have you always expected to retire when you are 60 or 65 years old but noticed that your workload and the nature of your job have changed so much that it is more of a chore than a joy? Would you like to retire but feel a little scared at the prospect?

There's no doubt about it, practising medicine is a fulfilling profession. However, if it has taken most of your time and energy for years, the thought of never seeing another patient may fill you with joy tinged with panic. When you no longer have the stress of it all, will you miss it? You may say you can't wait. But deep inside you have a lurking doubt. You know that you'll miss being a doctor and wonder what to do instead.

Which of your needs are fulfilled by being a doctor?

A doctor has status in the community. Being a doctor is great for your self-esteem; your opinion is valued and respected. You have security too, both financial and personal. There is also support; in theory, you have supportive colleagues who will encourage you to progress within the medical profession and achieve your career goals. If you want to meet any or all of these four needs then it is important to consider how you will do this outside medicine.

Think about your life

It is the end of another long day and you've finally arrived home exhausted.

Perhaps your briefcase is full of work to do before you go to bed. You've got years to go until you're officially due to retire. Have you planned how you'll spend your days when you are no longer doing busy clinics, long operating lists, or endless surgeries?

Do you reassure yourself and think, 'No problem. I'll take a few weeks' holiday and enjoy myself. I deserve a rest after all those years of being over-worked'? Is the rest of the plan vague or have you some specific things you'll do?

Whether it's your choice or someone else's, you may experience a gamut of emotions when you finally decide to take the plunge. You may feel a sense of sorrow, sadness, anger and guilt; a period of grieving for a part of your life that is over.

Your new life

Eventually you will be ready to move on to your new life as 'a doctor retired from clinical practice'. What do you imagine this will be like for you? It may depend on your attitude and motivation and how you plan to use your time. For some people it will be too easy to do nothing except be a couch potato. For others it will be a chance to discover that there are a multitude of fresh doors along their corridor of life waiting to be opened.

Starting your new life

Can you look forward to this part of your life as the start of something new and exciting? It will be a chance to do things you never had time to do while working as a busy doctor. It will be a possibility to increase your skills, to learn something, to discover a talent, or to travel to destinations both out-side and inside yourself. Whatever takes your fancy, this is the time to turn your dreams into reality.

Don't simply retire from something; have something to retire to.
                                                          Harry Emerson Fosdick

Why wait?

Perhaps retirement is still a long way off for you. What's stopping you making changes currently? How about living some of your dreams now, making sure that your needs are fulfilled by activities outside as well as inside medicine.

> Dr X found time to play the piano regularly when he decided to stop bringing work home with him in the evening. How did he achieve this? He stopped putting papers in his briefcase at the end of the day. The next morning, he felt refreshed when he returned to his desk to do the tasks.

Can you find a way to start doing what you want in parallel with your medical life? What's stopping you? It is possible to be a doctor and have a life too.[2]

Another kind of gardening

If you start to plant the seeds of your intentions for your retirement today, you will have taken the first step towards nurturing your new life. Just like your garden, you may keep on doing little bits, but you may not see much happening immediately. The following summer, however, you will be able to enjoy all sorts of amazing shrubs and flowers. The seeds you plant now will ensure that one day you'll be able to enjoy a happy and fulfilling retirement, whenever that may be.

We must be willing to let go of the life we have planned, so as to have the life that is waiting for us.

EM Foster

References

1   Lewis J (2002) Continuing working after retirement age. *BMJ Career Focus*. **324**:S163.
2   Kersley S (2001) Striking the balance. *BMJ Career Focus*. **323**:S2.

Part Four

Case Studies

Disclaimer: The following 'case studies' are based on general situations experienced by many doctors. None relates to a particular individual. Any resemblance to a specific person is purely coincidental.

> *Too many people, too many demands, too much to do; competent, busy, hurrying people – it just isn't living at all.*
>
> Anne Spencer Morrow Lindberg

19 The overwhelmed GP

Presenting symptoms

It's all too much.

Past history

You are a busy GP. It's the beginning of another week. You dread going to work. You are always exhausted. The day is never long enough to do everything you plan. It's always the same. From the moment you walk through the door of the surgery, you are bombarded with requests to sign forms and answer queries. There are phone calls which may result in extra patients to be fitted into an already busy clinic. There are aggressive patients demanding that something has to be done and telling you pointedly that they know their rights. There are an enormous number of repeat prescriptions to sign, with not enough time to review whether all the medication is absolutely necessary. At least those patients aren't filling appointment slots. What is soul destroying is that the situation never seems to improve. You used to think it was just a 'bad week' and the next one would be better. Now you realise, with a sinking heart, this is it. This is what it's like to be a GP in UK society today. At least this is what it is for you.

There are a few colleagues who seem to be coping well. From your perspective it's difficult to understand how they manage to keep a cheerful expression. They even seem to be able to have a game of tennis on their half day, and have been heard to mention that they went out at the weekend with their wife and children. As far as you are concerned these sort of things are almost forgotten luxuries. There's too much to do, always, to even consider any leisure activities. Your partner doesn't understand, however many times you've tried to explain how important it is, that your work has to take priority over anything else and they should have understood what living with a doctor would be like.

However, you don't think you can cope with your life as it is much longer. You don't sleep very well any more and have been overeating and drinking more alcohol than you know is good for you. As a doctor it's very difficult to know who you can turn to, who you can talk to about how you feel. You believe that everyone else apart from you copes well. You know you have to deal with whatever life throws at you.

You have always been a caring person and want to make a difference to people's lives. Because you were good at science at school, your teachers encouraged you to do medicine. It's been a rewarding career both financially and emotionally until the last few years when you've wondered what it's all about and begun to feel very disillusioned with it all. You have always enjoyed the intellectual process of coming to a diagnosis, treating your patients and the satisfaction of seeing them recover. However, even that enjoyment has disappeared recently. You are fantastic at caring for others but have neglected to care for yourself. These days you find it difficult to remember why you entered the medical profession. What you do all day bears little resemblance to your dreams of life as a doctor.

Examination

Outwardly you look well, even though somewhat tired. Your partner nags you about your weight. You believe that as far as the patients are concerned, you manage the workload adequately if not extremely well. Your patients seem to love you, although there have been a few complaints recently which you believe is the climate of increasing litigation towards doctors rather than any personal failing in your ability to practise adequately. You are smartly dressed and exude an aura of confidence. You rarely show any irritation with your patients or colleagues.

Home life is becoming rather stressful. When you eventually arrive home, you meet an irate partner and a cold supper, and you tend to have a short fuse. Your family relationships are suffering. Inside you are in turmoil. You know this situation isn't right and that it can't go on much longer. You have some antidepressants in your bag and wonder whether to take them.

Investigations

You need time to think about what has been happening lately. Find a quiet place to do this. Yes it seems impossible but your life depends on you changing the situation. You need to think about what are the most important areas of your life to you.

Place the following in order of importance to you:

- career
- family
- close relationship
- friends

- community
- spirituality
- self-care,
- money.

Then ask yourself:

- Is the order related to how you actually spend your life?
- Isn't it time to get your priorities right?
- Do you neglect your own needs as you look after those of your patients?
- When did you last do whatever it is that you love to do?
- What can you do for a few minutes as a start, something which will give you a buzz, make your heart sing again?

Write down your thoughts, re-read what you've written several times and consider them carefully. How are you going to change things?

Diagnosis

Chronic overwhelm.

Treatment

Prescription for change

Don't wait for the system to change. You have to take action to do something for you and your life.

You can make a difference by changing yourself. The important thing is to start – today. Begin by doing something, anything, differently. If you don't know what to do, clear your desk or throw away the pile of journals that you won't ever have time to read. Let go of believing you might miss reading something important. If it's that important it will appear elsewhere or someone will tell you about it.

Take time to sit quietly to think about and imagine your ideal life, in your mind's eye. Be aware of what you see, hear and smell. What does that feel like? What small steps are you prepared to take to move towards this dream? Decide on a very small action and get going with that today.

For example, stop interruptions while you are seeing patients. Specify a period when you do not want to be interrupted by phone calls or persistent queries. How much time will you start with? Half an hour? Ten minutes? Two minutes? Explain to the receptionist, and the others in the practice, that from now on you are unavailable for any interruptions during the specified time.

Instead of continuous or random interruptions you could instead desig-nate a specific period of time for requests and phone calls when you will be available for patients and others. In this way callers can be told when to phone you. During these times, be open and willing to be there for them.

Start to say 'no' when asked to do something extra which you don't want to do. Decide what you are definitely not going to do any more. Then, with-out getting into any discussion about why, just say 'no' and mean it. When you say 'no' to something, what are you saying 'yes' to?

Think about to whom you can assign some of the routine work. Delegate more. Get others to do the non-medical tasks. If necessary employ an extra assistant for this. Don't make any more excuses about why you can't do this and that. Make a start today with something, however small.

Shift the situation, bit by bit, day by day, until you make a complete recov-ery. You can change, just be willing.

Prognosis

Excellent, if the prescription is dispensed soon.

Challenge

Imagine you are the doctor described. What will you modify to reduce your actual or potential overwhelm?

20 The disillusioned consultant

Presenting symptoms

You are indispensable, so all your time and energy is used for your patients and you are too busy to look after yourself.

Past history

After years of struggle, long hours and endless studying for higher examinations you arrive, at last, at the golden destination. You reach the pinnacle of your medical career; the prize you strived for is yours. You are a hospital consultant.

However, even though you are highly regarded by both your patients and your colleagues, you feel let down by the long hours of work, by the lack of support from the system, and by the frustrations of inadequate facilities.

You also have nagging doubts about not being good enough, about being a fraud, about not being quite ready for this. Although being a consultant is no longer, necessarily, a job for life, the appointment feels like a life-long commitment, a life-long sentence. It is not only the job but all that goes with it. Is this the place you really want to live in for the next 30 years? You don't want to be saddled with the massive mortgage. You want to have the time to do fun things, the things you promised yourself you would do when you could manage to pay for them. Now that you can afford them you haven't the energy or excitement any more.

Was it for this that you worked so hard? Has it been worth the sacrifices? You neglected your partner, your friends, your family and your own wellbeing along the way. You've survived the arduous journey and reached the place you dreamed of and now wonder if it is the right destination. You have a demanding private practice as well as an everlasting NHS list of patients waiting to consult you. You are the person with your name over the patient's bed. The responsibility stops with you. The threat of litigation is like a little gremlin sitting constantly on your shoulder, shaking a finger at you and reminding you to do the extra test to be sure that every eventuality is covered.

Life is more stressful than ever. You are far too busy to take a break, so when holidays are arranged you end up working over Christmas and at other times you would like to have as time off. You always pull the short straw because you are the most junior consultant.

You are in demand to speak at international meetings about your latest research, so conferences have to take the place of holidays. It's more stress for you but you dare not say no. Your colleagues tell you that you have to join the circuit, that it's important to build your reputation.

It goes on and on. Years pass. The workload increases. Even at weekends, you keep on working. You see private patients and operate late into the night to boost your income to pay for the house and the private school fees. Your partner comments that you look tired but you ignore this and tell yourself that you can cope. You convince yourself that this way of life is only short-term, and yet the pressure continues. You know that you will have to slow down and take a holiday. But nothing changes. When you take a few days off, the workload accumulates so much while you are away that you dread going back afterwards.

Sometimes you think, very fleetingly, about retiring early. You do the sums and come to the conclusion that you have to work until you are 65 because of the heavy financial commitments you have. On the other hand you wonder what you'll find to do with yourself, because work is everything. There is nothing else in your life. Even though you complain, you realise that your life will be empty if there was no work to fill it.

Rather alarmingly you notice, then ignore, the occasional chest pains felt recently, when you are particularly rushed or stressed. Luckily you have some ancient glyceryl trinitrate tablets which you found at the back of a drawer. You take one if the pain is bad and tell yourself you have indigestion. You don't have any time to see your own GP, even if you had one. Why should you, when you know what's wrong? You never got around to registering when you moved to this city when you were appointed as a consultant. There seemed no point back then as there were always colleagues around to have a quick word with after meetings. But deep down you are scared.

As your reputation and private practice grew, so too has your NHS load and the frustrations of the guidelines and targets which bear little connection to clinical need. You are too busy looking after others to have time for any self-care. You vary between missing meals completely and eating large restaurant meals with pharmaceutical reps when negotiating funding for your latest research project. Exercise is a word you relate to books rather than to moving your body. You convince yourself you are fit enough as you get in and out of your car to do clinics in different hospitals. Your family seems to inhabit another world into which you rarely enter.

Examination

You are bewildered about what has happened. You realise you would not want to be treated by someone who is as tired and drawn as you. You see a face in the mirror of someone exhausted and stressed, and wonder where your joy for life went.

Investigations

Wheel of life

Draw a circle and divide it into eight equal segments. Label each one as follows:

- career
- money
- health
- friends and family
- significant other/partner
- spirituality and personal growth
- fun and recreation
- physical environment.

The eight sections in the wheel of life represent the state of balance in your life. The centre of the circle is a zero score, the circumference is a score of ten. Indicate your level of satisfaction in each area of your life by drawing a line across at the appropriate point within the segment. Your line does not have to touch those in adjacent segments.

Which part of your life needs the most attention? Are you having a bumpy ride? Do you like the situation? Note your answers and consider them carefully.

Diagnosis

Disillusionment.

Treatment

Prescription for change

Start with self-care. Your mind, body and spirit all need nurturing. Since all aspects of your life are interconnected you have a choice. Consider how to increase your fulfilment in the areas of you life which you ignore at the moment. Think how to make the best parts of your life even better. For example, if you improve your self-care by eating healthier food, your general wellbeing will improve and you will enjoy your work more.

Prognosis

Excellent, if the prescription is dispensed and taken soon. A little change for the better each day can lead you to complete recovery.

Suggestions

Look after yourself much, much better. What can you do today to improve your physical and emotional wellbeing? Some suggestions follow:

- eat healthily
- stop smoking
- limit alcohol
- take regular exercise.

Whatever you decide, 'just do it'. Decision without action is pointless. Find someone to make changes with you – a friend or a coach to support and motivate you through these changes. Indulge yourself. Don't make any more excuses about why you can't do this. Make a start today with something, however small.

Challenge

Imagine you are the doctor described. What will you change to improve your self-care? What has stopped, or is stopping, you from making those changes? What can you do differently today to start to make your life better?

Action may not always bring happiness; but there is no happiness without action.
Benjamin Disraeli

21 The doctor's other half

The doctor's wife ... must realize proudly that her husband is in the privileged class – privileged to have a duodenal ulcer, coronary thrombosis, and a lonely life. She must never be jealous, a virtue that harks back to the pre-stethoscope days when the doctor laid his beard-ed face on the lily-white bosom and listened with one ear for rales and with the other for the patient's husband. She must be sympathetic with her husband, for no one else ever will be.

Earle P Scarlett

Presenting symptoms

Your other half is a doctor and you wonder if you can cope with that lifestyle any more. You thought you'd found a soul mate but now you doubt it.

Past history

Life as a doctor's partner has turned out differently from what you imagined. Perhaps you met and fell for each other as students, or maybe you were work colleagues or even met through the internet or a dating agency. However it happened, you met and fell for a doctor. Your friends envied you so much. You longed to have the status of 'doctor's partner', but over the years the reality has changed. Life is no longer as it was when the quotation above was made. Times have changed and you are not sure if you can put up with the lifestyle any more.

You've changed where you live so many times because your partner is on training rotations which involve hospitals far apart. Each time this happens you wonder whether to move with him or her or whether to stay put and concentrate on your own career. If you move it might mean your own work prospects are curtailed. It becomes increasingly difficult to make social contacts each time you move. Your partner works long irregular hours so your social life together is virtually non-existent. Even when you have something arranged, it's likely that your partner either has an emergency to deal with at the time, or comes home too tired for anything.

You wonder what happened to the considerate person you knew when you first met. Now you wonder whether your partner fancies someone else more than you. When at home they expect everything to be organised around their needs because your partner is used to telling others what to do and having the requests carried out.

Many of your friends in similar situations have split up and you wonder if your relationship is doomed too. You are too busy yourself to have much time for your own needs.

You don't know what's happened to your life or the dreams of a wonderful life together.

Examination

You are an intelligent creative person with so much potential which has been lost since you hoped for togetherness in the 'doctor's partner' role. There are parts of you which remain in embryonic form, even though you are a mature adult.

Investigations

If you are neglecting your own needs as well as trying to look after those of being part of a couple, ask yourself when you last did whatever it is that you love to do.

Diagnosis

Relationship deterioration.

Treatment

Prescription for change

Take time. It's not too late to make some changes. Successful relationships depend on various factors. One of these is clarity of boundaries. It's important to say 'no' and mean it when you don't want to put up with something any more. You can be a person in your own right in spite of, or as well as, being part of a couple or a family. Make time to do what you love to do, even if your partner doesn't share the same enthusiasm. Do it without them. For example, this might mean visiting friends or going out to the theatre or cinema on your own.

Each week allocate some time to doing something which you love to do. Perhaps this could be painting or playing a musical instrument or exercising. Doing something regularly can lead you to complete recovery because it will enable you to find again the person hidden beneath the role of 'doctor's other half'.

Fill the gaps in your life by nurturing yourself.

Prognosis

Excellent, if the prescription for change is dispensed today.

Challenge

Start to look after yourself much, much better. What can you do today which will improve your physical and emotional wellbeing? Practise saying 'no' this week to things you no longer want to do. Take time to do something you really enjoy. Remember what it felt like before you were a 'doctor's partner' and try to recapture that feeling again. Find someone to support you to make the changes – a friend or a coach to encourage you. Go on, indulge yourself!

Don't make any more excuses about why you can't do this. Make a start today with something, however small.

If you are the doctor's partner described, decide to do something to improve your life. Decide what has stopped, or is stopping, you, and what change, however small or large, you can make, starting today, to make your life better.

If you are a doctor, in a relationship with someone like the person described, begin to recognise that your partner is also a person who needs to be seen and understood beyond the role of 'doctor's partner'.

22 The independent soul, the sole doctor

Presenting symptoms

You have always done really well professionally and are well respected for your knowledge and expertise and yet there is a feeling of emptiness. You may have just celebrated a special birthday and noticed you forgot to find a partner while you were striving for a successful career. Where have the years gone to? Is it too late to settle down with someone special and perhaps have some children?

When the heart speaks, the mind finds it indecent to object.

Milan Kundera

Past history

You recently realised that you have been concentrating so much on passing your specialist exams, getting the right jobs, doing the research to write the papers which will further your career, that you neglected the rest of your life.

Examination

You appear to be an efficient professional person, although there is possibly an air of sadness about you. You seem slightly aloof at times, as though it might be quite difficult to share a joke with you or exchange much personal information.

Investigations

Recognising this condition is the beginning of the treatment. Once you decide what you want, try drawing a mind map to consider what options you have and how you might go about achieving what you want.

Diagnosis

Connection deficit.

Treatment

Prescription for change

Decide what you desired outcome is. If you want to find a partner then ask friends and family and find out how they met. These days more and more professional people connect through the internet or sites run by newspapers.

If you prefer to meet someone in a less focused way, explore ways to bring other things aside from medicine into your life. Revisit hobbies or other things you used to enjoy, or join a course to learn something you've always wondered about but never had the time. Paint, sing or dance. When you change the body you are, the person you are, and how you feel, will change too

Prognosis

Excellent, if you can start to have fun and take life in a lighter way with a smile instead of heavily with a frown.

Holding on to anger, resentment and hurt only gives you tense muscles, a headache and a sore jaw from clenching your teeth. Forgiveness gives you back the laughter and the lightness in your life.

Joan Lunden

23 The overstressed doctor

Presenting symptoms

You feel worse each day. You are more and more tired and irritable. You don't want to get up in the morning and have little motivation. You wonder what life is all about. You've been drinking more alcohol than you used to do, but convince yourself that you can stop at any time, no problem. You know you'll have to seek help one of these days, but worry about confidentiality. You believe that whoever you see locally will talk to others and you don't know how to find someone to consult in another area. You have thoughts about ending it all if things don't improve soon.

Past history

Since going to medical school your whole identity has been encapsulated in the role of 'doctor'. This has taken over your life. Every waking hour is filled either by the endless work or worrying about what you did, what you should have done, or what you would do next time. Your self-esteem is at rock bottom. Work is the only thing in your life. It has priority over everything else:

- your self-care
- your friends and family
- your relationship with your partner
- your spiritual needs and community.

Patients with chronic diseases and others who don't recover return to you over and over again, so you have a distorted view of your success. It's easy to forget you have cured and helped more people than you have 'failures'. You believe that those who don't recover reflect your incompetence. This leads you to work longer and longer hours with less time for other things.

Examination

You are utterly exhausted and exhibit the classic signs and symptoms of a carer who cares for everyone but forgets about themself. You are definitely a healer who needs healing.

Investigations

Answer the following questions.

- When did you last have a proper lunch break, with food and some time away from work?
- If you actually took a day off, which you rarely do, what would you do for yourself?
- When did you last have fun or a good laugh?

Diagnosis

Build-up to burn-out.

Treatment

Prescription for change

Don't wait until it's too late. Make some changes. Start to take action today so that you will change the answers to the questions. If it's difficult to do on your own, talk to a friend, partner, colleague or coach – someone you can trust to support and encourage you. Don't delay. Stop the process before it builds to full-blown burn-out.

- How can you start to care for yourself more?
- What new boundaries will you put in place?
- Who will you say 'no' to?

Think about the following example. If you were asked to do something extra at work which is absolutely vital, you would shift things around to find some time. Put your own self-care in the same league. Free up time to look after yourself.

Decide what you will do differently from now on. A little change each day can lead you to complete recovery. Make the start to fill the gaps in your life.

Prognosis

Excellent, if the *prescription for change* is dispensed today, and the first steps taken urgently.

You may delay, but times will not.

Benjamin Franklin

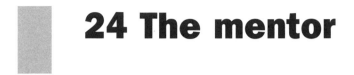

24 The mentor

Presenting symptoms

Exhaustion from the demands of being a mentor feeling unable to continue because of the attitude of the people to whom you give the benefit of your wealth of experience.

Past history

Other doctors often ask your advice about how to deal with certain sorts of patients or difficult situations. You've always been willing to tell them what to do and how to deal with the circumstances they find themselves in. They listen respectfully to your wise words and seem to find them useful. However, sometimes you have felt irritated by the way some of your good counsel has not been implemented.

You were asked to be part of the new mentoring scheme set up by your deanery. You know you are good at what you do and have a lot of knowledge and experience to teach others, especially newly qualified doctors and new consultants. You didn't want to attend the training course for this because you have years of experience and can already do what's necessary.

You went along to the training course but did not engage with the discussion or the other participants. It was a good chance to catch up on some journal reading.

You started with your mentees a few months ago but the experience isn't quite what you expected. Your mentees resent being designated to you and fail to keep appointments. They don't do what you ask them to do before your next meeting and you are exhausted and drained by the experience. You resent the extra hours you put into this scheme without any extra pay, and also the time it takes to travel to the other hospitals in the group to meet your mentees. When they don't turn up for their appointment the exercise seems even more futile.

All this results in having to take even more work home each evening, to keep up with your own clinical and administrative work. It's getting ridiculous. Your family don't seem to understand the pressure you are under at all and your relationship with them is deteriorating rapidly. You know you can't carry on like this much longer and that you should be able to deal with this yourself, but it's too difficult.

Examination

You look tired and stressed. You don't smile. You look at your watch regularly and say you've got a lot to do so can't talk for very long.

Investigations

To find out whether you are looking after yourself as well as possible, for a few days keep a log of how you spend your day.

- Note whether what you do is work, family, community or self-care related.
- Make a note by each activity about the level of stress you feel when doing it.
- Notice what if anything this log shows you.
- Reflect on if, or when, you would have liked some support from others.

Diagnosis

Lack of self-care.

Treatment

Prescription for change

Start to recognise your need to look after yourself as much or even more than you look after your mentees. Unless you care for yourself and your own needs you will not be the great mentor you want to be.

Think about what is really important for you and your life. For example, if you have young children, how important is it to spend time with them? Things like this are precious. You cannot be superman or superwoman, however much you want to be. Look at your time management . What are you doing that you don't have to do? Either stop doing those things altogether or delegate much more often and appropriately.

Be very clear about your role as mentor

If you find that taking on this extra role is tiring and you find the sessions with your mentee exhausting, then you may be telling rather than mentoring or coaching. As a coach or mentor you don't have to have all the answers; your mentee already knows what they want. You are there to facilitate their personal development.

In relation to your role as mentor be clear about:

- fitting the mentoring hours in with your other commitments
- when you will mentor
- where you will mentor
- who you will mentor
- being more efficient to cope with the extra duties involved
- looking after yourself.

Prognosis

With the *prescription for change* the prognosis is excellent.

25 The mentee

Presenting symptoms

You have just started a new job and feel overwhelmed by the amount you have to do each day.

Past history

You are beginning to wonder what to do. Your colleagues go home before you and seem to be more efficient. You have always been scared of making mistakes and go over everything you do many times. You arrive home exhausted each day. All you can do is eat and sleep and your social life has dropped to zero. You know your biological clock is ticking, especially if you are female and sometimes you worry you won't ever meet someone special and have children too. Your life is full of endless work, exams to study for, papers to write … .

By the time you've fulfilled all your career ambitions you will be in your late 30s, too old to do all the other things in life (at least that is what *you* believe).

You applied to join a mentoring scheme set up by the trust or the deanery and hoped this might be useful. You've been given the name of a potential mentor but so far haven't had the time to contact them.

Examination

You look tired and unhappy.

Investigations

Ask yourself why you haven't yet taken advantage of the local mentoring scheme. It could be the support you need at the moment to get you through the next few months.

Diagnosis

Mentor deficiency.

Treatment

Prescription for change

This can have dramatic results. Get in touch with the mentor. Speak to them on the phone. If it's too far to go to meet them face to face, arrange to speak on the telephone for a few sessions. This is just as effective and saves you time and energy.

When you find the right mentor you will have someone who will support and listen to you and encourage you to find ways to work more efficiently so that you can leave on time each day. You will be able to find ways to stop doing some tasks and perhaps to delegate some others.

By talking to a mentor you will find you change your perception about the situation. As you take on a more positive view of it you will be better able to adjust to what can be changed and accept those things which can't be changed. Your mentor has probably been through similar life experiences too, so hearing about their experiences might be useful.

As a mentee, remember your mentor is telling you what worked for them. This may or may not be right for you. You have a choice. A great mentor will enable you to find your own way forward to deal with the stress in your life.

Prognosis

Excellent if the *prescription for change* is taken without further delay.

26 The enlightened doctor

Presenting symptoms

A yearning for a totally different life experience.

Sometimes, being a doctor dulls your positive emotions. You often feel frustration, anger, resentment and depression. You recognise that it's good to be tuned in to all sorts of sensations, the good as well as the bad, the positive as well as the negative. However, you also know how to feel wonderful, and how this is the antidote to the negative emotions. You adore being overwhelmed with a sense of joy, exhilaration and excitement.

Past history

A couple of months ago you noticed an advertisement in the paper about a charity walk in the desert in Africa. You try to explain to your friends and colleagues how reading this made something happen inside you. It was the antithesis of your 'ideal holiday'.

You will camp, not wash for a week, wear dirty clothes, purify your drinking water with iodine tablets and walk 15 miles a day in hot and dusty conditions. Yet something about the advertisement spoke directly to you. It seemed to say, 'Come on, you can do it'. You wonder if you are completely crazy. However, the desire to take part has become a passion and you think about it day and night. You wake up with vivid dreams of what it might be like. You spend every free minute planning money-raising ideas, a get-fit schedule, and making lists of what to take with you (and surprise yourself being able to find a few free minutes).

Examination

You are a person with a mission. There is a sparkle in your eyes and the sound of your heart beginning to sing.

Diagnosis

Charity challenge fever.

Treatment

Prescription for change

Just do it! When you next see a poster for a challenge, decide to take part; put aside any objections which come into your mind. You can succeed and you will feel marvellous as a result, knowing that you can do almost anything.

Prognosis

Well done getting this condition. It will benefit not only you but also those others you inspire to do the same.

Excellent, let your spirit lead you. Taking part in a challenge is wonderful. You will feel on top of the world. The following are some of the benefits of taking part.

- You learn about the charity and what it does.
- You make a significant contribution to their funds through fundraising activities.
- You take the training seriously and become much fitter.
- You gain a sense of community with the other participants.
- You work as a member of a team helping one another.
- You have a spiritual experience.

The night sky in the desert is twinkling black velvet; and there is the vastness of the sandy plains and rocks. An enormous vista as far as the eye can see is an amazing feeling. You feel on top of the world – content, happy and exhilarated. When you complete a challenge you know you can do anything.

So what challenge will you take? Take a look at www.atd-expeditions.co.uk. This company organised the charity trek I completed in the Namibian desert. The organisation was superb. They specialise in treks for various charities all over the world, caring for the participants and the environment, and they support local conservation projects. Another similar organisation is to be found at www.discoveradventure.com.

Challenges are what make life interesting; overcoming them is what makes life meaningful.

Joshua J Marine

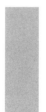

27 The unsettled doctor

Presenting symptoms

You want to make changes but don't know what.

Past history

You are at a turning point in your life. There has been much pressure on you from your boss to follow a particular career path. You are looking at an application form for a sought-after job but it isn't what you really want to do. Friends and colleagues tell you not to be so silly. You are the favoured candidate and this is an opportunity not to be missed. You know it doesn't feel right for you. You wonder whether to stay in your profession or leave.

Examination

You rush about with very little purpose rather like a headless chicken, because you don't know which way to go. You feel as though you are on a hamster wheel and you don't know how to get off.

Investigations

Even if you don't know the specifics, you can make a list of features that you want. For example, if where you live is where you want to live.

Diagnosis

Uncertainty about your medical future.

Treatment

Prescription for change

Decide what is important in your life. You can do this by thinking about what you really love to do and what you can do to bring that into your work. If you stay in your present job, make your mind up about what you could do to improve things. Talk to your colleagues and tell them how you feel. If you go to a new job make sure you know what the benefits to you would be and what would be the disadvantages.

Imagine yourself still in your existing job in a year's time and consider how it will be, and how you will feel, then. Do the same for the possible new job. Which appeals to you most? What other options do you have? Take a big sheet of paper and write down every possibility you think of, however outrageous.

Drawing a mind map is helpful. Put the words 'Where to now?' in the centre and then draw lines coming from this leading to your options. From each word other things will occur to you. See what happens and what links with what.

Go for a walk or sit quietly and listen to yourself. You will become aware of the answer that is right for you. It's your life – only you know how to live it.

Food for thought

You want to make changes in your life but don't get around to doing anything about them. Why is that? What's stopping you? What is the worst thing that could happen if you did what you want? Are you prepared to 'get out of the box' and think about your situation differently?

Imagine how you would like your ideal life to be. Take one very small part of this and introduce it into your life now. Start to behave 'as if' all is as you would like it to be. Other changes will start to happen. If, for example, in your ideal life you would go swimming once a week, then fit in some swimming now even for half an hour every two weeks.

Everyone who is overworked and putting up with a bad situation, may hope that someone out there will change things. It feels easier to stay in familiar discomfort than to take the big step, the leap into the unknown, so have the courage to say 'enough is enough' and make the changes yourself, otherwise nothing will ever change.

It's time to find some creative solutions to the situation you've had enough of. Start with some first steps to make it happen. Become very clear about what you will no longer tolerate and come up with ways to change these. Then, even the seemingly insurmountable can be overcome.

28 The doctor who has to re-take professional exams

Presenting symptoms

You spend every hour of every day trying to revise for your professional exams. It's bad enough being on call and working nights. You are zombie-like because of a chronic lack of sleep. Coping with all that, do you need the stress of taking your higher professional exams too?

Past history

The date of the exam is looming and you believe you will never finish all the studying you think you need to do. You spend hours each day sitting at your desk, books open, until some time later realising you've fallen asleep. You design complicated revision plans but regularly fail to keep to the strict regime you've set for yourself. You are not sleeping well and start to panic. You don't want to fail the exam but convince yourself this will happen. You are a perfectionist and expect to know everything.

Examination

You look tired.

Diagnosis

Chronic examination-itis.

Treatment

Prescription for change

You think you know nothing and will fail again. Take a reality check. Is that really true? Who is this exam for? It is for people like you who have been working in the specialty for a few years and who deal with the day-to-day challenges.

Ask yourself why you failed before. Was it to do with your exam technique rather than your lack of knowledge? You know many of the answers; perhaps you haven't presented them the way the examiners want them. How can you improve your technique? Is your handwriting legible? Do you plan your answers for a few minutes before you start to write? Do you divide the available time so that you have enough time to write something for each required question?

Tips for re-sitting exams

Would you like to pass next time? What can you do? Change your attitude. Believe in yourself. Indulge in positive self-talk. Change your thinking from 'I don't know anything' to 'I know enough to pass this exam'; from 'I am nervous' to 'I am confident'.

Look at your body language

Are you slumped in your chair, shoulders rounded, arms folded with a sad expression? Sit up straight with your shoulders back and put a huge smile on your face. How does that change the way you feel?

Things you can do

- Look through old papers.
- List the subject headings and tick them off as you revise.
- Do essay plans – one a day means you will have done five by Friday.
- Expand one essay plan each week into a full essay.
- Reward yourself.
- Ask for constructive criticism from a colleague.

Very few people achieve 100% in an exam. Even the examiners say this is impossible! You don't need to know it all to succeed. You have to be good enough, not perfect.

What will be useful?

- A broad knowledge of the subject.
- A good exam technique.
- The ability to plan your time to answer the required number of questions.
- Positive self-talk.

Good luck for the next time!

Is this a metaphor for other parts of your life? Let go of your need to be perfect. Relax. Life always offers new challenges. You can never know it all. Don't despair. You will always know something. Work out where and from whom you need help or support.

29 A New Year story

It's the end of the conference dinner. Most of the meal has been taken up with the man opposite and his colleagues talking 'shop'. It's the one thing they have in common with each other. It's like an ego-building exercise. They vie with one another to suggest that each one has more stress than the next and more difficulty dealing with the management. They all deplore the lack of money for their department and the rules imposed from faceless politicians. It's as though whoever made mention of anything else might lose credibility. How could they possibly be doing their work properly if they had time for other activities? Not unexpectedly, this belief means that the members of this group work obsessively long hours and always find reasons why they can't do what they used to, years ago.

It seems almost as though work is used as an excuse not to face the challenges in other parts of their lives. I'm bored with all the specialist talk. I decide it's time to break the mood, to open up the conversation a bit. I smile across the table. The tired man opposite me smiles back and looks surprised.

'How are things with you?' I ask.

'Can't wait to retire. Only another couple of years.'

'What will you do then?'

'Oh, the usual. Buy the boat. Potter around on the river. Take it over to France.'

'How come you are waiting until you retire? What's stopping you from doing that now?'

'Busy. Much too busy. You've no idea. Targets. Management decisions. Possible litigation. I'm completely exhausted by the time I get home. I couldn't possibly start going out on a boat then.'

He sighs deeply and looks at me.

'Actually I do understand', I said. 'I retired early from medicine. I wanted to do other things. I encourage others now. Do you realise that if you really wanted to, you could start to sail a bit even now. There's no need to wait until you retire. You just have to make a start', I reassure him.

'Maybe you're right. My poor old colleague had his retirement all planned out, then, blow me down, a month after the farewell party he had a stroke. Uses a wheelchair now and he can't do many of the things he planned. Never know, do we, we just never know what's around the corner.

'Do you know what?' he continues, 'What you said has really got to me. I've suddenly decided what to do. I'm going to buy the latest edition of the boating magazine and look at the adverts. Yes, I'm going to buy that boat next week. I can hardly believe what I'm saying to you, but I know I'll do it.'

'Here's my number. Do give me a ring in a couple of weeks and let me know what's happening.'

A few weeks later he phones me.

'Listen, it was all very well you persuading me to buy the boat but I still haven't any time to sail it. So what do I do now? I'm not sure whether I need whatever it is you offer. You know I feel awful saying this but I've been a great success all my medical life and yet I can't seem to get myself organised enough to get out in this fantastic boat. I'm extremely busy so I would find it difficult to find the time to come to see you.'

'Let's arrange a time to talk. This way we can both assess whether we could work together to achieve the changes you want to make. By the way, I work on the telephone so finding time for coaching needn't be a problem. Freeing up time is something we can work on, if you wish!'

I smile to myself and wonder if he'll contact me again.

He phones at the appointed time. I ask him to spend five to ten minutes telling me about himself and how he would like his life to be.

He tells me he is in his early 50s, married for the second time, and is a surgeon in a large district general hospital. He feels undervalued and overworked. He hates the added administrative work and the pressures to reach targets. To get the work done he has to start his operating lists or ward rounds early in the morning so leaves his house before his children are up. His ward rounds are extremely long because he is terrified of litigation so is obsessive about checking everything. His temper is shorter than it used to be and he knows that he gets unduly annoyed with the anaesthetist and the theatre staff who remind him at the end of the day that they want to go home.

He arrives home himself after seeing his private patients. His children have gone to bed and his supper has dried out. He is too tired to talk to his wife and the last thing he wants to hear about is her day or her problems. It's a lifestyle he's been following for years.

'So do something with that,' he laughs cynically down the phone line.

I ask him to tell me what his life will be like if he carries on as he is doing. He groans and tells me he thinks he'll probably end up with a heart attack. Unfazed, I ask him who 'he' is apart from the surgeon.

'If you could look into the future at yourself living a wonderful life, what would you see there? Where would you be? What would you be doing? What would you feel like?'

There is silence for a few moments.

'Very interesting questions. You're certainly making me think. I can hardly remember who I am apart from the surgeon bit of me. I used to enjoy painting years ago, oils and so on, and when I retire I plan to learn how to sail and go off at weekends up the river or along the coast. That is something to do one day. I've made a small step towards it by buying the boat.'

He pauses for a moment then adds, 'Do you know, sometimes I wonder if I'll ever reach retirement, or if the stress of this life will kill me before then.'

'What do you do to care for yourself? Do you take any exercise? Do you eat healthy food? Do you spend time in nature or wherever makes you feel calm? What do you do to relax?'

He thinks for a moment. 'I joined a gym in January last year, it was a New Year resolution to get fitter and lose some weight. Waste of money, that was. I've only been there a couple of times and now a year has gone by. You are right about nature. I'd much prefer to walk in the country or even cycle than go to a gym. If only I wasn't so busy at work.'

'Do you know something about "systems theory"?' I ask him. 'This suggests that all the aspects of our lives are interconnected. If you change one part others change too, almost effortlessly.'

'Tell me more.' He sounds interested.

'Well the best way to understand it is to try it,' I laugh. 'What change could you make this week, for a start? Forget about work for the moment. We've been talking about self-care. What small thing would you be prepared to do this week to look after yourself better?'

'Exercise. I like the idea of riding my bike. Yes, I'll do that. I'll take my folding bike to the hospital and ride around the grounds in the middle of the day. Instead of having a big lunch, I'll take some sandwiches, and go over to the park opposite to eat them.'

I laugh. 'Anything which might stop you doing that?'

'Well there may be a lunchtime meeting with a sponsored lunch. I may not get around to taking sandwiches from home'

'That's OK. So, what can you promise to do?'

'I will promise to have a bike-ride three times in the next week. I'll buy sandwiches in the canteen, so I don't have to waste time making any.'

'Excellent. How long do you plan to ride?' I ask.

'For fifteen minutes each time.'

'Great.'

I ask him to tell me what value he's had from our conversation and if he has any questions. After a pause, he replies.

'I was very cynical, I'll be honest with you. But even during this short conversation I realise how powerful your questions are. They certainly made me think. I feel much supported. I know the suggestions came from me.

What you asked got me thinking. I found the answers inside myself. I feel very focused now.'

Within three months he is sailing each week. The relationship with his wife has improved and he sees his children regularly.

When we meet again at the conference dinner the following year I hardly recognise him. He looks fit and well, and greets me with a big smile. As we shake hands he tells me, 'Talking to you last year was a catalyst. I've certainly changed my life since then. I can't express the value of that to me and my family. It's been my best year yet.'

Part Five

Life coaching for change

Without change, something sleeps inside us, and seldom awakens. The sleeper must awaken.

Frank Herbert

If we don't change, we don't grow. If we don't grow, we aren't really living.

Gail Sheehy

It is not necessary to change. Survival is not mandatory.

W Edwards Deming

30 Let your heart sing

To find the universal elements enough; to find the air and water exhilarating; to be refreshed by a morning walk or an evening saunter ... to be thrilled by the stars at night; to be elated over a bird 's nest or wildflower in spring – these are some of the rewards of the simple life.

John Burroughs

What lies behind us and what lies before us are tiny matters compared to what lies within us.

Ralph Waldo Emerson

Stop and listen

What does the voice inside reveal to you? It is telling you what you want very much. Can you hear what it says above the roar of your day-to-day cacophony? Would you like to open your heart to living a life you really want? Which door did you close when you opened the one to become a doctor? What would you find if you opened it again?

Is your life too routine, too busy and too stressful? Are you engulfed in the day-to-day overwhelm of general practice? If you continue along the same path what will you regret if or when you reach the age of 95? Have you forgotten what it's like to have fun, to have a laugh?

You don't stop laughing because you grow old. You grow old because you stop laughing.

Michael Pritchard

Do you want to do something wild and wonderful? Is your answer a 'don't be so silly' or 'what would people think of me'?

Would you love to re-visit hobbies, play music, sing, walk, jog, paint, write, dance, photograph or whatever, but believe you don't have the time?

Are you scared to feel that almost forgotten buzz again from doing something really exciting? How about trusting your instinct, your inner voice, which urges you to give something a try? You may say, 'What if I fail? What if they think I'm crazy...?'. Have you tried reassuring yourself with a 'never mind that … at least I had a go!'?

Whose life are you living? Are you sure? Who sets the agenda you follow? How can you change?

Daydream

To accomplish great things, we must dream as well as act.

Anatole France

Close your eyes. Imagine being at one with the universe, at ease, happy, fulfilled, relaxed. Who are you? What are you doing? Where are you? How do you feel? What's different?

Listen

What gives you, an extra-ordinary sense of excitement, a buzz, an awareness of 'this is what life is about', that you need more of again?

Believe

Has your life as a doctor suppressed your natural creativity? Is it the right time now to allow your imagination to run free? What beliefs about yourself or the 'system' stop you having a fabulous life? Are you scared of what others might say or think? Is that the way you want to live? You can't predict how the other person will react if you behave differently. They, like you, have a choice. You may even be their inspiration if you start to 'walk your talk', if you actually do what you've been dreaming about for ages.

Change your thoughts and you change your world.

Norman Vincent Peale

Do it your way

To live a creative life, we must lose our fear of being wrong.

Joseph Chilton Pearce

Maybe the time has come to put you first for a change and 'feel the fear and do it anyway'.[1] Now is your opportunity to have what you want in your life.

Get out of your rut

Find a rope to haul yourself out of your hole and seek whatever support and encouragement you need to change your life.

It's not that some people have willpower and some don't. It's that some people are ready to change and others are not.

James Gordon

Keep going

Your decision and enthusiasm to make a change will give you momentum. Decide on your goal. Be proactive. Work out the steps to get there and you'll be well on the way. Keep going and you will get to where you want to go.

Hold on

Julia Cameron recommends two wonderful tools to keep you on track. These are 'morning pages' and taking yourself on an 'artist's date'.[2]

Every day cover at least three pages in your journal with a flow of consciousness writing. Write your thoughts about what's happening and your reaction to the changes you're making, or just write rubbish. Think of 'morning pages' as a limbering up exercise for your mind.

For your 'artist's date', make a commitment to do something on your own, just for you. This could be, for example, an outing, a walk or sitting quietly in the garden.

Take action

If you really want more joy and happiness, then truly believe in yourself and know that you have the power to create the life you want. Stop waiting for others to do things differently. You can change your life yourself, but *you* have to do something. You have to take the first step, however small.[3]

They always say time changes things, but you actually have to change them yourself.

Andy Warhol

Keep going

Do I hear you murmuring, 'Been there, done that, started a load of projects but can't stick at anything'? What can keep you going? Will you use your diary, a computer programme and charts to tick? Who can be there for you? Someone who will encourage you to do what you want and give you positive encouragement? Your partner, friend, relation, mentor or coach? Someone to travel along this bit of your life's journey with you for a while?

Go confidently in the direction of your dreams. Live the life you have imagined.

Henry David Thoreau

Celebrate

What will you do when you are on the top of your world?

I celebrate myself, and sing myself.

Walt Whitman

References

1   Jeffers S (1991) *Feel the Fear and Do It Anyway*. Rider, London.
2   Cameron J (1995) *The Artist's Way*. Pan Books, London.
3   Covey S (1999) *The Seven Habits of Highly Effective People*. Simon & Schuster, New York.

31 What on earth is life coaching?

Go confidently in the direction of your dreams. Live the life you have imagined.

Henry David Thoreau

Do you sometimes wonder what life as a doctor is all about and whether the satisfaction and enjoyment from it is balanced by the stress and overwork? Have you ever thought about or questioned whether acclaim from your colleagues is worth the time physically and emotionally away from your family, your partner and most important of all, yourself?

Within the chapters of this book you've been encouraged to think of ways to change so that you truly can live the life you want, both as a doctor and as a human being.

You've been challenged, among other things, to:

- find more time[1]
- look after yourself better[2]
- stop procrastinating[3]
- communicate more effectively[4]
- improve your personal relationships.[5]

The fundamental messages are as follows.

- It is possible to make changes for the better.
- Define your specific goals.
- Recognise and maintain boundaries.
- Clarify personal responsibility.
- Say 'no' if you don't want something.
- Start big tasks with small manageable chunks.
- Explore different ways to find solutions.
- Take action.

So far, so good. Perhaps you really do want something different in your life, and yet a year on you are in the same place. You are as frustrated as you were and think that you have to put up with it all. Consider what your life would be like next year or in five years, if you continue in the same way. Is it more comfortable to stay in your discomfort than to take a risk and do something different? Are you ready to step out of your comfort zone?

What are you waiting for?

Are you waiting for someone else to make the first move? What's stopping you from being proactive? Is it fear? What are you frightened of? What's the worst thing that could happen? If what you fear happened, what would you do? Are you letting that stop you?

It helps to have someone on your side. Who can support you and give positive encouragement? Is there is a friend or a member of your family who can do this?[6] If they are part of the problem, or have their own agenda which might discourage you, perhaps you could ask a mentor or a coach for objective encouragement.

What is coaching?

The term 'coaching', with the prefix of 'life', 'personal', 'executive' or 'corporate', is said to have been coined by Thomas Leonard (1956–2003) in the early 1990s. The model comes from sports coaching. The principles and philosophy of coaching incorporate the ideas of Maslow (self-actualisation), Lucke and Locke (goal setting) and Steven Covey (seven habits).

Coaching is about:

- believing in possibilities
- being accountable
- challenging assumptions
- having a sounding board
- being motivated
- having a catalyst for change
- devising strategies
- thinking creatively
- setting and achieving goals
- being action oriented
- considering different options
- deciding which action to take.

The following are some of the tools coaches use:

- non-judgemental listening
- open questioning
- brainstorming
- mind mapping
- positive affirmations
- visualisation
- goal setting
- action steps
- journaling
- encouragement.

What is the difference between coaching, counselling and mentoring? There are similarities and connections between all of these.

Coaching is about moving forward from where you are in your life to where you want to be. The coach helps you achieve your own goals. The agenda is yours, the coach challenges, motivates and encourages action.

Counselling is for understanding and coming to terms with your past and movement out of a crisis situation.

Mentoring is guidance from someone, often in the same profession who can advise, encourage and support you in your day-to-day work. Some mentoring is called developmental and is very similar to coaching.

Coaching doctors and others

Coaching is widely known within the business community – 'it bridges the growing chasms between what managers are being asked to do and what they have been trained to do…'.[7] Even in the BMJ, coaching has been discussed, described or mentioned.[8]

However, within the medical culture there seems to be a reluctance to seek support even when it may be required.

Dr A was pleased when colleagues noticed that his desk was clear and tidy for the first time in living memory but also that he was less stressed and listened to them much more effectively. He asked for their opinion instead of trying to enforce his own ideas. Even his wife noticed that he was better company. He was reluctant, however, to admit that the changes had happened after he had worked with a coach.

Who is coaching for?

Coaching is for you, if you are a successful consultant, GP, hospital or community doctor who is overloaded by the demands and challenges of your profession. In spite of the fact that you look after your patients faultlessly, something is missing in your life. You wish you felt the enthusiasm you had when you first qualified. Perhaps you believe that it would be difficult to make life better so you carry on and you neglect yourself and your needs, your partner, your family and your community. It seems easier to stay where you are instead of making the changes you want, and yet there is a little voice inside telling you that life doesn't have to be like this.

It is possible to be a doctor and have a life too.

Coaching is a catalyst for change.

A journey of a thousand miles begins with a single step.

Confucius

References

1   Kersley S (2002) What would you do if you had the time? *BMJ Career Focus*. **324**:S53.
2   Kersley S (2002) Looking after number one. *BMJ Career Focus*. **324**:S85.
3   Kersley S (2002) Do you procrastinate? *BMJ Career Focus*. **324**:S164.
4   Kersley S (2002) Do your colleagues understand you? *BMJ Career Focus*. **324**:S117.
5   Kersley S (2002) Relationship: what relationship? *BMJ Career Focus*. **325**:S60.
6   Lagnado M (2002) Friends and family are good (and cheap) life coaches. *BMJ*. **324**:1099.
7   Morris B (2000) So you're a player. Do you need a coach? *Fortune Magazine*. **141**:144.
8   Atik Y (2000) Personal coaching for senior doctors. *BMJ Career Focus*. **320**:S2.

And finally ...

Life is like a spreadsheet: when you change one thing everything else automatically changes too.

Susan E Kersley

Appendix 1 Frequently asked questions

How do I find a coach?

- Use search engines to look for 'life coach'.
- By personal recommendation. More and more people are hiring coaches these days. It's a good way to find anyone from a plumber to a coach. If you've experienced coaching which you have found useful, don't keep it a secret, recommend your coach to your friends and colleagues.
- International Coach Federation (ICF): www.coachfederation.org
- Coach University: www.coachu.com
- Coachville: www.coachville.com

Why hire a coach?

If you are ready to make changes in your life but lose interest and enthusiasm when things go wrong, and want to find someone unconnected with your day-to-day life, on to whom you can bounce ideas, then a coach can be useful. A coach will listen, ask questions to make you think, and help you find the way forward. A coach has just one agenda: yours.

Does a coach tell me how to solve my problems?

No. A coach enables you to find your own answers. Deep inside, you already know what to do, but something stops you from doing it. You can talk to your coach about what's stopping you, what options there might be, how the challenge might be understood in a new way, and come to realise that it's possible to face up to and overcome your fears in order to achieve what you want.

What happens when I contact a coach?

Most coaches offer a free introductory discussion so the two of you can decide if you would benefit from working together. You will get a sense of what coaching is, and whether it might be useful. You also have the chance to ask the coach any questions you may have and for the coach to explain how they organise the sessions.

Most coaches work on the telephone so it doesn't matter where you live. Choose a coach who seems right for you.

What happens next?

If you decide to proceed, then the coach will tell you how they work. Some require you to sign on for a minimum time; others leave it to you. If you are responsive to coaching you may make big changes very quickly. However, it's useful to make a commitment to at least three months of coaching if you want lasting change to occur.

The coach will send you an intake form or questionnaire to help you focus on what you want to achieve. You may also be asked to complete a 'call preparation form' before each session.

How are the sessions organised?

This varies according to the individual coach. Sessions may be from half an hour or longer. You can make big shifts even in a relatively short time. A challenging question can change your life! By the end of the session you will have promised to take some action before you speak to your coach again.

How much does it cost?

What would living a better life be worth to you? Coaches charge professional fees.

Recommended reading

Buzan T (1996) *The Age Heresy*. Ebury Press, London.

Cameron J (1995) *The Artist's Way*, Pan Books, London.

Covey S (1992) *The Seven Habits of Highly Effective People*. Simon & Schuster, New York.

Covey S (1994) *First Things First*. Simon & Schuster UK Ltd, London.

Forster M (2000). *Get Everything Done*. Hodder and Stoughton, London.

Hay L (1988) *You Can Heal your Life*. Eden Grove Editions, London.

Jeffers S (1987) *Feel the Fear and Do It Anyway*. Rider, London.

Kiyosaki R (2002) *Rich Dad Poor Dad*. Time Warner Books, London.

Leonard T (1998) *The Portable Coach*. Scribner, New York.

Macnab F *The 30 Vital Years: the positive experience of ageing*. Wiley, Chichester.

Miedaner T (2000) *Coach Yourself to Success*. Contempory Books, Chicago.

Richardson C (1998) *Take Time for Your Life*. Broadway Books, Chicago.

Whitlow J (2002) *Coaching for Performance*. Nicholas Brealey Publishing, London.

Whitmore J and Sandahl P (1998) *Co-Active Coaching*. Davies-Black, Mountain View, CA.

Resources

The Open College of Art: www.oca-uk.com

The Open University: www.open.ac.uk

University of the Third Age: www.u3a.org.uk

Appendix 2
The International
Coach Federation

The information below is reprinted, with permission, from the ICF website: www.coachfederation.org.

What is the International Coach Federation (ICF)?

The ICF is an organisation with more than 4000 members and 177 chapters in 31 countries. It is the largest worldwide non-profit professional association of personal and business coaches and provides Professional, Master and Internal Corporate Coach certifications. It establishes and administers standards for credentialing professional coaches and coach training agencies.

Coaching is an interactive process that helps individuals and organisations develop more rapidly and produce more satisfying results. Coaches work with clients in areas including, but not limited to, career, transition, life/personal, executive, small business and organisational/corporate. As a result of coaching, clients may set better goals, take more action, make better decisions and more fully use their natural strengths.

What is the ICF philosophy of coaching?

The ICF adheres to a form of coaching that honours the client as the expert in their personal and/or professional life and believes that every client is creative, resourceful and whole. Standing on this foundation, the coach's responsibility is to:

- discover, clarify and align with what the client wants to achieve
- encourage client self-discovery
- elicit client-generated solutions and strategies
- hold the client as responsible and accountable.

What is the ICF definition of coaching

Professional coaching is an ongoing partnership that helps clients produce fulfilling results in their personal and professional lives. Through the process of coaching, clients deepen their learning, improve their performance, and enhance their quality of life.

In each meeting, the client chooses the focus of conversation, while the coach listens and contributes observations and questions. This interaction creates clarity and moves the client into action. Coaching accelerates the client's progress by providing greater focus and awareness of choice. Coaching concentrates on where clients are today and what they are willing to do to get where they want to be tomorrow.

Is there an ethical code for coaches?

The following is the Pledge of Ethics made by an ICF member coach:

> As a professional coach, I acknowledge and honour my ethical obligations to my coaching clients and colleagues and to the public at large. I pledge to comply with ICF Standards of Ethical Conduct, to treat people with dignity as free and equal human beings, and to model these standards with those whom I coach. If I breach this Pledge of Ethics or any ICF Standards of Ethical Conduct, I agree that the ICF in its sole discretion may hold me accountable for so doing. I further agree that ICF's holding me accountable for my breach may include loss of my ICF membership or my ICF certification.

What are the ICF Standards of Ethical Conduct?

- I will conduct myself in a manner that reflects well on coaching as a profession and I will refrain from doing anything that harms the public's understanding or acceptance of coaching as a profession.
- I will identify my level of coaching competence to the best of my ability and I will not overstate my qualifications, expertise or experience as a coach.
- I will, at the beginning of each coaching relationship, ensure that my coaching client understands the terms of the coaching agreement between us.
- I will not claim or imply outcomes that I cannot guarantee.
- I will respect the confidentiality of my client's information, except as otherwise authorised by my client, or as required by law.

- I will obtain permission from each of my clients before releasing their names as clients or references.
- I will be alert to noticing when my client is no longer benefiting from our coaching relationship and thus would be better served by another coach or by another resource and, at that time, I will encourage my client to make that change.
- I will avoid conflicts between my interests and the interests of my clients. Whenever the potential for a conflict of interest arises, I will, on a timely basis, discuss the conflict with my client to reach informed agreement with my client on how to deal with it in whatever way best serves my client.
- I will, on a timely basis, disclose to my client all compensation from third parties that I may receive for referrals of, or advice given to, that client.
- I will honour every term of the agreements I make with my clients and, if separate, with whoever compensates me for the coaching of my clients.
- I will not give my clients or any prospective clients information or advice I know to be confidential, misleading or beyond my competence.
- I will acknowledge the work and contributions of others; I will respect copyrights, trademarks and intellectual property rights and I will comply with applicable laws and my agreements concerning these rights.
- I will use ICF membership lists only in the manner and to the extent that I'm so authorised by the ICF or the applicable ICF chapter or ICF committee.
- I will coach in a manner compatible with the ICF definition of coaching and, whenever asked by my clients about my ethical standards, I will inform them of my pledge and agreement to comply with the ICF Pledge of Ethics and ICF Standards of Ethical Conduct.

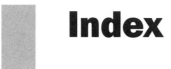

Index

abundance 66–9
acknowledgement, communication
  90
action 31, 143
  goals 74, 76
  happiness 114
  wellbeing 87–8
activities/hobbies 26
art 22, 32
assumptions 100
  unproven 27, 30
attitude 23, 29–30, 66, 86
autonomy 9–12
awareness 85
  time 44–5

balance, life 14–15, 83–4
barriers 27–8
beliefs 27, 142
  challenging 46
  limiting 38
benefits, change 16–17
body language 26, 86
body/mind/spirit
  healthy 59, 87–8
  interconnectedness 85
box, getting out of 9
breaks, taking 84

case studies 105–37
  catalyst 134–7
  challenges 128–9
  change 130–1
  charity walk 128–9
  disillusioned consultant 111–14
  enlightened doctor 128–9
  exams 132–3
  independent soul 118–19
  indispensability 111–14
  mentee 126–7

mentor 123–5
New Year story 134–7
overstressed doctor 120–2
overwhelmed GP 107–10
professional exams 132–3
relationships 115–17
retirement 134–7
sole doctor 118–19
spouses 115–17
stress 120–2
unsettled doctor 130–1
catalyst 10
  case study 134–7
celebrate 144
challenges, case study 128–9
challenging beliefs 46
change 15–18
  benefits 16–17
  case study 130–1
  cost 32
  difficulty 15
  necessity? 139
  need for 17
  possibility 31–2
  proactivity 15
  readiness to 143
  seeds of 22
  starting 16
  steps to 23–35
  timing 17, 22, 58, 80–1
  wanting 23
charity walk, case study 128–9
choice 39
choir 26
clarity, communication 95
clearing out clutter 33–4, 61–2
clinics
  guidelines 100
  ideal 98–100
  review 100

seeing fewer patients   97–100
clutter, clearing out   33–4, 61–2
coaching, life   *see* life coaching
coaching model   5
comfort zone   38
communication   27–8, 89–96
    acknowledgement   90
    clarity   95
    deep listening   93
    effective   94–5
    email   92
    feedback   92
    importance   90, 92
    improving   89, 91, 93
    inhibition   89
    meetings   91–2
    notice boards   92
    obstacles   93–4
    relationships   72–3
    standards   95–6
    stupidity   89
    viewpoints   89
complaining   13, 23
compromise, relationships   71
connections, relationships   70
consideration, relationships   71–2
cooperation, relationships   72
coping, relationships   70–1
cost, change   32
counselling, vs life coaching   4, 147
crisis   40

daydreaming   142, 145
    see also visualising
decision time   31–3
    indecision time   33–4
deep listening, communication   93
delay, time   122
delegation   5, 15, 26, 45, 46–7
diet   57, 59, 83, 87
disillusioned consultant, case study
    111–14
doctors' lives   13–15
dreams   8

effective communication   94–5
email, communication   92
enlightened doctor, case study   128–9
'enough is enough'   48–9

environment   62–3
equipment   55–60
exams, case study   132–3
excuses   51–2, 53–4
expectations   79, 80–1

fear   16, 142
feedback, communication   92
fewer patients, seeing   97–100
first step   30
focus   10
forgiveness   119
frequently asked questions   151–3
fun   65, 68
future
    creating   87
    looking to   19–20
    waiting for   36

geographical environment   62–3
giving   68
goals   10–11, 12
    achieving   74–6
    action   74, 76
    top tips   74–6
greetings   21–2, 86, 137

happiness, action   114
healthy body / mind / spirit   59, 87–8
heart sing   141–4
hobbies / activities   26
home environment   62

ICF   *see* International Coach
    Federation
ideal clinics   98–100
identity, personal   20–2
idleness   133
improvement factors   3, 6, 8
indecision time   33–4
independent soul, case study   118–19
indispensability, case study   111–14
indulgence   34–5
inhibition, communication   89
inner guidance   61
inner value   97
inner voice   37, 77, 141–2
interconnectedness, body / mind /
    spirit   85

International Coach Federation (ICF) 154–6

journals, keeping 10, 24–5, 28, 75, 85, 143
journey, 'wake up call' 39–40

kaleidoscope 34
keep going 143–4

laughing 141
see also smiling
learning 52–3
life balance 14–15, 83–4
life coaching 145–8
vs counselling 4, 147
and doctors 3–7
ICF 154–6
relevance 6
limiting beliefs 38
listening 142
communication 93
lists, 'draining' 64
lists, 'to do' 44

managing time 43–50, 67
medical model 4–5
medical way of life 14
meetings, communication 91–2
mentee, case study 126–7
mentor, case study 123–5
mentoring 147
mind/body/spirit, healthy 59, 87–8
mind maps 39
mindset, positive 11, 24, 86
models
coaching model 5
medical model 4–5
money 67
cost of change 32

New Year story, case study 134–7
'no', saying 6, 38, 46, 48, 53
notice boards, communication 92
number one 55–60

obstacles, communication 93–4
opportunity 36, 40
outer value 97

overstressed doctor, case study 120–2
overwhelmed GP, case study 107–10

patients, seeing fewer 97–100
personal identity 20–2
personal record 10
positive mindset 11, 24, 86
positives, looking at 38–9
prescription for change 9
presenting, television 25
proactivity, change 15
procrastination 17, 18, 27–8, 33–4, 47, 51–4
professional exams, case study 132–3
progress 39

questions, frequently asked 151–3

readiness to change 143
record, personal 10
regular tasks 49
relationships 63–4, 70–3
case study 115–17
retirement 101–3, 134–7
case study 134–7
risk
taking 27
value 73
routine, changing 52
rubbish, clearing out 33–4, 61–2

sailing 25, 134–7
seeds of change 22
seeing fewer patients 97–100
self-care 81
self first 84
self-knowledge 19–22
simple life 141
smiling 26, 86, 137
see also laughing
sole doctor, case study 118–19
spirit/body/mind, healthy 59, 87–8
spouses, case study 115–17
spreadsheet 62, 149
standards
communication 95–6
maintaining 95–6

starting   10–11, 28–30
starting change   16
steps to change   23–35
strength, support   81
stress
   case study   120–2
   overstressed doctor   120–2
stupidity, communication   89
supervision   81
support   11, 14, 32–3, 49–50, 53,
   79–80, 85, 86
   strength   81
   weakness   81

television presenting   25
time
   awareness   44–5
   delay   122
   managing   43–50, 67
   wasting   44–5
time out   86
timing, change   17, 22, 58, 80–1
'to do' lists   44

unsettled doctor, case study   130–1
ups and downs   11

value
   inner/outer   97
   risk   73
viewpoints, communication   89
visualising   10–11, 12, 18, 24–6,
   141–2, 145
   see also daydreaming

'wake up call'   36–40
wanting change   23
wasting time   44–5
weakness, support   81
websites   7, 88, 129, 151, 153, 154
wellbeing   83–8
   action   87–8
women doctors   5